Clinical Hypertension and Vascular Diseases

Series Editor: William B. White

More information about this series at http://www.springer.com/series/7673

William B. White

Editor

Blood Pressure Monitoring in Cardiovascular Medicine and Therapeutics

Third Edition

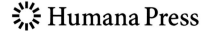 Humana Press

Editor
William B. White, M.D., F.A.S.H., F.A.H.A., F.A.C.P.
Calhoun Cardiology Center
University of Connecticut School of Medicine
Farmington, CT, USA

Clinical Hypertension and Vascular Diseases
ISBN 978-3-319-22770-2   ISBN 978-3-319-22771-9   (eBook)
DOI 10.1007/978-3-319-22771-9

Library of Congress Control Number: 2015958778

Springer Cham Heidelberg New York Dordrecht London

Printed on acid-free paper

Humana Press is a brand of Springer
Springer International Publishing AG Switzerland is part of Springer Science+Business Media (www.springer.com)

Foreword

This *Third Edition of Blood Pressure Monitoring in Cardiovascular Medicine and Therapeutics* extends the tradition of excellence in this area and is now entering its 16th year. The editor, Dr. William B. White, has assembled a group of well-respected authors to cover the entire spectrum of how ambulatory blood pressure monitoring (ABPM) has changed the face of clinical trials and clinical medicine. It also helps the reader understand how to interpret data in different clinical settings. For those with an interest in blood pressure variability and 24 h ABPM, this book is an indispensable resource. ABPM is now recommended for initial evaluation of hypertension by some national guidelines, while all guidelines recommend its use for conditions such as masked hypertension, white coat hypertension, and adequacy of blood pressure control while sleeping.

The technology available in the most recent monitors is quite sophisticated and can assess changes in vascular compliance as well as overall blood pressure patterns. For this reason both the clinical and research use of these devices have expanded dramatically over the past 6–8 years since the book's last edition was published. The third edition covers all aspects of blood pressure monitoring including review of the epidemiology and methodology used in outcome and blood pressure studies, comprehensive assessment of home blood pressure monitoring research and its translation into clinical practice, and a discussion of its use in the general management of patients.

The pathophysiology of circadian rhythms is discussed with five chapters dedicated to this topic covering the spectrum of chronobiology. A new chapter on relevance of blood pressure variability as a potential determinant of cardiovascular morbidity and mortality is an important addition to this edition of the book. Additionally, a new chapter covering the importance of neurohormonal activity, sodium and other cations, as well as renin–angiotensin system, obstructive sleep apnea, and the environment on blood pressure variability has been added. Another new and interesting chapter deals with ABPM and stroke outcomes. Moreover, there is a new chapter on the use of ABPM in clinical practice. This is a case-based chapter with nearly a dozen different clinical examples demonstrating the utility of ambulatory monitoring as an adjunct to the rest of the diagnostic work-up.

A whole section of the book has been dedicated to *special populations* including children, older people, and those with kidney disease as well as ischemic heart disease and outcomes based on ambulatory blood pressure readings.

There is no question that this is the quintessential text on blood pressure monitoring in clinical medicine and is second to none for its authoritative chapters and practical advice to clinicians as well as its perspective on understanding the ABPM results of a given patient. I highly recommend it to all who have an interest in this topic as "The Book on the Subject."

Chicago, IL, USA   George L. Bakris, M.D., F.A.S.H.

Preface

The third edition of *Blood Pressure Monitoring in Cardiovascular Medicine and Therapeutics* is devoted to the topic of circadian variation in cardiovascular disease, with a special emphasis on blood pressure and the clinical evaluation and treatment of hypertension. Clinical investigation related to home and ambulatory monitoring of the blood pressure has led to significant improvements in our ability to confirm hypertension as well as to identify clinical entities in patients with hypertension and vascular complications. This research is important not only because hypertension is so ubiquitous among adults around the globe, but also because the attributable cardiovascular morbidity and mortality associated with the hypertensive disease process are so substantial.

Since the first edition of this book in 2000 and its second edition in 2007, research efforts in basic and clinical hypertension have progressed, and work devoted to the measurement of blood pressure and blood pressure variability has been a major part of this scientific advancement with new measurement devices, novel drug and device therapies, and outcomes research in observational studies and clinical trials. During the past 8 years, numerous important research papers in the fields of ambulatory and home blood pressure monitoring have been published, and regular consensus conferences have been held at the European and/or International Society of Hypertension meetings as well as at the American Society of Hypertension annual meeting and expositions. Thus, it remains important and clinically relevant to have an updated third edition of my book that cohesively aggregates research findings involving blood pressure monitoring in clinical medicine and in cardiovascular therapeutics.

The volume has been organized into four major sections which cover broad areas in blood pressure measurement or monitoring as it relates to epidemiology, methodology, clinical associations and outcomes, and practical utility. The five chapters in Part I describe the methodology of clinical, home, and ambulatory blood pressure monitoring in research and clinical practice. Dr. Myers presents a concise chapter on different means to accurately measure the blood pressure in the medical care environment based on his many years of work in this area in Toronto. A comprehensive assessment of home blood pressure monitoring research as it translates into clinical practice including review of the epidemiologic data and other outcome findings, the importance of blood pressure variability, and discussing its use for the general management of patients was provided by Dr. Parati and colleagues from Milan. My former colleague, Dr. Mansoor from St. John's, Antigua, explains the importance of the environment and physical activity recordings in cardiovascular disease. These techniques may be helpful for obtaining meaningful data during ambulatory blood pressure recordings in clinical trials. Advances in actigraphy research have allowed investigators to pinpoint changes in physical activity that may directly impact on blood pressure variability. Vanessa Barber and I from Farmington, Connecticut, have updated an overview of ambulatory monitoring of the blood pressure, including descriptions of device validation, patterns of blood pressure variation discovered with the advent of this technique, and usefulness of the methodology in clinical hypertension practice. Drs. Atkins and O'Brien have updated their chapter on the importance of device validation and their reliability. While seemingly an unexciting topic, the importance of device validation cannot be overestimated as it is a requirement for investigators to confirm the overall validity of these recorders being used in clinical trial research and clinical practice.

The five chapters in Part II bring in new information related to our understanding of the pathophysiology of the circadian biology of cardiovascular disorders. A number of prior authors from the second edition as well as new authors and topics comprise this section. Drs. Smolensky, Portaluppi, and Hermida begin with an overview of the chronobiology of blood pressure regulation in humans. This chapter lays the groundwork for the rest of this section with its comprehensive discussion of the progress that has been made in research involving the chronophysiology of human disease with major emphases on hypertension, coronary artery disease, and stroke. Dr. Asayama and colleagues from Leuven have written a new chapter on relevance of blood pressure variability as a potential determinant of cardiovascular morbidity and mortality. During the past two decades, there has been substantial controversy over the independent relevance of short-term blood pressure variability derived from ambulatory monitoring versus longer-term variability that is associated with weekly or monthly clinical visits—these topics are covered in this balanced chapter. Dr. Burnier and coworkers from Lausanne have also written a new chapter covering the importance of neurohormonal activity, sodium and other cations, renin–angiotensin system, obstructive sleep apnea, and the environment on blood pressure variability. Drs. Angeli and Verdecchia from Perugia have once again provided a state-of-the-art chapter on the prognostic value of ambulatory blood pressure monitoring based on their long-term research in this field as well as through other databases from around the world. To wrap up this section, Dr. Gorelick and colleagues from Grand Rapids, Michigan, have written a new chapter for the book on ambulatory blood pressure and stroke—the authors are experts in vascular neurology who have had a long-standing interest in the relationships among blood pressure, stroke, and cognitive function, and their chapter is a welcome addition to this book.

There are eight chapters in Part III which focus on ambulatory blood pressure in special populations of patients with hypertension: Drs. Gulati and White from Hartford and Farmington, Connecticut, cover the older patient with systolic hypertension from the perspective of clinical cardiology and their longitudinal work on small vessel brain disease as it relates to out-of-office blood pressure; Dr. Flynn from Seattle comprehensively covers children and adolescents from the perspective of a leader in pediatric nephrology and hypertension; Drs. Hermida and Ayala from Vigo, Spain, comprehensively evaluate data during pregnancy from the perspective of experts in physiology and maternal–fetal medicine; Dr. Peixoto and coworkers from New Haven, Connecticut, and Rio de Janeiro provide us with a substantially updated and complete chapter on patients with chronic kidney disease and those on dialysis from the perspective of experts in clinical nephrology.

There are also four new chapters in Part III: a focus on ambulatory blood pressure in patients with ischemic heart disease and heart failure by Drs. Campbell and Javed from Little Rock and New Orleans from their perspective as experts in heart failure and hypertension; Dr. Viera from Chapel Hill, North Carolina, has an update on masked hypertension based on his own research as well as that of others in this important new field, while Dr. Krakoff from New York has written an update on white coat hypertension from the perspective of a hypertension specialist and a long-time researcher in out-of-office blood pressure monitoring. Finally, Dr. Lemmer from Heidelberg has written a new chapter on the importance of gender from the perspective of a clinical pharmacologist using examples from both animal models and clinical data.

In Part IV, there are three chapters, with two new authors for the book's third edition. The focus of the section is on the applications of home and ambulatory monitoring in clinical research and hypertension management. Drs. Stergiou and Ntineri from Athens have written a very comprehensive review of the use of home (or self) monitoring of the blood pressure in clinical research with a particular focus on therapeutic trials—at the time of publication of the prior edition of this book, there were very few studies published in this area. We welcome this new chapter by dedicated experts in this area. Drs. White and Malha from Farmington and New York have developed an updated, extensive review of the usefulness of ambulatory blood pressure monitoring during antihypertensive drug development as well as in novel trials of device therapy, such as renal denervation. Ambulatory blood pressure monitoring elucidates the efficacy of new antihypertensive therapies versus placebo as well as in comparator trials of two therapies. It also is an important tool to assess device therapy of hypertension to reduce the impact of observer bias. In the final chapter, Dr. Townsend, a hypertension specialist from Philadelphia, has written a new chapter on the use of ambulatory blood pressure monitoring in clinical practice. This is case-based chapter with nearly a dozen different clinical examples demonstrating the utility of ambulatory monitoring as an adjunct to the rest of the diagnostic work-up.

The clinicians and investigators who contributed to this textbook have written comprehensive and up-to-date information from a field in hypertension and vascular medicine that is dynamic and in which knowledge is advancing at a rapid pace. Just 20 years ago, most research in the field of ambulatory monitoring of the blood pressure was descriptive and did not correlate the data to target organ disease or cardiovascular outcomes. Hence, practicing physicians were not provided with enough solid information to have an impact on the day-to-day management of their patients. This certainly is no longer the case as after nearly 30 years of outcomes studies that include target organ disease and events, ambulatory blood pressure monitoring has matured into a highly useful methodology for clinical hypertension research as well as an important aid in the management of patients with hypertension and vascular disease. In fact, policymakers in many countries have supported its use in the evaluation and treatment of newly diagnosed patients with hypertension.

I am truly grateful for all of the outstanding chapters provided by my contributing authors, which greatly enhanced my job as volume editor. Diane Webster, my long-time assistant at the University of Connecticut School of Medicine, provided outstanding support in helping to organize the manuscripts during the course of their production as well as to review references, author information, permissions, and titles. Special thanks to Vanessa Barber, a talented research assistant in our clinical research center who not only coauthored a chapter with me but also spent a large amount of time and effort assessing the 21 chapters for overlap and redundancy as well as format. Finally, I would like to extend my ongoing gratitude to my wife, Nancy Petry, a highly accomplished researcher, author, and editor in the field of behavioral medicine and devoted mother of our dear children Hannah and Noah White, for her love and support during the past decade.

Farmington, CT, USA   William B. White, M.D.

Contents

Contributors

Fabio Angeli, M.D. Division of Cardiology and Cardiovascular Pathophysiology, Hospital "S.M. della Misericordia", Perugia, Italy

Kei Asayama, M.D., Ph.D. Studies Coordinating Centre, Research Unit Hypertension and Cardiovascular Epidemiology, KU Leuven Department of Cardiovascular Sciences, University of Leuven, Leuven, Belgium

Department of Planning for Drug Development and Clinical Evaluation, Tohoku University Graduate School of Pharmaceutical Sciences, Sendai, Japan

Department of Hygiene and Public Health, Teikyo University School of Medicine, Tokyo, Japan

William S. Asch, M.D., Ph.D. Section of Nephrology, Yale University School of Medicine, New Haven, CT, USA

Neil Atkins Medaval Ltd., Dublin, Ireland

Diana E. Ayala, M.D., M.P.H., Ph.D. Bioengineering & Chronobiology Laboratories, Atlantic Research Center for Information and Communication Technologies (AtlantTIC), University of Vigo, Vigo, Spain

Vanessa Barber Clinical Research Center, University of Connecticut School of Medicine, CT, USA

Olivier Bonny, M.D., Ph.D. Department of Pharmacology and Toxicology, Universite de Lausanne, Lausanne, Switzerland

Michel Burnier, M.D. Department of Medicine, Service of Nephrology and Hypertension, Centre Hospitalier Universitaire Vaudois, Lausanne, Switzerland

Patrick T. Campbell, M.D. Heart Failure and Transplant Cardiology, Transplant Institute Baptist Health, Little Rock, AR, USA

Muhammad U. Farooq, M.D. Division of Stroke and Vascular Neurology, Mercy Health Hauenstein Neurosciences, Grand Rapids, MI, USA

Joseph T. Flynn, M.D., M.S. Division of Nephrology, Seattle Children's Hospital, Seattle, WA, USA

Philip B. Gorelick, M.D., M.P.H. Mercy Health Hauenstein Neurosciences, Grand Rapids, MI, USA

Department Translational Science & Molecular Medicine, Michigan State University, College of Human Medicine, Grand Rapids, MI, USA

Vinay Gulati, M.D. Division of Cardiology, Hartford Hospital, Hartford, CT, USA

Tine W. Hansen, M.D., Ph.D. The Steno Diabetes Center, Gentofte and Research Center for Prevention and Health, Copenhagen, Denmark

Azusa Hara, Ph.D. Studies Coordinating Centre, Research Unit Hypertension and Cardiovascular Epidemiology, KU Leuven Department of Cardiovascular Sciences, University of Leuven, Leuven, Belgium

Ramón C. Hermida, Ph.D. Bioengineering and Chronobiology Laboratories, Atlantic Research Center for Information and Communication Technologies (AtlantTIC), University of Vigo, Vigo, Spain

Fahad Javed, M.D. Ochsner Heart and Vascular Institute, New Orleans, LA, USA

Lawrence R. Krakoff, M.D. Icahn School of Medicine at Mount Sinai, New York, NY, USA

Björn Lemmer, M.D. Faculty of Medicine Mannheim, Institute of Experimental & Clinical Pharmacology & Toxicology, Ruprecht-Karls University of Heidelberg, Mannheim, Germany

Yan Li, M.D., Ph.D. Center for Epidemiological Studies and Clinical Trials and Center for Vascular Evaluations, Shanghai Institute of Hypertension, Shanghai Key Laboratory of Hypertension, Ruijin Hospital, Shanghai Jiaotong University School of Medicine, Shanghai, China

Ian Macumber, M.D. Division of Nephrology, Seattle Children's Hospital, Seattle, WA, USA

Line Malha, M.D. NYU School of Medicine, New York, NY, USA

George A. Mansoor, M.Sc., M.B.B.S. Mount Saint John Medical Center, St. Johns, Antigua and Barbuda

Jiangyong Min, M.D., Ph.D. Division of Stroke and Vascular Neurology, Mercy Health Hauenstein Neurosciences, Grand Rapids, MI, USA

Martin G. Myers, M.D. Schulich Heart Program, Division of Cardiology, Sunnybrook Health Sciences Centre, Toronto, ON, Canada

Department of Medicine, University of Toronto, Toronto, ON, Canada

Angeliki Ntineri, M.D. Third University Department of Medicine, Hypertension Center STRIDE-7, Sotiria Hospital, Athens, Greece

Eoin O'Brien, M.D. The Conway Institute, University College Dublin, Dublin, Ireland

Juan Eugenio Ochoa, M.D., Ph.D. Department of Cardiovascular Neural and Metabolic Sciences, San Luca Hospital, IRCCS Istituto Auxologico Italiano, Milan, Italy

Gianfranco Parati, M.D. Department of Health Sciences, University of Milano-Bicocca, Milan, Italy

Department of Cardiovascular Neural and Metabolic Sciences, San Luca Hospital, IRCCS Istituto Auxologico Italiano, Milan, Italy

Aldo J. Peixoto, M.D. Department of Internal Medicine, Section of Nephrology, Yale University School of Medicine, New Haven, CT, USA

Francesco Portaluppi, M.D., Ph.D. Hypertension Center, S. Anna University Hospital, University of Ferrara, Ferrara, Italy

Sergio F.F. Santos, M.D., Ph.D. Division of Nephrology, State University of Rio de Janeiro (UERJ), Rio de Janeiro, RJ, Brazil

Michael H. Smolensky, Ph.D. Department of Biomedical Engineering, Cockrell School of Engineering, The University of Texas at Austin, Austin, TX, USA

Jan A. Staessen, M.D., Ph.D. VitaK Research and Development, Maastricht University, Maastricht, The Netherlands

Studies Coordinating Centre, Research Unit Hypertension and Cardiovascular Epidemiology, KU Leuven Department of Cardiovascular Sciences, University of Leuven, Leuven, Belgium

George S. Stergiou, M.D. Third University Department of Medicine, Hypertension Center STRIDE-7, Sotiria Hospital, Athens, Greece

Raymond R. Townsend, M.D. Perelman School of Medicine, University of Pennsylvania, Philadelphia, PA, USA

Paolo Verdecchia, M.D. Department of Internal Medicine, Hospital of Assisi, Assisi, Italy

Anthony J. Viera, M.D. Department of Family Medicine and Hypertension Research Program, University of North Carolina at Chapel Hill, Chapel Hill, NC, USA

Fang-Fei Wei, M.D. Studies Coordinating Centre, Research Unit Hypertension and Cardiovascular Epidemiology, KU Leuven Department of Cardiovascular Sciences, University of Leuven, Leuven, Belgium

Center for Epidemiological Studies and Clinical Trials and Center for Vascular Evaluations, Shanghai Institute of Hypertension, Shanghai Key Laboratory of Hypertension, Ruijin Hospital, Shanghai Jiaotong University School of Medicine, Shanghai, China

William B. White, M.D. Calhoun Cardiology Center, University of Connecticut School of Medicine, Farmington, CT, USA

Gregoire Wuerzner, M.D. Department of Medicine, Service of Nephrology and Hypertension, Centre Hospitalier Universitaire Vaudois, Lausanne, Switzerland

Part I
Techniques for Monitoring Blood Pressure

Chapter 1
Monitoring Blood Pressure in the Office

Martin G. Myers

Historical Perspective

The measurement of blood pressure (BP) originated in a field with a horse and a cleric. In 1733, the Reverend Stephen Hales used a water-filled glass tube inserted into the left crural artery of a horse to demonstrate that the circulating blood was under a pressure of about 2.5 m of water. However, it was not until 1896 that Riva-Rocci developed the first practical method to record systolic BP using a cuff inflated on the upper arm attached to a mercury column to record the pressure at which the pulse was obliterated. In 1905, Korotkoff modified the technique by introducing auscultation over the brachial artery to detect the systolic and diastolic BP during deflation of the cuff on the upper arm. Thus, began the modern era of BP measurement.

For the next century, the mercury sphygmomanometer was the standard technique for recording BP in the office setting. A BP reading became part of the routine examination. Typically, the physician would first take the patient's medical history and then move to an adjacent room where the physical examination which included a BP measurement was performed. Detailed guidelines were developed by organizations such as the American Heart Association in an attempt to standardize the measurement technique, especially after research indicated that readings could be affected by a variety of factors. In his classic text, *High Blood Pressure* [1], published in 1968, Sir George Pickering described various causes of measurement

M.G. Myers, M.D. (✉)
Schulich Heart Program, Division of Cardiology, Sunnybrook Health Sciences Centre, 2075 Bayview Avenue, Toronto, ON, Canada, M4N 3M5

Department of Medicine, University of Toronto, Toronto, ON, Canada
e-mail: martin.myers@sunnybrook.ca

© Springer International Publishing Switzerland 2016
W.B. White (ed.), *Blood Pressure Monitoring in Cardiovascular Medicine and Therapeutics*, Clinical Hypertension and Vascular Diseases,
DOI 10.1007/978-3-319-22771-9_1

error, mostly related to the patient and physician but also to the surroundings. The concept of "casual" versus "basal" BP was proposed, including measures to reduce the effect of the patient's anxiety on BP, such as multiple readings taken without conversation. Unknown at the time, these were likely the first attempts to deal with office-induced hypertension, now known as the "white coat effect."

Although Pickering made many important contributions to our understanding of BP, he was an early proponent of BP as a continuous variable with no specific cut-point separating a normal BP from hypertension. In several chapters of *High Blood Pressure*, he reviewed the epidemiologic data showing the relationship between increasing levels of BP and cardiovascular morbidity and mortality. He also noted the different cut-points proposed for defining hypertension, covering a range from 120/80 to 180/110 mmHg. It soon became clear that the selection of 140/90 mmHg for defining hypertension based upon manual BP readings was quite arbitrary. Moreover, the prevailing belief at that time was that diastolic BP was most important with systolic hypertension simply being a manifestation of a rigid aorta and, in itself, not associated with cardiovascular risk.

General Conditions for BP Measurement

There are several aspects of BP measurement which need to be considered regardless of the type of sphygmomanometer used to take the reading.

On the first visit, BP should be recorded supine and standing to detect any postural changes. Also, readings should be taken in both arms, either simultaneously, if feasible, or sequentially in the same arm. For routine visits, readings are usually taken with the patient seated in a chair with the back supported and legs uncrossed. More than one reading is recommended, especially if the initial BP is borderline or high. The mean BP should be noted, although individual readings may also be of interest if there is a marked decrease after the first one, which could reflect increased anxiety on the part of the patient. The patient should be in a quiet place and must not talk before or during the reading, neither to the doctor/nurse nor on a mobile phone, if left alone. Resting for about five minutes before the readings is recommended for most types of measurements, particularly those which involve the presence of a heath professional during the readings. An appropriate size cuff with a bladder which encircles the upper arm should be used for all devices.

Devices for Manual BP Measurement (Table 1.1)

In what is probably the single most important development in the measurement of blood pressure, the mercury sphygmomanometer is no longer the preferred method for recording BP in routine clinical practice [2, 3]. There are two main reasons for this change. The first relates to concerns about the adverse effects mercury has on

Table 1.1 Commonly used devices for blood pressure measurement in the office setting

Manual
Mercury sphygmomanometer
Aneroid sphygmomanometer
Semi-automated
Home BP recorders adopted for office use
Fully automated
BpTRU
Omron HEM-907
Microlife WatchBP Office

the environment, which has led the European Community and other countries to restrict its use [4]. The second reason is that measurement of BP with a mercury sphygmomanometer is subject to multiple types of bias and error which are not shared by modern electronic devices.

Recording BP manually using a mercury or aneroid-type sphygmomanometer involves a health professional auscultating the Korotkoff sounds over the brachial artery, while inflating the cuff to at least 20 mmHg above the anticipated systolic BP and then deflating it at a rate of 2 mmHg per heartbeat. These steps require special training, normal hearing, no conversation, strict adherence to the inflation and deflation protocol, precise recording of the point at which the Korotkoff sounds appear and then disappear, and taking of multiple readings and then accurate transcription of the readings. Many of these requirements are frequently disregarded in routine clinical practice. Examples include not allowing the patient to rest for 5 min before the first measurement, talking with the patient, overly rapid deflation of the cuff, and rounding off readings to the nearest zero value (digit preference). Minimizing the role of humans in recording BP eliminates many potential sources of error which leads to a more accurate reading [5].

One advantage of the mercury sphygmomanometer itself is that it does not require calibration or periodic servicing other than verifying that there has not been any loss of mercury and that the cuff, tubing, and deflation mechanism are functioning properly. The mercury sphygmomanometer continues to be used in the validation of other devices such as electronic, oscillometric sphygmomanometers, so hypertension centers should maintain at least one mercury device for this purpose. Some experts also recommend using a mercury sphygmomanometer in patients with special conditions such as atrial fibrillation, although there is little evidence that a manual BP reading taken by a health professional in such circumstances is more accurate than readings taken with other devices such as an automated, electronic sphygmomanometer. What may be most important is to obtain multiple readings, regardless of the BP measurement technique, in order to account for the variable heart rate.

Next to the mercury sphygmomanometer, the most widely used manual BP recorder in clinical practice has been the aneroid device which also has the advantage of being portable and relatively inexpensive. However, the actual mechanism inside the aneroid sphygmomanometer responsible for obtaining the pressure reading requires periodic maintenance and re-calibration, a procedure which is often not followed [6]. Other manual mercury sphygmomanometers such as the Hawksley Random Zero were developed in an effort to circumvent some of the shortcomings of the standard mercury device, but these have been found to have other sources of measurement error which have precluded their use [7].

In recent years, more sophisticated, non-mercury, manual sphygmomanometers for office use have been developed. Models which have passed independent validation include the Accoson Greenlight 300 [8], Heine Gamma G7 [9], Nissei DM-3000 [10], Rossamax Mandaus I [11], and Welch-Allyn Maxi Stabil 3 [12]. Each of these devices requires the involvement of a health professional. To date, none of these recorders has achieved widespread use in clinical practice.

Impact of Manual BP in Management of Hypertension

The involvement of a health professional in the measurement of BP can affect the accuracy and reliability of the readings [13]. The failure to follow guidelines for BP measurement, as noted above, tends to provoke a white coat effect, especially in patients who may already be anxious about seeing a physician. Stimuli such as conversation can cause substantial increases in BP, potentially leading to a misdiagnosis of "white coat hypertension" [14]. On average, manual office BP in routine clinical practice is about 10/7 mmHg higher than manual BP recorded in a research study according to guidelines (Table 1.2). It is estimated that 15–25 % of patients diagnosed with mild–moderate hypertension will be normal when BP is recorded outside of the office setting such as with 24-h ambulatory BP monitoring (ABPM) or home BP [15, 16]. The presence of a white coat effect in patients already receiving drug therapy may also lead to additional, unnecessary medication, a condition called pseudo-resistant hypertension [17]. Longitudinal, clinical outcome studies have consistently reported that manual BP, even when recorded according to guidelines in a research setting, correlates poorly with target organ damage. Much stronger correlations have been seen with ABPM and home BP [18, 19].

Table 1.2 Differences between manual BP recorded in routine clinical practice and manual BP obtained following standard guidelines in research studies

	Type of blood pressure measurement (mmHg)		
First author	N	Routine clinical practice	Guidelines BP in research study
Myers [40]	147	146/87	140/83
Brown [43]	611	161/95	152/85
Myers [27]	309	152/87	140/80
Graves [44]	104	152/84	138/74
Gustavsen [45]	420	165/104	156/100
Head [46]	6817	150/89	142/82
Mean difference		10/7	

Semi-automated Sphygmomanometers in Office Practice

Concerns about the accuracy of manual office BP in diagnosing hypertension have resulted in recent guidelines recommending against the use of manual BP measurement in the office for the diagnosis and management of hypertension [2, 3]. One option has been to rely upon 24-h ABPM for diagnosing hypertension and home BP for management of hypertension after therapy has been started. However, many physicians have been reluctant to abandon office BP and have chosen to use semi-automated, electronic devices as a replacement for mercury and aneroid sphygmomanometers.

Most semi-automated devices are modifications of oscillometric home BP recorders, which have been adapted for use in the office setting. The use of semi-automated recorders in major studies [20], such as the Omron-HEM 705 in the Anglo-Scandinavian Outcomes Trial (ASCOT), has prompted both primary care physicians and hypertension specialists to switch from manual BP recorders to semi-automated devices which have been validated for accuracy. Typically, the doctor or nurse follows procedures used previously with manual BP except that readings are taken without auscultation and manual cuff inflation/deflation, which reduces measurement error and observer bias. Some semi-automated recorders take two or three readings at pre-specified intervals after the start button is pressed.

Three studies [21–23] have compared the mean awake ambulatory BP or home BP with office BP readings taken with a semi-automated recorder with the patient alone in an examining room (Table 1.3). With the office BP readings being taken 2, 3, or 5 times, the mean value exceeded the out-of-office BP by 12/5, 7/4, and 4/5 mmHg, respectively. In a fourth study [24], three semi-automated BP readings taken in a hypertension clinic in the presence of a nurse or doctor were compared to home BP readings recorded using the same device by the patient. Once again, the mean semi-automated office BP was higher (9/5 mmHg) than the mean home BP. Thus, replacement of manual BP recorders with semi-automated, oscillometric sphygmomanometers does not eliminate the white coat effect, even if readings are taken with the patient resting quietly alone. Nonetheless, semi-automated devices have been quite popular in that they are readily available and relatively inexpensive. To date, there have been no studies comparing conventional manual BP with semi-automated BP in routine clinical practice, which makes it difficult to document the specific advantages the semi-automated method is presumed to have.

Table 1.3 Studies comparing semi-automated BP (mmHg) readings with awake ambulatory BP ([a]) or home BP ([b])

Study author	No. of patients	Semi-automated BP	Awake ambulatory BP or home BP
Myers et al. [21]	27	157/83	145/78[a]
Myers et al. [22]	139	146/86	142/81[a]
Stergiou et al. [24]	30	137/83	128/83[b]
Al-Karkhi et al. [23]	162	140/86	133/83[b]

Automated Office Blood Pressure Measurement

The most recent guidelines focus primarily on semi-automated electronic devices as the sphygmomanometer of choice for office BP readings. The ESH/ESC 2013 recommendations [2] did go one step further and recommended (fully) automated recorders capable of taking multiple BP readings with the patient resting alone. This type of BP measurement has been called "automated office BP (AOBP)." Canadian guidelines now recommend AOBP readings in routine clinical practice [25].

The importance of AOBP in clinical practice first became evident in 2005 when Beckett and Godwin reported on AOBP readings recorded in 481 treated hypertensive patients recruited from primary care practices in the community [26]. In this population, mean AOBP (140/80 mmHg) was significantly lower than the mean of the last three routine manual BP readings (151/83 mmHg) recorded by the patients' own family physicians. These findings were subsequently confirmed in a series of 309 patients referred for 24-h ABPM who had a mean AOBP of 132/75 mmHg compared to the last routine manual office BP of 152/87 mmHg recorded by the patient's own family physician [27].

The main advantage of AOBP over semi-automated electronic devices is that AOBP does not require any active involvement of the patient or a health professional. The presence of a doctor or nurse when BP is measured increases the BP reading in some patients, presumably by adding to the anxiety generated by the visit itself. Having the patient take their own readings using a semi-automated device circumvents this factor, but the readings are still, on average, higher. One study [22] compared five AOBP readings taken with the fully automated BpTRU device with five readings taken by the patient while resting alone using a semi-automated sphygmomanometer. The latter BP was 5/4 mmHg higher than the AOBP, which was similar to the mean awake ambulatory BP.

The Pros and Cons of AOBP

As noted in the European and Canadian guidelines [2, 3, 25], an AOBP measurement has three basic components; the use of a fully automated sphygmomanometer which is capable of taking multiple readings with the patient resting quietly alone. There are currently three validated devices specifically designed for AOBP: the BpTRU [28], the Omron HEM-907 [29], and the Microlife WatchBP Office [30]. To date, most of the research into AOBP has been conducted using the BpTRU. Each of these devices is capable of taking 3–5 readings at 1 min intervals with no more than a one minute period required before the first reading is taken. The BpTRU takes five readings timed from the start of the first reading to the start of the second, whereas the other two devices record BP with a full minute from the end of one reading to the start of the next. Thus, an average AOBP reading can be taken over 5–6 min. Initially, there was some concern about the time required to take multiple

AOBP readings in a busy clinical practice. However, if guidelines for recording a proper (manual or semi-automated) office BP are followed, the patient should remain quiet for 5 min before the first of at least two readings are taken. Thus, AOBP would only take longer if the doctor or nurse does not adhere to the current guidelines for office BP measurement which is likely often the case.

Studies [31, 32] using manual BP measurement have reported that as little as 10 s between readings may be all the time required to obtain an accurate measurement. Experiments conducted with the BpTRU and Omron HEM-907 have shown that readings taken at 1-minute intervals are comparable to readings taken at 2-min intervals [33]. Earlier studies using the BpTRU recorded BP at 2-min intervals, but 1 min is now recommended for an AOBP measurement [34]. Also, in most studies on AOBP, the patient was kept seated alone in a quiet room. However, AOBP values are also similar when readings are taken with the patient resting quietly in an office waiting room versus an examining room (35,36). Conventional manual BP is affected by the surroundings in which readings are taken. Such is not the case with AOBP. Readings taken with the BpTRU with the subjects resting quietly in a community pharmacy were similar to AOBP recorded in the office of their family physician [37]. Moreover, AOBP obtained in a hypertension specialist's office was similar to AOBP taken in an ABPM unit [38]. Thus, a valid AOBP reading should be possible provided the patient is resting alone without talking or otherwise interacting with other people, especially health professionals.

Finally, the higher cost of AOBP recorders has been an impediment to their greater use in clinical practice. Recently, less expensive models have appeared which should make financial considerations much less of an issue when it comes to selecting the optimum sphygmomanometer for office use.

Relationship Between AOBP and ABPM

ABPM has become the gold standard for determining the risk of experiencing a cardiovascular event in relation to an individual's BP. AOBP has been compared with the mean awake ambulatory BP in various populations and settings (Table 1.4). Mean AOBP is similar to the mean awake ambulatory BP in unselected hypertensive patients attending the offices of their own family physicians. This relationship was present in both treated and untreated patients. Mean AOBP was also similar to the awake ambulatory BP in patients with suspected hypertension referred for ambulatory BP monitoring, a population more likely to have a white coat effect. This similarity in BP readings is present regardless of whether or not the patients are receiving antihypertensive drug therapy. In all studies, the manual BP recorded during routine visits to the patient's own family doctor outside of the context of a research study was substantially higher than both the AOBP and awake ambulatory BP [13, 39]. The ambulatory BP also exhibited a significantly stronger correlation with the AOBP than the routine manual office BP [13].

Table 1.4 Comparison of automated office BP (AOBP) with the awake ambulatory BP in different patient populations

Study author	No. of Subjects	Setting	AOBP	Awake ambulatory BP
Beckett et al. [26]	481	Family practice	140/80	142/80
Myers et al. [27]	309	ABPM unit	132/75	134/77
Myers et al. [38]	62	Hypertension clinic	140/77	141/77
Myers et al. [47]	254	ABPM unit	133/80	135/81
Godwin et al. [48]	654	Family practice	139/80	141/80
Myers et al. [22]	139	ABPM unit	141/82	142/81
Myers et al. [39]	303	Family practice	136/78	133/74
		Mean	137/79	138/79

Even though the measurement of BP is an integral part of primary care, comparatively little research has been done into the validity of readings taken during routine office visits compared to BP recorded with strict adherence to guidelines in research studies (Table 1.2). In one study [40], the mean manual office BP obtained in 147 patients by their own family physicians was 6/4 mmHg higher than comparable office readings taken by the same doctors as part of a research study. Moreover, left ventricular mass index, a measure of target organ damage related to BP, correlated significantly ($r=0.27$) with the special manual BP taken for research purposes, but there was no correlation ($r=0.06$) with the routine manual BP. This phenomenon is known as the "Hawthorne Effect" and is used to describe changes in behavior which tend to occur when an individual (e.g., doctor or nurse) is under observation, such as recording BP as part of a research study [41].

The Conventional versus Automated Measurement of Blood Pressure in the Office Study

Until recently, there was considerable reluctance to abandon conventional manual BP measurement in favor of more modern techniques such as the oscillometric recorders used for ABPM, home BP, and AOBP. The proponents of manual BP maintained that virtually all of the data upon which the diagnosis and management of hypertension are based were obtained using the mercury sphygmomanometer. The pendulum finally shifted to electronic devices in 2011 when the British National Institute for Health and Clinical Excellence's (NICE) evidence-based guidelines [42] recommended that a diagnosis of hypertension should be based upon 24-h ABPM and not the office BP. For many physicians, this dramatic departure from conventional thinking led to considerable confusion. The result was a shift to electronic devices to record BP in the office with the assumption that this approach would alleviate many of the concerns about manual BP documented in the NICE monograph. However, there is little evidence that changing the device without removing other causes of measurement error is sufficient to justify the continued use of office BP for the diagnosis and management of hypertension.

Concurrently, investigators decided to examine the impact that introducing AOBP into routine primary care practice might have on the accuracy of office BP. In the Conventional versus Automated Measurement of Blood Pressure in the Office (CAMBO) study [39], 67 practices (555 patients) in five cities in Eastern Canada were randomly allocated to either use of the BpTRU to record the patient's BP or continued use of manual sphygmomanometers. In order to minimize the "Hawthorne Effect" [41] as a factor, there were no other interventions such as educating staff on proper management of hypertension.

At the first office visit after enrollment, the mean AOBP had decreased by 14/3 mmHg compared to the mean routine manual office BP (150/81 mmHg) recorded by the patient's own family physician prior to entry into the study. The mean AOBP (136/78 mmHg) was only slightly higher than the mean awake ambulatory BP (133/74 mmHg). There was a relatively small decrease in office BP at the first office visit in the control, manual BP group, presumably due to the Hawthorne Effect, with clinic staff obtaining lower BP readings.

The results of this cluster randomized clinical trial in a real-world setting confirmed the earlier findings in previous series of hypertensive patients in a variety of settings.

Principles of Automated Office BP

An important aspect of office BP measurement is the need to minimize extraneous factors which might affect the accuracy of the reading and lead to misdiagnosis of hypertension. Office BP is highest and least accurate with greater involvement of the patient and physician or nurse [7]. Manual BP in routine clinical practice is the best example of this with BP being on average 10/7 mmHg higher than readings taken according to guidelines in the context of a research study (Table 1.2). When these guidelines are followed, the "research" office BP more closely approximates the awake ambulatory and home BP but is still about 5–10/5 mmHg higher [27], giving a cut-point for hypertension of 140–145/90 versus 135/85 mmHg for the out-of office readings. The apparent equivalence of AOBP and both awake ambulatory BP and home BP (Table 1.4) makes the cut-point for defining hypertension using AOBP the same for all three methods (135/85 mmHg).

There are three basic principles to follow in order to obtain a proper AOBP reading: *Multiple readings* with a *fully automated sphygmomanometer* with the patient *resting alone* in a quiet place. If these principles are followed, AOBP will be an improvement over conventional manual BP measurement by providing more accurate readings which are devoid of a white coat effect and which are suitable for most types of office practice in countries with sufficient resources.

Table 1.5 Recommendations for office BP measurement

• Conventional manual BP measurement should be discouraged
• Use automated electronic sphygmomanometers which have been independently validated for accuracy
• Human involvement in BP measurement should be kept to a minimum in order to reduce observer error and bias and to decrease the patient's anxiety
• Multiple readings should be taken with fully automated electronic sphygmomanometers with the patient resting quietly alone (AOBP)
• Hypertension diagnosed in the office should be confirmed with 24-h ABPM or home BP if ABPM is not available

Conclusions

The determination of an individual's BP status is currently in a transition phase. Reliance upon the mercury sphygmomanometer during the past century has now progressed to the use of automated electronic devices to record BP in the office, at home, and over 24-h. Longitudinal cardiovascular outcome studies have consistently shown ABPM to be the best predictor of future risk based upon an individual's BP status with home BP being an acceptable alternative if ABPM is not available. Under these circumstances, the role of office BP in the diagnosis and management of hypertension has been questioned. Now that office BP is no longer synonymous with manual BP measurement, it is being viewed in a more favorable light, provided that validated electronic devices are used and certain procedures are followed (Table 1.5). The accumulating evidence supports AOBP measurement as the best method for determining BP status in the office, with a more definitive diagnosis of hypertension still requiring 24-h ABPM or home BP. Thus, all three types of BP measurement are complementary with each method continuing to have a role in the management of hypertension.

References

1. Pickering G. High blood pressure. London: J&A Churchill; 1968.
2. Mancia G, Fagard R, Krzysztof N, et al. 2013 ESH/ESC guidelines for the management of arterial hypertension. J Hypertens. 2013;31:1281–357.
3. Weber ME, Schiffrin EL, White WB, et al. Clinical practice guidelines for the management of hypertension in the community – a statement of the American Society of Hypertension and the International Society of Hypertension. J Hypertens. 2014;32:3–15.
4. Scientific Committee on Emerging and Newly Identified Health Risks. Mercury sphygmomanometers in healthcare and the feasibility of alternatives. SCENIHR, 2009. (http://ec.europa.eu/health/scientific_committees/emerging/scenihr_09-13/opinions_en.htm)
5. Myers MG. Eliminating the human factor in office blood pressure measurement. J Clin Hypertens. 2014;16:83–6.
6. Mion D, Pierin AMG. How accurate are sphygmomanometers. J Hum Hypertens. 1981;12:245–8.

7. O'Brien E, Mee F, Atkins N, O'Malley K. Inaccuracy of the Hawksley random zero sphygmo-manometer. Lancet. 1990;336:1465–8.
8. Graves JW, Tibor M, Murtagh B, Klein L, Sheps SG. The Accoson Greenlight 300, the first non-automated mercury-free blood pressure measurement device to pass International Protocol for blood pressure measuring devices in adults. Blood Press Monit. 2004;9:13–7.
9. Dorigatti F, Bonso E, Zanier A, Palatini P. Validation of Heine Gamma G7 (G5) and XXL-LF aneroid devices for blood pressure measurement. Blood Press Monit 2007;12:29-33.
10. Tasker F, De Greeff A, Shennan AH. Development and validation of a blinded hybrid device according to the European Hypertension Society protocol: Nissei DM-3000. J Hum Hypertens. 2010;24:609–16.
11. Tasker F, de Greff A, Liu B, Shennan AH. Validation of a non-mercury ascultatory device according to the European Society of Hypertension protocol: Rosssmax Mandaus II. Blood Press Monit. 2009;14:121–4.
12. Reinders A, Jones C, Cuckson A, Shennan A. The Maxi Stabil 3: Validation of an aneroid device according to a modified British Hypertension Society protocol. Blood Press Monit. 2003;8:83–9.
13. Myers MG. The great myth of office blood pressure measurement. J Hypertens. 2012;30:1894–8.
14. Lynch JJ, Long JM, Thomas SA, Malinow KL, Katcher AH. The effects of talking on blood pressure of hypertensive and normotensive individuals. Psychosom Med. 1981;43:25–32.
15. Pickering TG, Hall JE, Appel LJ, et al. Recommendations for blood pressure measurement in humans and experimental animals Part 1: blood pressure measurement in humans a statement for professionals from the subcommittee of Professional and Public Education of the AM Heart Association Council on High Blood Pressure Research. Hypertension. 2005;45:142–61.
16. Parati G, Stergiou GS, Asmar R, et al. European Society of Hypertension guidelines for blood pressure monitoring at home: a summary report of the Second International Consensus Conference on Home Blood Pressure Monitoring. J Hypertens. 2008;26:1505–26.
17. Myers MG. Pseudoresistant hypertension attributed to white-coat effect. Hypertension. 2012;59:532–3.
18. Hansen TW, Kikuya M, Thijs L, et al. Prognostic superiority of daytime ambulatory conventional blood pressure in four populations: a meta-analysis of 7030 individuals. J Hypertens. 2007;25:1554–64.
19. Stergiou GS, Siontis KCM, Ioannidis JPA. Home blood pressure as a cardiovascular outcome predictor. Hypertension. 2010;55:1301–3.
20. Dahlhof B, Sever PS, Poulter NR, et al. Prevention of cardiovascular events with an antihypertensive regimen of amlodipine adding perindopril as required versus atenolol, adding bendroflumethazide as required, in the Anglo-Scandinavian Cardiac Outcomes Trial - Blood pressure lowering arm (ASCOT-BPLA): a multicenter randomized controlled trial. Lancet. 2005;366:895–906.
21. Myers MG, Meglis G, Polemidiotis G. The impact of physician vs automated blood pressure readings on office-induced hypertension. J Hum Hypertens. 1997;11:491–3.
22. Myers MG, Valdivieso M, Chessman M, Kiss A. Can sphygmomanometers designed for self-measurement of blood pressure in the home be used in office practice? Blood Press Monit. 2010;15:300–4.
23. Al-Karkhi I, Al-Rubaiy R, Rosenqvist U, Falk M, Nystrom FH. Comparisons of automated blood pressures in a primary health care setting with self-measurements at the office and home using the Omron i-C10 device. Blood Press Monit 2015;20:98–103.
24. Stergiou GS, Efstathiou SP, Alamara CV, Mastorantonakis SE, Roussias LG. Home or self blood pressure measurement? What is the correct term? J Hypertens. 2003;21:2259–64.
25. Daskalopoulou SS, Rabi DM, Zarnke KB, et al. The 2015 Canadian Hypertension Education Program recommendations for blood pressure measurement, diagnosis, assessment of risk, prevention, and treatment of hypertension. Can J Cardiol 2015;31:549–568.

26. Beckett L, Godwin M. The BpTRU automatic blood pressure monitor compared to 24-h ambulatory blood pressure monitoring in the assessment of blood pressure in patients with hypertension. BMC Cardiovasc Disord. 2005;5:18.
27. Myers MG, Valdivieso M, Kiss A. Use of automated office blood pressure measurement to reduce the white coat response. J Hypertens. 2009;27:280–6.
28. Mattu GS, Perry Jr TL, Wright JM. Comparison of the oscillometric blood pressure monitor (BPM-100$_{Beta}$) with the auscultatory mercury sphygmomanometer. Blood Press Monit. 2001;6:153–9.
29. White WB, Anwar YA. Evaluation of the overall efficacy of the Omron office digital blood pressure HEM-907 monitor in adults. Blood Press Monit. 2001;6:107–10.
30. Stergiou GS, Tzamouranis D, Protogerou A, Nasothimiou E, Kapralos C. Validation of the Microlife WatchBP Office professional device for office blood pressure measurement according to the International Protocol. J Hypertens. 2008;26 (Suppl 1):S481.
31. Yarrows SA, Patel K, Brook R. Rapid oscillometric blood pressure measurement compared to conventional oscillometric measurement. Blood Press Monit. 2001;6:145–7.
32. Eguchi K, Kuruvilla S, Ogedegbe G, Gerin W, Schwartz JE, Pickering TG. What is the optimal interval between successive blood pressure readings using an automated oscillometric device. J Hypertens. 2009;27:1172–7.
33. Myers MG, Valdivieso M, Kiss A, Tobe SW. Comparison of two automated sphygmomanometers for use in the office setting. Blood Press Monit. 2009;14:45–7.
34. Myers MG, Valdivieso M, Kiss A. Optimum frequency of automated blood pressure measurements using an automated sphygmomanometer. Blood Press Monit. 2008;13:333–8.
35. Greiver M, White D, Kaplan DM, Katz K, Moineddin R, Doabchian E. Where should automated blood pressure measurements be taken? Blood Press Monit. 2012;17:137–8.
36. Armstrong D, Matangi M, Brouillard D, Myers MG. Automated office blood pressure – being alone and not location is what matters most. Blood Press Monit 2015;20:204–208.
37. Chambers LW, Kaczorowski J, O'Reilly S, Ig Nagni S, Hearps SJC. Comparison of blood pressure measurements using an automated blood pressure device in community pharmacies and family physicians' offices: a randomized controlled trial. CMAJ Open 2013.DOI:10.9778/cmajo.2013005.
38. Myers MG, Valdivieso M, Kiss A. Consistent relationship between automated office blood pressure recorded in different settings. Blood Press Monit. 2009;14:108–11.
39. Myers MG, Godwin M, Dawes M, et al. Conventional versus automated measurement of blood pressure in primary care patients with systolic hypertension: randomized parallel design controlled trial. BMJ. 2011;342:d285.
40. Myers MG, Oh P, Reeves RA, Joyner CD. Prevalence of white coat effect in treated hypertensive patients in the community. Am J Hypertens. 1995;8:591–7.
41. Sedgwick P. The Hawthorne effect. BMJ. 2011;344:d8262.
42. National Institute for Health and Clinical Excellence: Hypertension NICE Clinical Guidelines 127. National Clinical Guidelines Centre. London, UK, August, 2011.
43. Brown MA, Buddle ML, Martin A. Is resistant hypertension really resistant? Am J Hypertens. 2001;14:1263–9.
44. Graves JW, Nash C, Burger K, Bailey K, Sheps SG. Clinical decision-making in hypertension using an automated (BpTRU) measurement device. J Hum Hypertens. 2003;17:823–7.
45. Gustavsen PH, Hoegholm A, Bang LE, Kristensen KS. White coat hypertension is a cardiovascular risk factor: a 10-year follow-up study. J Hum Hypertens. 2003;17:811–7.
46. Head GA, Mihallidou AS, Duggan KA, et al. Definition of ambulatory blood pressure targets for diagnosis and treatment of hypertension in relation to clinic blood pressure: prospective cohort study. BMJ. 2010;340:1104–11.
47. Myers MG. A proposed algorithm for diagnosing hypertension using automated office blood pressure measurement. J Hypertens. 2010;28:703–8.
48. Godwin M, Birtwhistle R, Delva D, et al. Manual and automated office measurements in relation to awake ambulatory blood pressure monitoring. Fam Pract. 2011;28:110–7.

Chapter 2
Home (Self) Monitoring of Blood Pressure

Gianfranco Parati and Juan Eugenio Ochoa

Introduction

Elevated blood pressure (BP) levels represent the most important modifiable risk factor for cardiovascular disease and for disease burden in developed countries [1]. Consistent evidence has shown that BP reduction with antihypertensive therapy reduces cardiovascular events, particularly in patients with moderate to severe hypertension [2]. An accurate assessment of BP levels and early identification and treatment of hypertension is thus essential for reducing the cardiovascular risk associated with this condition [3]. Since most evidence on the cardiovascular risk associated with elevated BP, as well as on the benefits of lowering BP levels, comes from studies using office BP (OBP) measures [4, 5], this technique is regarded as the reference standard for assessment of BP in clinical practice [3]. However, OBP is affected by important intrinsic limitations (i.e., inherent inaccuracy of the technique and the inability to track BP changes during subjects' usual activities and over a long period of time) and by extrinsic factors (i.e., observer's bias, digit preference, interference by the "white coat effect") that lead to over- or underestimation of subjects' BP values. In turn, this leads to misclassification of BP levels, i.e., masked hypertension, white coat hypertension, and false BP control or false resistant hypertension in treated subjects. In recognition of this, current guidelines for

G. Parati, M.D. (✉)
Department of Health Sciences, University of Milano-Bicocca,
Piazza Brescia 20, Milan 20149, Italy

Department of Cardiovascular Neural and Metabolic Sciences, San Luca Hospital, IRCCS
Istituto Auxologico Italiano, Milan, Italy
e-mail: gianfranco.parati@unimib.it

J.E. Ochoa, M.D., Ph.D.
Department of Cardiovascular Neural and Metabolic Sciences, San Luca Hospital, IRCCS
Istituto Auxologico Italiano, Milan, Italy

© Springer International Publishing Switzerland 2016
W.B. White (ed.), *Blood Pressure Monitoring in Cardiovascular Medicine and Therapeutics*, Clinical Hypertension and Vascular Diseases,
DOI 10.1007/978-3-319-22771-9_2

hypertension management advise combining OBP with information on out-of-office BP levels measured by means of ambulatory BP monitoring (ABPM) or home BP monitoring (HBPM) [3, 6–11], with the aim to better identify the presence of high BP levels and to define the need to start/modify antihypertensive treatment. Currently, 24-h ABPM is considered the gold standard for out-of-office BP monitoring, [10, 12]; however, because of its costs and need of trained clinic staff and specialized equipment, its use is in most cases (with the exception of NICE guidelines) recommended for selected groups of hypertensive patients [3, 4, 6, 13, 14]. Although HBPM cannot provide the extensive information on daily life BP behavior available with 24-h ambulatory recordings, it may represent an excellent complement to both OBP and ABPM in assessing BP levels for several reasons. In particular, the wide availability of automated and easy-to-use devices for home BP monitoring, which are acceptable for both patients and physicians, supports the extensive implementation of HBPM in clinical practice. Moreover, when performed on a regular basis, repeated BP measures obtained by patients at home (i.e., home BP monitoring of BP levels over 7 days before the clinical visit) offer the possibility to obtain accurate and frequent information on out-of-office BP not only during a single day, but also over several days, weeks, or months in a usual life setting, also allowing evaluation of dynamic BP changes over wider time windows, and to quantify the degree of BP variability (BPV) [8] (Table 2.1). All of these features not only allow a better identification of elevated BP levels, but also assessment of BP control in treated subjects, thus aiding in guiding therapeutic decisions. Besides, at variance from OBP, HBPM requires the active involvement of patients in managing their high BP conditions, which enhances patients' compliance and adherence to antihypertensive treatment, thus potentially increasing the rates of BP control. Because HBPM combines improved accuracy with the advantages of low cost and easy implementation, it is recommended whenever feasible for routine use in the clinical management of hypertension. The present chapter is aimed at reviewing the main features of HBPM, its prognostic significance, clinical advantages, and potential applications for the management of hypertension. In its last part, the chapter addresses the role of home-based blood pressure telemonitoring and information technologies for the management of hypertensive patients.

Methodological Aspects of HBPM

Measurement conditions and procedures: Although automated and semi-automated HBPM devices based on the oscillometric technique are widely used by hypertensive patients, their application is not always accompanied by the required knowledge or sufficient training to ensure a proper BP self-measurement at home. The resulting problems often include use of inaccurate devices and errors in measurement methodology and in interpretation of HBP values [15]. Care is thus required to guarantee that HBP measurements are kept under close supervision by physicians, in order to prevent an excessive frequency of self-BP readings due to anxiety as well as improper

Table 2.1 Comparison of features of three main methods for BP measurement

Feature	OBP	ABPM	HBPM
No. of readings	Low	High	Medium
White coat effect	Yes	No	No
Operator dependency	Yes	No	No
Need of device validation	No[a]	Yes	Yes
Daytime BP	+	+++	++
Night-time BP and dipping	-	+++	-/+[b]
Morning BP	±	++	+
24-h BP variability	-	++	±
Long-term BP variability	-	±	++
WCH and MH diagnosis	-	++	++
Placebo effect	++	-	-
Reproducibility	Low	High (24-h average values)	High (average of several values)
Prognostic value	+	+++	++
Patient involvement	-	-	++
Patient training	-	±	++
Physician involvement	+++	++	+
Patients' acceptance	++	±	++
Monitoring of treatment effects	Limited information	Extensive information on 24-h BP profile, cannot be repeated frequently	Appropriate for long-term monitoring, limited information on BP profile
Hypertension control improvement	+	++	+++
Cost	Low	High	Low
Availability	High	Low	High

Modified from Parati et al. [8], by permission

WCH white coat hypertension, *MH* masked hypertension, *OBP* Office Blood Pressure, *ABPM* ambulatory BP monitoring, *HBPM* home BP monitoring

[a]Yes if oscillometric device is used

[b]New HBPM devices may perform night-time BP measures

self-management of drug treatment by patients. Overall, conditions and procedures for proper HBP performance are similar to those recommended for OBP measurements [9]. Specifically, the patient should be relaxed in the sitting position, with the back supported, without crossing legs, in a quiet room and at least 5 min of rest should precede the measurement. The arm should be supported on a table and the cuff positioned at the heart level (when the arm-cuff is below or above the heart level, BP will be overestimated or underestimated, respectively). At the time of the first visit, when prescribing HBPM, BP measurements should be comparatively performed in both arms. If inter-arm BP difference exceeds 10 mmHg for SBP and/or 5 mmHg for DBP and persists after repeated measurements, the arm with the higher BP should be selected for future BP measurements both in the office and at home [9]. Attention should be given to selection of cuff size according to arm circumference, so that the bladder dimensions are adequate for accurate BP measurement.

Device selection: Monitors that measure BP at the upper arm (brachial artery) have been shown to be the most accurate and reliable in measuring peripheral BP levels. Although some automatic devices for BP measurement at the wrist or at the finger level have been developed, it should be mentioned that they are subject to important limitations mainly related to peripheral vasoconstriction, alterations in BP waveform going from central to more distal sites of recording, and the possibility of varying hydrostatic height difference between the peripheral cuff and the heart level, which may lead to significant inaccuracies in BP measurement. This is why use of wrist cuff devices is currently discouraged. Finally, it should be mentioned that despite the multitude of devices available on the market for HBPM, only some of them have fulfilled independent validation criteria for use in clinical practice (updated lists of validated BP-measuring devices are provided at dedicated websites such as www.dableducational.org, www.ipertensionearteriosa.net or www.bhsoc. org). In summary, on the background of the available evidence, current guidelines for HBPM recommend the use of validated, automated, electronic, oscillometric, upper arm-cuff devices, particularly those offering the possibility to store, transmit, or print measurements [9].

Frequency and timing of HBPM: When performed in a standardized fashion, BP measures collected by patients at home have been shown to be more accurate and reproducible than office and ambulatory BP levels [16–18]. To achieve the maximum benefits from HBPM, the optimal HBPM schedule to be used for clinical decision making should be able to offer a quantification of the prevailing level of HBP, aimed at yielding reproducible information on HBP values, with prognostic relevance. Since the reliability of HBPM increases with the number of BP readings available for analysis, a minimum of 12 measurements and up to 25 measurements are needed to achieve clinically relevant information on HBP levels. Recent secondary analysis of a large, randomized, clinical trial compared strategies for home- or clinic-based BP monitoring to determine the optimal methodology for obtaining clinically meaningful BP measurements [19]. In this trial, participants were asked to record BP values every other day at the same time. A minimum of three values over two weeks was required and only values spaced over 12 h were included. The study concluded that the best approach for correctly classifying BP control should be an average of several BP measurements including both measurements from the clinic- and home-based settings [19–21]. However, the important variations in terms of frequency of self-BP measures, the frequency of reporting home-monitored values, clinicians' involvement, duration, and setting have been widely variable among studies, thus preventing authors from deriving consistent conclusions. Current guidelines recommend measuring BP levels at home over 7 days, with at least two morning and two evening measurements [9]. For clinical decision making, the average of all these values should be used with the exception of the first day, which should be discarded [9]. This 7-day schedule is recommended immediately before each visit to the physician's office, either at diagnosis or during follow-up. In recognition that long-term HBPM might allow a closer assessment of the stability of HBP control, improve patients' involvement and compliance with treatment, and maintain their BP measurement skills, it was suggested that 1–2 measurements per week might be useful also during the between-visit period [9]. Of note, programmable HBPM devices have been recently introduced that provide measures of night time BP levels comparable to those obtained by means of 24-h ABPM [22–24], thus widening the clinical applications of HBPM.

How Are Hypertension and BP Control Defined Based on HBPM?

Hypertension has a strong, continuous relationship with cardiovascular risk. Traditionally, OBP measurements have been used for cardiovascular risk stratification and for defining targets of therapy. The classification of BP categories (i.e., optimal BP <120/80; pre-hypertension 120–139/80–89; and hypertension ≥140/90 mmHg) as well as definition of BP targets to be achieved by treatment, has been based on epidemiological studies using OBP measurements [3, 25]. These values cannot be directly extrapolated to HBPM, because meta-analyses of several studies on unselected populations or hypertensive patients [26, 27], comparing HBP and OBP distribution curves, have demonstrated HBP values to be lower than corresponding OBP values. Longitudinal studies in general populations [28–37] and in hypertensive subjects [38–40] as well as clinical trials on the use of HBPM have confirmed that the cut-off limit to define hypertension based on HBP should be lower than that used for OBP [41, 42]. Although the relationship between BP values self-measured at home and the incidence of CV morbidity and mortality should be further clarified by prospective studies, there is an agreement to diagnose hypertension when HBP is ≥135/85 mmHg (corresponding to an OBP of ≥140/90 mmHg). Prospective data are still needed, however, to formally recommend the proposed thresholds of <120/80 mmHg and <130/85 mmHg to define optimal and normal HBP, respectively. A couple of studies suggested that HBP thresholds for hypertension in high-risk patients might be lower than 135/85 mmHg [30, 39]. Although the target HBP to be achieved with treatment should logically be below the threshold used to diagnose hypertension (i.e., <135/85 mmHg), these target HBP levels are still unknown, being currently explored by the ongoing HBPM studies [43]. Although attaining therapeutic goals may be difficult in some patients, it should be remembered that, even if BP is not fully controlled, each mmHg of reduction in HBP is important, as it contributes to the prevention of CV complications.

Prognostic Value of HBPM

As a general remark, it has to be acknowledged that the evidence available to support the prognostic value of HBPM is less than for ABPM, also because of the smaller number of outcome studies available so far [8, 9]. When averaged over a period of a few days, home BP measures have been shown to significantly predict the development of major nonfatal cardiovascular events (myocardial infarction, stroke) [28–35, 38, 44–52] as well as cardiovascular (fatal cardiovascular events) and all-cause mortality [28, 34, 35, 39, 47, 48, 53]. In most available studies, the prognostic value of HBPM has been found superior to that of OBP measurements with one exception, where a similar predictive value was observed for both techniques [38] (see Fig. 2.1 and Table 2.2).

Longitudinal and cross-sectional studies have reported that target organ involvement, including left ventricular mass index (LVMI), carotid intima-media thickness,

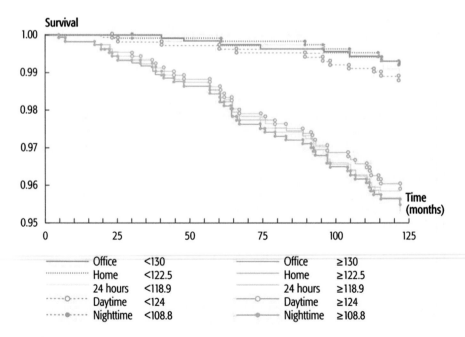

Fig. 2.1 Kaplan–Meier curves for survival free of CV disease in subjects with office, *home*, and ambulatory SBP values above and below median values. Modified from Sega et al. [35], by permission

Table 2.2 Home blood pressure measurements and outcomes

Study	Population	Time of measurements	Average number of measurements	Outcome
Ohkubo et al. (1998) (Ohasama) [28], Hozawa et al. (2000) (Ohasama) [47]	General population aged ≥40 years	Morning	21	Cardiovascular, non-cardiovascular, and all-cause mortality
Ohkubo et al.2004 (Ohasama) [29]	General population aged ≥40 years	Morning	1–25	Total stroke morbidity
Asayama et al. (2005) (Ohasama) [30]	General population aged ≥40 years	Morning	25	Total stroke morbidity
Ohkubo et al.2004 (Ohasama) [31]	General population aged ≥40 years	Morning	25	Total, hemorrhagic, and ischemic stroke morbidity
Asayama et al. 2004 (Ohasama) [32]	General population aged ≥40 years	Morning and evening	47	Total stroke morbidity
Nishinaga et al. 2005 (Kahoku) [33]	Community dwelling elderly aged ≥65 years	Morning and evening	20	Cardiovascular, non-cardiovascular and all-cause mortality
Okumiya et al. 1999 (Kahoku) [48]	Community dwelling elderly aged ≥75 years	Morning and evening	20	Disability, cardiovascular and all-cause mortality, cardiovascular and stroke morbidity,
Bobrie et al. 2004 (SHEAF study) [38]	Treated hypertensives aged ≥60 years	Morning and evening	27	Cardiovascular and all-cause mortality, total cardiovascular morbidity
Sega et al. (2005), Mancia et al. (2006) (PAMELA study) [34, 35]	General population aged 25–74 years	Morning and evening	2	Cardiovascular and all-cause mortality
Agarwal et al. 2006 (CKD Veterans) [39]	Veterans with CKD	Morning, afternoon and evening	Not available	Morbidity of end stage renal disease, all-cause mortality
Fagard, et al. 2005 (Flanders) [46]	General population aged ≥60 years	Morning	3	Major cardiovascular events (cardiovascular death, myocardial infarction and stroke)
Stergiou et al. 2007. (Didima) [53]	General population aged ≥18 years	Morning and evening	12	Total cardiovascular morbidity and mortality
Niiranen et al. 2014 [49]	Two cohorts of General population aged 34–64 years; and newly diagnosed and untreated hypertensive men and women aged 35–54 years	Morning and evening	14	composite of cardiovascular mortality, myocardial infarction, stroke, heart failure hospitalization, and coronary intervention

Modified from Parati et al. [8], by permission

and microalbuminuria, is more strongly correlated with HBP measurements than with OBP measurements in patients with hypertension [51, 54–60] as well as in patients with chronic kidney disease (CKD) on hemodialysis (HD) [61], in elderly people, in women with pre-eclampsia, and in hypertensive patients with diabetes [8]. In the case of patients with CKD, HBP has been shown to be a better predictor of progression of CKD (as assessed with eGFR) [40, 62], including its progression to end stage renal disease (ESRD) [39] and of cardiovascular events and mortality [63] than OBP. In particular, in ESRD, HBPM may be more informative than pre- and post-dialysis OBP readings as it provides BP measurements that are more representative of the BP load over the interdialytic period. Indeed, several studies in ESRD have found HBP to be prognostically superior than OBP also in predicting subclinical organ damage (i.e., LVH) [61] and cardiovascular events (i.e., all-cause and CV mortality) [64, 65].

Role of HBPM in the Diagnosis and Management of Hypertension: Identification of Masked Hypertension and White-Coat Hypertension

As discussed above, HBPM and ABPM provide out-of-office BP measurements detecting BP changes in real life conditions and preventing the alarm reaction associated with OBP [66]. It is thus not surprising that BP levels measured in the clinic setting are in general higher than ambulatory BP measurements performed out of the clinic environment [67]. This is considered a major explanation for the frequently observed disagreements between OBP and out-of-office BP measurements when classifying hypertensive subjects [30]. Indeed, when considering the threshold values to define hypertension using OBP ($\geq$140/90 mmHg) and HBP or 24h ABP ($\geq$130/80 mmHg), a given individual may fall into one of four BP categories: sustained normotension (normal office BP and normal home or 24h ABP), sustained hypertension (high OBP and high home or 24h ABP), white coat hypertension (high office BP and normal home or 24h ABP), or masked hypertension (normal office BP and high home or 24h ABP) (Fig. 2.2).

Evidence on the ability of HBPM to identify WCH and MH [56, 68] was provided in a report of the Pressioni Arteriose Monitorate e Loro Associazioni (PAMELA) study in which the initial diagnosis of WCH (i.e., identified as office BP >140/90 mmHg and 24-h BP mean <125/79 mmHg or home BP <132/82 mmHg) was reassessed 10 years later. Overall, the study showed similar results in the ability of HBPM and ABPM for identifying WCH, sustained hypertension, true normotension, and masked hypertension, even if a substantial percentage of subjects changed from one category to another, including progression to sustained hypertension (Fig. 2.3).

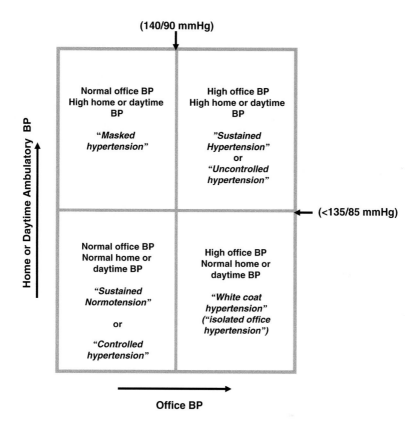

Fig. 2.2 Schematic relationship between office and home or daytime ambulatory BP. Classification of patients based on the comparison of office and home or daytime ambulatory blood pressure (BP). When focusing on ABP, current guidelines recommend to use 24h rather than daytime ABP, in order to include also night-time BP values Taken from Parati et al. [8], by permission

Role of HBPM in the Assessment of BP Control in Treated Hypertension

In the light of the available evidence supporting the prognostic and clinical advantages offered by HBPM, current international and national guidelines recommend the use of HBPM as part of the routine diagnostic and therapeutic approach to hypertension, particularly in treated patients [8, 69–74]. By providing accurate and frequent BP measures at regular time intervals over several days, weeks, or months, in a setting of typical daily living, HBPM is able to accurately track changes in BP levels induced by antihypertensive treatment and becomes a better indicator of BP control than OBP measurements alone [8]. HBPM may be an excellent tool to assess and improve the achievement of BP control, particularly in patients with apparent resistant hypertension in whom BP cannot be easily controlled even with several classes of antihypertensive medications. In support of this concept, several studies

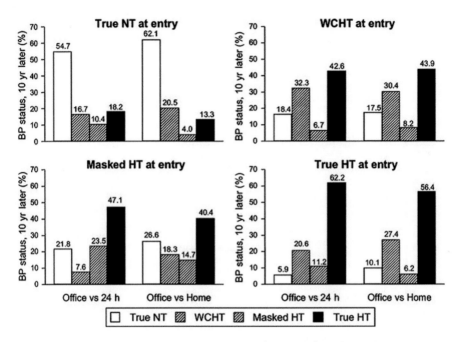

Fig. 2.3 Mean percentage changes in BP status among normotension (NT), white coat hypertension (WCHT), and masked hypertension (MHT) over the 10-year period of the study. Data referring to true hypertension (true HT) are shown for comparison. Taken from Mancia et al. [68], with permission

exploring the benefits of HBPM for the long-term management of patients on antihypertensive therapy have shown that when properly implemented, HBPM may significantly increase achievement of BP control when compared to conventional OBP [75, 76], while reducing the need of follow-up medical visits [77]. The benefits of HBPM in this regard may be derived from several factors. First, the use of HBPM improves adherence to prescribed treatment (see below). Secondly, in subjects who receive antihypertensive treatment, OBP measurements alone may be inaccurate in assessing true BP control. For instance, the alerting reaction to the medical visit may continue to be present in anyone treated for hypertension, regardless of the number of drugs being taken [78]. It is not uncommon to find patients with mild hypertension based on HBPM or ABPM who yet appear to have severe hypertension in the clinic, due to a white coat effect in this condition [79], or treated subjects who, despite achieving adequate out-of-office BP control with antihypertensive drugs, continue to present elevation in office BP levels because of a persistent emotional reaction to the medical visit. This phenomenon, which is equivalent to WCH in untreated patients, has been addressed as "white coat resistant hypertension" (WCRH) or false resistant hypertension in order to emphasize its occurrence in subjects receiving antihypertensive treatment [14].

Observational and interventional studies in treated hypertensives implementing OBP measures along with ambulatory or home BP monitoring have shown overwhelmingly that up to one-third of treated hypertensives may be mistakenly classified as having resistant hypertension, when they actually have "false resistant hypertension" due to a persisting white coat effect [80]. A condition of greater clinical concern is masked resistant hypertension (MRH) or false BP control (i.e., BP appear to be controlled based on OBP, but is elevated when out-of-office BP levels are recorded)—this condition has been also reported to occur in about 30 % of treated subjects [81, 82].

The high prevalence of MRH and WCRH among treated hypertensive individuals further reinforces the clinical relevance of identifying these conditions. On the one hand, identification of WCRH would prevent undesirable modifications of antihypertensive treatment, i.e., an unnecessary increase in dose or number of antihypertensive drugs, and reduction of the chance of adverse effects associated with improperly prescribed multidrug therapy that often interferes with patients' quality of life, leading in the end to poor compliance with treatment. At the same time, it would reduce the expenditures associated with unnecessary additional pharmacological treatment and/or unnecessary interventional device-based strategies (i.e., carotid baroreceptor activation [83] and renal denervation [84]) for the management of resistant hypertension. Indeed, given the elevated costs and the invasive nature of these approaches, as well as their potential adverse effects when improperly indicated, discarding WCRH based on out-of-office BP measures is currently considered among the eligibility criteria before proceeding with interventional treatment of resistant hypertension [85]. In contrast, identification of MRH would indicate the need to implement early modifications on antihypertensive treatment in order to prevent development/progression of subclinical organ damage and cardiovascular events associated with this condition.

Regarding the ability to identify masked hypertension and white coat hypertension, several studies have comparatively explored the performance of HBPM against the reference standard for out-of-office BPM represented by ABPM. Although MH was first studied with ABPM [86], it has been demonstrated that HBP can be as reliable as ABPM in identifying this phenomenon as well as the associated target-organ damage associated with MH [87]. Evidence has also been provided that HBPM is as reliable as ABPM in identifying WCH [87] and useful in identifying "truly" hypertensive patients likely to benefit from implementation of antihypertensive therapy from those with WCH in whom antihypertensive treatment is probably not needed [41]. In a recent study conducted in a group of subjects on stable treatment with ≥ 3 antihypertensive drugs using ABPM as reference method [88] in which resistant hypertension was defined as elevated OBP ($\geq 140/90$ mmHg) and true resistant hypertension as concomitant elevation in-office and out-of-office BP (SBP and/or DBP $\geq 135/85$ mmHg for HBP or awake ABP), there was agreement between ABP and HBP in diagnosing clinic or "white coat" resistant hypertension in 82 % of the cases (59 % with and 23 % without clinic resistant hypertension; kappa 0.59). Regarding the diagnosis of true resistant hypertension, there was agreement between ABP and HBP in 74 % of the cases (49 % with and 25 % without true resistant hypertension; kappa 0.46). The sensitivity, specificity, and positive and negative predictive values for HBP in detecting white coat resistant hypertension were 93 %,

63 %, 81 %, and 83 %, respectively. The respective values for HBP in detecting true resistant hypertension were 90 %, 55 %, 71 %, and 82 %, indicating that HBP may be a useful tool in the evaluation of false and true resistant hypertension [88].

Based on the above data, it may be concluded that a proper assessment of BP control and classification of treated hypertensive patients with the combined use of office, ambulatory, and ideally home BP measurements are essential for defining the need of performing additional diagnostic procedures (i.e., screening tests for secondary causes of resistant hypertension) and/or implementing more aggressive pharmacological or interventional strategies (Fig. 2.4) [89].

While emphasizing the above advantages of HBPM in assessing BP control by treatment, we have also to acknowledge that HBPM may not provide information on BP levels during night-time sleep, which have shown to be of major clinical relevance because of their demonstrated prognostic value [35, 44, 90–93]. However, in recent years validated, memory-equipped devices have been designed that can be programmed to provide nocturnal BP readings comparable to those obtained with 24-h ABPM [22–24].

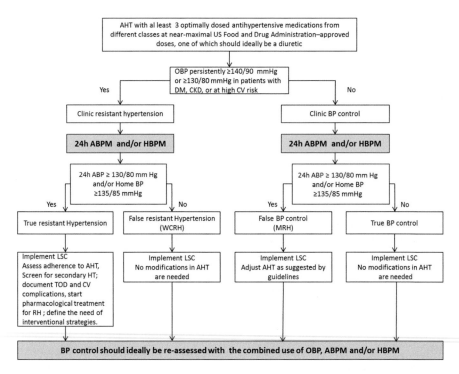

Fig. 2.4 Initial diagnostic approach to the patient with clinic resistant hypertension. *AHT* antihypertensive treatment, *HT* hypertension, *OBP* office blood pressure, *DM* diabetes mellitus, *CKD* chronic kidney disease, *CV* cardiovascular, *BP* blood pressure, *ABPM* ambulatory blood pressure monitoring, *HBPM* home blood pressure monitoring, *WCRH* "white coat" resistant hypertension, *MRH* "masked" resistant hypertension, *RH* resistant hypertension, *LSC* life style changes. Modified from Parati et al. [89], with permission

HBPM is admittedly less effective than ABPM in assessing the time distribution of BP control by treatment over 24 h. However, HBPM performed in the morning (before drug intake) and in the evening over different days may provide useful information about the efficacy of therapeutic coverage over 24 h and in the long term and may identify cases of morning hypertension attributable to insufficient duration of action of prescribed antihypertensive medications.

HBPM allows patients to perform repeated and regular BP measurements over extended periods of time and may be particularly advantageous in the case of treated hypertensive subjects with CKD, and particularly in those with ESRD. In hemodialysis (HD) patients, BP control poses unique challenges because of the marked reductions in intravascular volume immediately after HD and its progressive increases throughout the inter-dialytic period, which induce an extremely variable behavior of BP [94]. In this context, HBPM provides potential advantages such as the possibility of sampling BP at various times throughout the inter-dialytic period to aid in tracking daytime and day-to-day BP variations and providing BP measurements that are more representative of subject's actual BP burden.

HBPM: A Substitute or a Complement to ABPM and OBP Measures?

In view of the limitations characterizing OBP measurements, it becomes clear that an adequate assessment of BP control and a proper diagnosis of resistant hypertension cannot be based on just isolated OBP readings. Indeed, a recent position paper on ABPM of the European Society of Hypertension [14] recommends performing 24-h ABPM and/or HBPM for detecting the presence of WCH and identifying the presence of true hypertension and masked hypertension in all patients with uncomplicated, stage 1 and 2 hypertension before starting antihypertensive drug therapy. Based on the evidence from several studies supporting the clinical value of ABPM either for selecting patients for treatment or for assessing the effects of antihypertensive drug therapy, ABPM is currently considered the standard method for confirming the diagnosis of hypertension in clinical practice [12, 14] and for assessing BP control in treated hypertensive patients [3, 6, 14, 10]. However, ABPM is not always available everywhere and requires trained clinic staff and specialized equipment and software for its analysis [9].

When performed on a regular basis and following standardized protocols [9], repeated BP measures obtained by patients at home result in accurate and frequent out-of-office BP measurements not only during a single day, but also over several days, weeks, or months in the non-medical setting, hence providing more reliable measures not only on the degree, but also on the consistency of BP control over time [9].

In view of the available evidence supporting the superior prognostic value of home vs. office BP levels, as well as the clinical advantages of HBPM, current hypertension guidelines recommend more extensive use of HBPM not only for the initial diagnostic approach to hypertension (i.e., to identify "truly" hypertensive patients, likely to benefit from implementation of antihypertensive therapy [41]), but also for the long-term follow-up of treated hypertensive patients, even if they have controlled OBP, in order to better define the actual BP normalization rate achieved by various drug regimens [8, 9, 3, 25, 95]. Although HBPM shares many of the advantages of ABPM, including a cost-effective approach to the diagnosis of hypertension, it should not be considered as a substitute but rather as a complement to ABPM, since these methods are likely to pick up different types of BP behavior in a person's activities of daily living.

Role of HBPM in Improving Adherence to Treatment and Reducing Therapeutic Inertia

Poor adherence to therapy has been recognized as one of the most important factors contributing to uncontrolled hypertension. By encouraging patients to become actively involved in their care, and by positively affecting their perceptions about the management of hypertension, HBPM offers the possibility to improve patient's compliance and adherence to lifestyle changes and/or medical treatment [96]. Recent meta-analyses of randomized controlled trials have shown that compared to usual care based on OBP measurements, HBPM-guided antihypertensive treatment may significantly increase rates of achievement of BP control [75, 97] probably as a consequence of better compliance to treatment. In fact, HBPM is being increasingly implemented in clinical settings not only to guide antihypertensive therapy and to assess long-term BP control, but also as a means to improve patient's compliance and adherence to antihypertensive treatment [98]. Another important advantage of HBPM in clinical practice is that it may help to overcome therapeutic inertia, since more information is provided to practitioners that allow more appropriate clinical decisions.

Assessment of Day-to-Day Blood Pressure Variability

HBPM may offer clinically relevant information when considering BPV over long periods of time. Although most studies on the prognostic relevance of BPV have focused on short-term BP changes assessed from 24-h ABPM, evidence from recent studies and clinical trials has suggested that an increased BPV in the mid-term (day-to-day) and in the long-term (i.e., between weekly, monthly, or yearly visits) relates to adverse implications for CV prognosis [99–103]. Although an extensive assessment of BPV for intermediate periods could theoretically be obtained by performing ABPM over consecutive days (i.e., during 48 h or more), this approach is neither well-accepted by patients nor available in all clinical settings. An alternative method for assessment of day-by-day BPV consists of its calculation from BP measurements performed by patients at home over several days. Although HBPM cannot provide extensive information on nocturnal BP and BP profiles as ABPM does, a major advantage of this technique is that it provides information on the consistency of BP control over time earlier than when considering long-term visit-to-visit BPV, thus allowing early adjustment of antihypertensive treatment (and thus timely preventing development/progression of organ damage associated with inconsistent BP control). Besides, HBP monitors are widely available and are well-accepted by patients and are a more feasible approach for the evaluation of day-by-day BPV by applying different metrics: (1) Blood pressure standard deviation [104, 105], but with accounting for its dependence on mean BP levels, i.e., by calculating the coefficient of variation (SD × 100/BP mean) [104]; (2) morning maximum and minimum blood pressure (MMD); (3) "average real variability" (ARV), computed as the average of the absolute differences between consecutive BP measurements, focusing on the sequence of BP readings, thus reflecting reading-to-reading, within-subject variability in BP levels [106]; (4) variance independent of the mean (VIM), a method proposed to exclude the effect of mean BP from BPV by applying nonlinear regression analysis (i.e., plotting SD against mean) [99]. These indices of day-by-day BPV have been shown to be of prognostic value as indicated by a series of studies in which an increased day-by-day BPV independently of average home BP levels was predictive of development, establishment, and evolution of cardiac, vascular, and renal organ damage [107]. In a cross-sectional analysis of a population of never-treated participants with hypertension, an increased day-by-day BPV in home systolic BP (assessed as the maximum mean triplicate in home systolic BP over 14 consecutive days) was positively correlated with left ventricular mass index, increased carotid intima-media thickness, and urinary albumin/creatinine ratio over and above mean home SBP levels [107]. In a population of type 2 diabetes patients from Japan, increasing values of day-by-day variability (assessed as CV of morning and evening HBP measured over 14 consecutive days) were significantly higher in subjects presenting with macroalbuminuria (i.e., urinary albumin excretion ≥300 mg/g creatinine). Additionally, the CVs of morning systolic and diastolic BP and evening systolic BP were significantly correlated with urinary albumin excretion independently of other confounders [108]. A further report, also in type 2 diabetic patients, found higher values of SD of morning systolic HBP to be associated with increased arterial stiffness (i.e., higher pulse wave velocity) independent of other known risk factors [109]. Another study, conducted in a cohort of hypertensive patients, found home systolic BPV and max systolic BP to be associated with urinary albumin excretion [110]. In the frame of the Home Blood Pressure for Diabetic Nephropathy (HBP-DN) study, a prospective study in type 2 diabetic patients with microalbuminuria, higher values of SD of home systolic blood pressure (HSBP) were observed among subjects with the lowest values of estimated GFR (eGFR) [111]. Regarding the predictive value for cardiovascular events and mortality, the two main population studies exploring the prognostic value of mid-term BPV have found increasing values of day-by-day BPV to be associated with an increased risk of fatal and nonfatal cardiovascular events [101–103]. In the Ohasama study from Japan, increasing values of variability in systolic HBP were associated with a higher risk of the composite end point of cardiac and stroke mortality, but only with a significant risk of stroke mortality, when the outcomes were independently considered [101]. In another report from the Ohasama study, increasing values of variability in systolic HBP were associated with a higher risk of cerebral infarction in ever smokers, but not in never smokers [102]. When the prognostic value of novel indices of BPV derived from self-measured HBP was evaluated in the population of the Ohasama study, increasing values of VIM and ARV, but not of morning maximum and minimum blood pressure (MMD) determined on a median of 26 readings, were associated with an increased risk of cardiovascular and total mortality. However, when adjustment was performed by accounting for average BP and common confounders, the incremental predictive value of VIM, MMD, and ARV over and beyond HBP level was only marginal (i.e., from <0.01 to 0.88 %) [102]. In the Finn–Home study in a cohort of adults from the general population [103], increasing variability in systolic and diastolic HBP measures performed over seven consecutive days was associated with a higher risk of cardiovascular events after 7.8 years of follow-up, which remained significant even after adjusting for age and average HBP levels, thus supporting the additive value of HBP variability in predicting CV prognosis [103]. Contrasting results were reported after 12-years of follow-up in a Belgium population in which no predictive value for HBP variability was observed for either cardiovascular mortality or morbidity after accounting for average BP levels [112]. In relation to the effects of antihypertensive treatment, despite the wide availability of monitors for HBP monitoring, only few interventional studies in hypertension have implemented routine assessment of HBPV in order to address whether reducing day-by-day BP variability with antihypertensive treatment in addition to reducing average home BP levels is associated with improvements in cardiovascular protection.

The results of interventional studies addressing the effects of antihypertensive treatment on HBP variability have been inconsistent. While some have found treatment with a beta-blocker to be related with lower HBP variability [109], other studies conducted in diabetic patients or in the general population have reported higher values of HBP variability in the arm receiving beta-blockers [109, 112]. A longitudinal study conducted in a population of hypertensive patients from Japan (with systolic HBP>135 mmHg) explored whether reductions in HBP variability (determined on the basis of BP measures performed in the morning and the evening over seven consecutive days) were associated with changes in renal damage [assessed with urinary albumin excretion (UAE)] before and after 6 months of candesartan treatment. Although significant reductions were observed both in average BP levels and in HBP variability after 6 months of therapy, only treatment-induced reductions in average HBP but not in home BPV or in maximum home SBP were associated with reductions in UAE levels [110]. Another study reported lower values of systolic BPV in patients treated for <12 months with an angiotensin receptor blocker (ARB) but not with a calcium channel blocker (CCB) [113]. The only clinical study comparing the effects of different antihypertensive drug classes on BPV found a

CCB/ARB combination to be more effective in reducing systolic HBP variability, than a ARB/thiazide combination [114]. In the same study, significant reductions in pulse wave velocity (an index of arterial stiffness) induced by the ARB/CCB treatment (6 months) were independently correlated with changes in systolic HBP variability [114]. A recent non-randomized analysis of a population of diabetic subjects receiving different drug classes found lower values of morning HBP variability in subjects receiving calcium antagonists than in those receiving angiotensin converting enzyme (ACE) inhibitors or ARBs [115].

Telemonitoring of Home BP Monitoring

The wide availability and low cost of automated BP measuring devices and the emphasis put by healthcare systems on delivering patient-centered care have stimulated development of home-based telemonitoring. Such a system requires active involvement of patients who self-monitor their BP levels as well as pulse rate and send these values to a healthcare provider. However, in daily clinical practice, these data are usually reported in handwritten logbooks and oftentimes are inaccurate and/or illegible. This makes interpretation of HBPM values a difficult task, either when exploring BP behavior over the recording period and/or when estimating the BP changes in response to antihypertensive treatment. These issues may discourage physicians from using HBPM data for clinical decision-making. In recent years, the rapid development of e-health-related technologies has made it possible to develop home-based telemonitoring systems that allow transfer of data obtained by patients at home to a remote sever (through a stationary or mobile phone or internet connection) where HBPM values are stored and analyzed [116, 117]. Automatically generated reports of these data are easier to interpret by the physician or the health personnel and thus more useful to make therapeutic decisions, which may be communicated to the patient without the need for additional clinic visits. Several HBPT systems are available, some of which also allow sending reminders to patients indicating the time of BP measurement and/or of medication intake. Patients can alter their health behaviors or have adjustments made in their medication regimen between visits, avoiding the need to wait months between visits for adjustments. Home-based monitoring may also alert the provider about new changes in a patient's health that may be associated with uncontrolled hypertension. In addition to traditional face-to-face clinic visits, patient-centered care involves providing care outside the clinic as well, which has been linked to improved patient satisfaction and to innovative ways of providing healthcare [118]. Moreover, telephone contacts offer a medium to enable patients to be reached regardless of geographic location and have been shown effective in changing multiple patient behaviors [119, 120]. Considering the decreased transportation burden and time savings, home-based telemonitoring may be more convenient for patients [121] and may encourage the development of a sense of control and support for chronic disease self-management [122].

Improving Achievement of BP Control Rates with Home BP Telemonitoring

Recent reports of interventional studies and meta-analyses of clinical trials have provided evidence that addition of remote telemonitoring of home BP values is effective in improving compliance to treatment, blood pressure control, and related medical and economic outcomes in hypertensive patients [117, 123–126], especially in those with treatment-resistant hypertension due to poor compliance with multiple drug prescriptions [127] (Fig. 2.5).

Preliminary reports also suggest a possible utility of HBPT for self-titration of antihypertensive medication by patients [128]. However, despite these results, heterogeneity of published studies in terms of HBPM protocols (i.e., devices, frequency of measures, method for reporting BP levels) and study populations suggests that well-designed, large-scale, randomized, controlled studies are still required to demonstrate the clinical usefulness of this technique [117, 126].

The Role of Nurse and Pharmacist in Home Blood Pressure Telemonitoring Systems

Patient-centered hypertension management requires a team-oriented approach often involving multidisciplinary roles (nurses, pharmacists, physicians) with the patient at the core [129]. In recent trials, nurses with varying levels of training [120, 130–133],

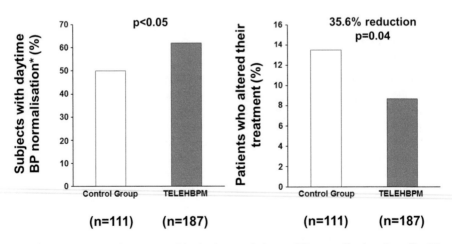

Fig. 2.5 Percentage of patients with daytime ambulatory BP normalization (systolic BP <130 mmHg and diastolic BP <80 mmHg). In this study, hypertensive patients were randomized to be conventionally managed based on office BP measurement (*white bars*, n = 111) or to be managed based on teletransmission of home BP values (*gray bars*: n = 187). Modified from Parati et al. [123], by permission

and clinical pharmacists [134–138], have been involved in this approach to patients' care. In particular, nurse-delivered interventions have been shown to contribute to improved patient outcomes [120, 132]. These nursing professionals are trained to address lifestyle and behavioral actions such as diet and exercise patterns, strategies for weight reduction, and smoking cessation, among others. Nurses at all practice levels are able to educate patients on proper home-based BP monitoring techniques, procedures for telemonitoring, and interpretation about appropriate BP thresholds. In addition, nurse practitioners (NP) are advanced practice-registered nurses with additional training enabling them to prescribe or manage pharmacotherapy. Their services involve ordering, conducting, and interpreting diagnostic and laboratory tests; prescribing pharmacologic agents and non-pharmacologic therapy; and teaching and counseling. Like the NP, clinical pharmacists with additional training and scopes of practice are able to prescribe and manage pharmacotherapy. Clinical pharmacists are an excellent source of counseling regarding safe, appropriate, and cost-effective medications use [139, 140]. Pharmacists may initiate, discontinue, or adjust pharmacotherapy based on clinical indications [135, 141, 139, 140].

Clinical pharmacist-administered behavioral and medication management interventions have been shown to improve BP control and the management of other chronic conditions leading to reductions in cardiovascular risk [141]. To date though, most of the evidence supporting the effects of pharmacist-driven interventions on BP levels has been provided in a traditional community-based setting rather than through telemonitoring [142, 143]. Of note, while the NP or clinical pharmacist may appear to be ideal interventionists with their pharmacotherapy privileges, cost-effectiveness is a major factor as LPNs and RNs may require significantly less monetary resources.

Cost-effectiveness of Home BP Telemonitoring-Based Programs

Although some financial aspects may limit the implementation of HBPT (i.e., costs of purchasing and maintaining the system, the need of trained personnel, requirement of telephonic/Internet connections), they may be partly counterbalanced by the reduction in the costs of patients' management compared with usual care. It is suggested that home-based monitoring may encourage more appropriate resource utilization by curtailing the need for unnecessary clinic visits (e.g., visits solely for a BP check), while simultaneously initiating needed visits when a patient's BP is out of target range. Several studies have demonstrated that home-based BP monitoring, especially when coupled with behavioral interventions, may be cost-additive or cost-neutral to the healthcare system in the short-term [144–146]. Of note, combining telemonitoring of BP levels plus behavioral modification and/or self-modification of treatment with the support of pharmacies could represent an excellent strategy not only to improve achievement of BP control, but also to further reduce healthcare costs and expenses. It has been generally felt that the initial expense will result in long-term savings through cardiovascular disease reduction. The few studies conducted exploring this issue have shown that home-based BP telemonitoring may not only improve achievement of BP control, but also reduce the adverse cardiovascular outcomes associated with elevated BP levels. However, additional research is still needed to better understand the cost-effectiveness and long-term effects of home-based BP monitoring in clinical outcomes.

Conclusions

HBPM is a simple, inexpensive methodology that offers significant clinical advantages over routine OBP measurements. Consistent evidence has indicated that home BP is a strong and modifiable risk factor with superior prognostic value over conventional OBP measurements in predicting initiation, establishment and progression of subclinical organ damage, and the development of fatal and non-fatal CV events and all-cause and CV mortality in hypertension. A number of randomized controlled trials (RCTs) have also provided evidence of the benefits and cost-effectiveness of programs based on implementation of home-based BP telemonitoring. During the diagnostic assessment of hypertension, it reduces misclassification of BP levels by identifying WCH and MH, and in treated hypertensive subjects telemonitoring allows a better assessment of the BP response to antihypertensive treatment and may help improving therapeutic decisions. At variance from OBP, HBPM requires the active involvement of patients in managing their high BP conditions, which enhances patients' compliance and adherence to antihypertensive treatment. Besides, provided that the practitioner has more information available to make clinical decisions, HBPM also helps to reduce therapeutic inertia. In turn, all of this may potentially increase rates of BP control. Finally, unlike ABPM, HBPM does not allow the assessment of BP during sleep or at work, nor the quantification of short-term BP variability, although it may allow to assess day-by-day BP variability, thus offering a means to quantify long-term BP variations which, as recently suggested, may have prognostic significance. Based on these clinical advantages over OBP measurements (in particular its improved accuracy, low cost and easy implementation), the use of HBPM has been strongly supported by current guidelines for hypertension management as a complement to office BP measures and ambulatory BP monitoring and as part of the routine diagnostic and therapeutic approach to hypertension management [3, 8, 11, 12, 25, 147].

Despite the several advantages and potential applications offered by HBPM, in particular in subjects with resistant hypertension, evidence from intervention randomized trials on hypertension management is still needed in order to address several important issues in this field, such as the definition of HBP targets to achieve with BP lowering strategies or the optimal strategy for a meaningful application of HBPM in clinical practice.

References

1. Lim SS, Vos T, Flaxman AD, Danaei G, Shibuya K, Adair-Rohani H, et al. A comparative risk assessment of burden of disease and injury attributable to 67 risk factors and risk factor clusters in 21 regions, 1990-2010: a systematic analysis for the Global Burden of Disease Study 2010. Lancet. 2012;380(9859):2224–60. Epub 2012/12/19.
2. Wright Jr JT, Bakris G, Greene T, Agodoa LY, Appel LJ, Charleston J, et al. Effect of blood pressure lowering and antihypertensive drug class on progression of hypertensive kidney disease: results from the AASK trial. JAMA. 2002;288(19):2421–31. Epub 2002/11/21.
3. Mancia G, Fagard R, Narkiewicz K, Redon J, Zanchetti A, Bohm M, et al. 2013 ESH/ESC guidelines for the management of arterial hypertension: the Task Force for the Management of Arterial Hypertension of the European Society of Hypertension (ESH) and of the European Society of Cardiology (ESC). Eur Heart J. 2013;34(28):2159–219. Epub 2013/06/19.
4. O'Brien E, Asmar R, Beilin L, Imai Y, Mallion JM, Mancia G, et al. European Society of Hypertension recommendations for conventional, ambulatory and home blood pressure measurement. J Hypertens. 2003;21(5):821–48. Epub 2003/04/26.
5. MacMahon S, Peto R, Cutler J, Collins R, Sorlie P, Neaton J, et al. Blood pressure, stroke, and coronary heart disease. Part 1, Prolonged differences in blood pressure: prospective observational studies corrected for the regression dilution bias. Lancet. 1990;335(8692):765–74. Epub 1990/03/31.
6. Parati G, Stergiou G, O'Brien E, Asmar R, Beilin L, Bilo G, et al. European Society of Hypertension practice guidelines for ambulatory blood pressure monitoring. J Hypertens. 2014;32(7):1359–66. Epub 2014/06/03.
7. Armstrong C. JNC8 Guidelines for the Management of Hypertension in Adults. Am Fam Physician. 2014;90(7):503–4. Epub 2014/11/05.
8. Parati G, Stergiou GS, Asmar R, Bilo G, de Leeuw P, Imai Y, et al. European Society of Hypertension guidelines for blood pressure monitoring at home: a summary report of the Second International Consensus Conference on Home Blood Pressure Monitoring. J Hypertens. 2008;26(8):1505–26. Epub 2008/07/16.
9. Parati G, Stergiou GS, Asmar R, Bilo G, de Leeuw P, Imai Y, et al. European Society of Hypertension practice guidelines for home blood pressure monitoring. J Hum Hypertens. 2010;24(12):779–85. Epub 2010/06/04.
10. Ritchie LD, Campbell NC, Murchie P. New NICE guidelines for hypertension. BMJ. 2011;343:d5644. Epub 2011/09/09.
11. Houle SK, Padwal R, Tsuyuki RT. The 2012-2013 Canadian Hypertension Education Program (CHEP) guidelines for pharmacists: an update. Can Pharm J. 2013;146(3):146–50. Epub 2013/06/26.
12. Pickering TG, Miller NH, Ogedegbe G, Krakoff LR, Artinian NT, Goff D. Call to action on use and reimbursement for home blood pressure monitoring: a joint scientific statement from the American Heart Association, American Society Of Hypertension, and Preventive Cardiovascular Nurses Association. Hypertension. 2008;52(1):10–29. Epub 2008/05/24.
13. Chertow GM, Levin NW, Beck GJ, Depner TA, Eggers PW, Gassman JJ, et al. In-center hemodialysis six times per week versus three times per week. N Engl J Med. 2010; 363(24):2287–300. Epub 2010/11/26.
14. O'Brien E, Parati G, Stergiou G, Asmar R, Beilin L, Bilo G, et al. European Society of Hypertension position paper on ambulatory blood pressure monitoring. J Hypertens. 2013;31(9):1731–68. Epub 2013/09/14.
15. Stryker T, Wilson M, Wilson TW. Accuracy of home blood pressure readings: monitors and operators. Blood Press Monit. 2004;9(3):143–7. Epub 2004/06/17.
16. Stergiou GS, Efstathiou SP, Argyraki CK, Gantzarou AP, Roussias LG, Mountokalakis TD. Clinic, home and ambulatory pulse pressure: comparison and reproducibility. J Hypertens. 2002;20(10):1987–93. Epub 2002/10/03.

17. Stergiou GS, Baibas NM, Gantzarou AP, Skeva II, Kalkana CB, Roussias LG, et al. Reproducibility of home, ambulatory, and clinic blood pressure: implications for the design of trials for the assessment of antihypertensive drug efficacy. Am J Hypertens. 2002;15(2 Pt 1):101–4. Epub 2002/02/28.

18. Warren RE, Marshall T, Padfield PL, Chrubasik S. Variability of office, 24-hour ambulatory, and self-monitored blood pressure measurements. Br J Gen Pract. 2010;60(578):675–80. Epub 2010/09/21.

19. Powers BJ, Olsen MK, Smith VA, Woolson RF, Bosworth HB, Oddone EZ. Measuring blood pressure for decision making and quality reporting: where and how many measures? Ann Intern Med. 2011;154(12):781-8, W-289-90. Epub 2011/06/22.

20. McManus RJ, Mant J, Bray EP, Holder R, Jones MI, Greenfield S, et al. Telemonitoring and self-management in the control of hypertension (TASMINH2): a randomised controlled trial. Lancet. 2010;376(9736):163–72. Epub 2010/07/14.

21. Kaambwa B, Bryan S, Jowett S, Mant J, Bray EP, Hobbs FD, et al. Telemonitoring and self-management in the control of hypertension (TASMINH2): a cost-effectiveness analysis. Eur J Prev Cardiol. 2014;21(12):1517–30. Epub 2013/08/31.

22. Ishikawa J, Shimizu M, Sugiyama Edison E, Yano Y, Hoshide S, Eguchi K, et al. Assessment of the reductions in night-time blood pressure and dipping induced by antihypertensive medication using a home blood pressure monitor. J Hypertens. 2014;32(1):82–9. Epub 2013/12/12.

23. Ushio H, Ishigami T, Araki N, Minegishi S, Tamura K, Okano Y, et al. Utility and feasibility of a new programmable home blood pressure monitoring device for the assessment of night-time blood pressure. Clin Exp Nephrol. 2009;13(5):480–5. Epub 2009/05/19.

24. Stergiou GS, Triantafyllidou E, Cholidou K, Kollias A, Destounis A, Nasothimiou EG, et al. Asleep home blood pressure monitoring in obstructive sleep apnea: a pilot study. Blood Press Monit. 2013;18(1):21–6. Epub 2012/12/25.

25. Lackland DT. Hypertension: Joint National Committee on Detection, Evaluation, and Treatment of High Blood Pressure guidelines. Curr Opin Neurol. 2013;26(1):8–12. Epub 2012/12/18.

26. Thijs L, Staessen JA, Celis H, de Gaudemaris R, Imai Y, Julius S, et al. Reference values for self-recorded blood pressure: a meta-analysis of summary data. Arch Intern Med. 1998;158(5):481–8. Epub 1998/03/21.

27. Thijs L, Staessen JA, Celis H, Fagard R, De Cort P, de Gaudemaris R, et al. The international database of self-recorded blood pressures in normotensive and untreated hypertensive subjects. Blood Press Monit. 1999;4(2):77–86. Epub 1999/08/18.

28. Ohkubo T, Imai Y, Tsuji I, Nagai K, Kato J, Kikuchi N, et al. Home blood pressure measurement has a stronger predictive power for mortality than does screening blood pressure measurement: a population-based observation in Ohasama. Jpn J Hypertens. 1998;16(7):971–5. Epub 1998/10/30.

29. Ohkubo T, Asayama K, Kikuya M, Metoki H, Hoshi H, Hashimoto J, et al. How many times should blood pressure be measured at home for better prediction of stroke risk? Ten-year follow-up results from the Ohasama study. J Hypertens. 2004;22(6):1099–104. Epub 2004/05/29.

30. Asayama K, Ohkubo T, Kikuya M, Metoki H, Obara T, Hoshi H, et al. Use of 2003 European Society of Hypertension-European Society of Cardiology guidelines for predicting stroke using self-measured blood pressure at home: the Ohasama study. Eur Heart J. 2005; 26(19):2026–31. Epub 2005/05/27.

31. Ohkubo T, Asayama K, Kikuya M, Metoki H, Obara T, Saito S, et al. Prediction of ischaemic and haemorrhagic stroke by self-measured blood pressure at home: the Ohasama study. Blood Press Monit. 2004;9(6):315–20. Epub 2004/11/27.

32. Asayama K, Ohkubo T, Kikuya M, Metoki H, Hoshi H, Hashimoto J, et al. Prediction of stroke by self-measurement of blood pressure at home versus casual screening blood pressure measurement in relation to the Joint National Committee 7 classification: the Ohasama study. Stroke. 2004;35(10):2356–61. Epub 2004/08/28.

33. Nishinaga M, Takata J, Okumiya K, Matsubayashi K, Ozawa T, Doi Y. High morning home blood pressure is associated with a loss of functional independence in the community-dwelling elderly aged 75 years or older. Hypertens Res. 2005;28(8):657–63. Epub 2006/01/06.
34. Mancia G, Facchetti R, Bombelli M, Grassi G, Sega R. Long-term risk of mortality associated with selective and combined elevation in office, home, and ambulatory blood pressure. Hypertension. 2006;47(5):846–53. Epub 2006/03/29.
35. Sega R, Facchetti R, Bombelli M, Cesana G, Corrao G, Grassi G, et al. Prognostic value of ambulatory and home blood pressures compared with office blood pressure in the general population: follow-up results from the Pressioni Arteriose Monitorate e Loro Associazioni (PAMELA) study. Circulation. 2005;111(14):1777–83. Epub 2005/04/06.
36. Asayama K, Ohkubo T, Kikuya M, Obara T, Metoki H, Inoue R, et al. Prediction of stroke by home "morning" versus "evening" blood pressure values: the Ohasama study. Hypertension. 2006;48(4):737–43. Epub 2006/09/06.
37. Tsuji I, Imai Y, Nagai K, Ohkubo T, Watanabe N, Minami N, et al. Proposal of reference values for home blood pressure measurement: prognostic criteria based on a prospective observation of the general population in Ohasama, Japan. Am J Hypertens. 1997;10(4 Pt 1):409–18. Epub 1997/04/01.
38. Bobrie G, Chatellier G, Genes N, Clerson P, Vaur L, Vaisse B, et al. Cardiovascular prognosis of "masked hypertension" detected by blood pressure self-measurement in elderly treated hypertensive patients. JAMA. 2004;291(11):1342–9. Epub 2004/03/18.
39. Agarwal R, Andersen MJ. Prognostic importance of clinic and home blood pressure recordings in patients with chronic kidney disease. Kidney Int. 2006;69(2):406–11. Epub 2006/01/13.
40. Rave K, Bender R, Heise T, Sawicki PT. Value of blood pressure self-monitoring as a predictor of progression of diabetic nephropathy. J Hypertens. 1999;17(5):597–601. Epub 1999/07/14.
41. Staessen JA, Den Hond E, Celis H, Fagard R, Keary L, Vandenhoven G, et al. Antihypertensive treatment based on blood pressure measurement at home or in the physician's office: a randomized controlled trial. JAMA. 2004;291(8):955–64. Epub 2004/02/26.
42. Verberk WJ, Kroon AA, Lenders JW, Kessels AG, van Montfrans GA, Smit AJ, et al. Self-measurement of blood pressure at home reduces the need for antihypertensive drugs: a randomized, controlled trial. Hypertension. 2007;50(6):1019–25. Epub 2007/10/17.
43. Saito S, Asayama K, Ohkubo T, Kikuya M, Metoki H, Obara T, et al. The second progress report on the Hypertension Objective treatment based on Measurement by Electrical Devices of Blood Pressure (HOMED-BP) study. Blood Press Monit. 2004;9(5):243–7. Epub 2004/10/09.
44. Fagard RH, Celis H. Prognostic significance of various characteristics of out-of-the-office blood pressure. J Hypertens. 2004;22(9):1663–6. Epub 2004/08/18.
45. Mancia G, Zanchetti A, Agabiti-Rosei E, Benemio G, De Cesaris R, Fogari R, et al. Ambulatory blood pressure is superior to clinic blood pressure in predicting treatment-induced regression of left ventricular hypertrophy. SAMPLE Study Group. Study on Ambulatory Monitoring of Blood Pressure and Lisinopril Evaluation. Circulation. 1997;95(6):1464–70. Epub 1997/03/18.
46. Fagard RH, Van Den Broeke C, De Cort P. Prognostic significance of blood pressure measured in the office, at home and during ambulatory monitoring in older patients in general practice. J Hum Hypertens. 2005;19(10):801–7. Epub 2005/06/17.
47. Hozawa A, Ohkubo T, Nagai K, Kikuya M, Matsubara M, Tsuji I, et al. Prognosis of isolated systolic and isolated diastolic hypertension as assessed by self-measurement of blood pressure at home: the Ohasama study. Arch Intern Med. 2000;160(21):3301–6. Epub 2000/11/23.
48. Okumiya K, Matsubayashi K, Wada T, Fujisawa M, Osaki Y, Doi Y, et al. A U-shaped association between home systolic blood pressure and four-year mortality in community-dwelling older men. J Am Geriatr Soc. 1999;47(12):1415–21. Epub 1999/12/11.
49. Niiranen TJ, Maki J, Puukka P, Karanko H, Jula AM. Office, home, and ambulatory blood pressures as predictors of cardiovascular risk. Hypertension. 2014;64(2):281–6. Epub 2014/05/21.

50. Ward AM, Takahashi O, Stevens R, Heneghan C. Home measurement of blood pressure and cardiovascular disease: systematic review and meta-analysis of prospective studies. J Hypertens. 2012;30(3):449–56. Epub 2012/01/14.
51. Fuchs SC, Mello RG, Fuchs FC. Home blood pressure monitoring is better predictor of cardiovascular disease and target organ damage than office blood pressure: a systematic review and meta-analysis. Curr Cardiol Rep. 2013;15(11):413. Epub 2013/09/24.
52. Niiranen TJ, Hanninen MR, Johansson J, Reunanen A, Jula AM. Home-measured blood pressure is a stronger predictor of cardiovascular risk than office blood pressure: the Finn-Home study. Hypertension. 2010;55(6):1346–51. Epub 2010/04/14.
53. Stergiou GS, Baibas NM, Kalogeropoulos PG. Cardiovascular risk prediction based on home blood pressure measurement: the Didima study. J Hypertens. 2007;25(8):1590–6. Epub 2007/07/11.
54. Stergiou GS, Argyraki KK, Moyssakis I, Mastorantonakis SE, Achimastos AD, Karamanos VG, et al. Home blood pressure is as reliable as ambulatory blood pressure in predicting target-organ damage in hypertension. Am J Hypertens. 2007;20(6):616–21. Epub 2007/05/29.
55. Tachibana R, Tabara Y, Kondo I, Miki T, Kohara K. Home blood pressure is a better predictor of carotid atherosclerosis than office blood pressure in community-dwelling subjects. Hypertens Res. 2004;27(9):633–9. Epub 2005/03/08.
56. Hara A, Ohkubo T, Kikuya M, Shintani Y, Obara T, Metoki H, et al. Detection of carotid atherosclerosis in individuals with masked hypertension and white-coat hypertension by self-measured blood pressure at home: the Ohasama study. J Hypertens. 2007;25(2):321–7. Epub 2007/01/11.
57. Niiranen T, Jula A, Kantola I, Moilanen L, Kahonen M, Kesaniemi YA, et al. Home-measured blood pressure is more strongly associated with atherosclerosis than clinic blood pressure: the Finn-HOME Study. J Hypertens. 2007;25(6):1225–31. Epub 2007/06/15.
58. Tsunoda S, Kawano Y, Horio T, Okuda N, Takishita S. Relationship between home blood pressure and longitudinal changes in target organ damage in treated hypertensive patients. Hypertens Res. 2002;25(2):167–73. Epub 2002/06/06.
59. Tomiyama M, Horio T, Yoshii M, Takiuchi S, Kamide K, Nakamura S, et al. Masked hypertension and target organ damage in treated hypertensive patients. Am J Hypertens. 2006;19(9):880–6. Epub 2006/09/01.
60. Gaborieau V, Delarche N, Gosse P. Ambulatory blood pressure monitoring versus self-measurement of blood pressure at home: correlation with target organ damage. J Hypertens. 2008;26(10):1919–27. Epub 2008/09/23.
61. Agarwal R, Brim NJ, Mahenthiran J, Andersen MJ, Saha C. Out-of-hemodialysis-unit blood pressure is a superior determinant of left ventricular hypertrophy. Hypertension. 2006;47(1):62–8. Epub 2005/12/14.
62. Suzuki H, Nakamoto H, Okada H, Sugahara S, Kanno Y. Self-measured systolic blood pressure in the morning is a strong indicator of decline of renal function in hypertensive patients with non-diabetic chronic renal insufficiency. Clin Exp Hypertens. 2002;24(4):249–60. Epub 2002/06/19.
63. Agarwal R, Andersen MJ. Blood pressure recordings within and outside the clinic and cardiovascular events in chronic kidney disease. Am J Nephrol. 2006;26(5):503–10. Epub 2006/11/25.
64. Alborzi P, Patel N, Agarwal R. Home blood pressures are of greater prognostic value than hemodialysis unit recordings. Clin J Am Soc Nephrol. 2007;2(6):1228–34. Epub 2007/10/19.
65. Agarwal R. Blood pressure and mortality among hemodialysis patients. Hypertension. 2010;55(3):762–8. Epub 2010/01/20.
66. Parati G, Mancia G. White coat effect: semantics, assessment and pathophysiological implications. J Hypertens. 2003;21(3):481–6. Epub 2003/03/18.
67. Little P, Barnett J, Barnsley L, Marjoram J, Fitzgerald-Barron A, Mant D. Comparison of agreement between different measures of blood pressure in primary care and daytime ambulatory blood pressure. BMJ. 2002;325(7358):254. Epub 2002/08/03.

68. Mancia G, Bombelli M, Facchetti R, Madotto F, Quarti-Trevano F, Polo Friz H, et al. Long-term risk of sustained hypertension in white-coat or masked hypertension. Hypertension. 2009;54(2):226–32. Epub 2009/07/01.
69. Mancia G, De Backer G, Dominiczak A, Cifkova R, Fagard R, Germano G, et al. 2007 Guidelines for the Management of Arterial Hypertension: The Task Force for the Management of Arterial Hypertension of the European Society of Hypertension (ESH) and of the European Society of Cardiology (ESC). J Hypertens. 2007;25(6):1105–87. Epub 2007/06/15.
70. Chobanian AV, Bakris GL, Black HR, Cushman WC, Green LA, Izzo Jr JL, et al. Seventh report of the Joint National Committee on Prevention, Detection, Evaluation, and Treatment of High Blood Pressure. Hypertension. 2003;42(6):1206–52. Epub 2003/12/06.
71. Williams B, Poulter NR, Brown MJ, Davis M, McInnes GT, Potter JF, et al. Guidelines for management of hypertension: report of the fourth working party of the British Hypertension Society, 2004-BHS IV. J Hum Hypertens. 2004;18(3):139–85. Epub 2004/02/20.
72. Whitworth JA, World Health Organization ISoHWG. 2003 World Health Organization (WHO)/International Society of Hypertension (ISH) statement on management of hypertension. J Hypertens. 2003;21(11):1983–92. Epub 2003/11/05.
73. Imai Y, Otsuka K, Kawano Y, Shimada K, Hayashi H, Tochikubo O, et al. Japanese society of hypertension (JSH) guidelines for self-monitoring of blood pressure at home. Hypertens Res. 2003;26(10):771–82. Epub 2003/11/19.
74. Pickering TG, Hall JE, Appel LJ, Falkner BE, Graves J, Hill MN, et al. Recommendations for blood pressure measurement in humans and experimental animals: Part 1: blood pressure measurement in humans: a statement for professionals from the Subcommittee of Professional and Public Education of the American Heart Association Council on High Blood Pressure Research. Hypertension. 2005;45(1):142–61. Epub 2004/12/22.
75. Cappuccio FP, Kerry SM, Forbes L, Donald A. Blood pressure control by home monitoring: meta-analysis of randomised trials. BMJ. 2004;329(7458):145. Epub 2004/06/15.
76. Rogers MA, Small D, Buchan DA, Butch CA, Stewart CM, Krenzer BE, et al. Home monitoring service improves mean arterial pressure in patients with essential hypertension. A randomized, controlled trial. Ann Intern Med. 2001;134(11):1024–32. Epub 2001/06/05.
77. McManus RJ, Mant J, Roalfe A, Oakes RA, Bryan S, Pattison HM, et al. Targets and self monitoring in hypertension: randomised controlled trial and cost effectiveness analysis. BMJ. 2005;331(7515):493. Epub 2005/08/24.
78. Myers MG. Pseudoresistant hypertension attributed to white-coat effect. Hypertension. 2012;59(3):532–3. Epub 2012/01/19.
79. Parati G, Ulian L, Santucciu C, Omboni S, Mancia G. Difference between clinic and daytime blood pressure is not a measure of the white coat effect. Hypertension. 1998;31(5):1185–9. Epub 1998/05/12.
80. de la Sierra A, Segura J, Banegas JR, Gorostidi M, de la Cruz JJ, Armario P, et al. Clinical features of 8295 patients with resistant hypertension classified on the basis of ambulatory blood pressure monitoring. Hypertension. 2011;57(5):898–902. Epub 2011/03/30.
81. Oikawa T, Obara T, Ohkubo T, Kikuya M, Asayama K, Metoki H, et al. Characteristics of resistant hypertension determined by self-measured blood pressure at home and office blood pressure measurements: the J-HOME study. J Hypertens. 2006;24(9):1737–43. Epub 2006/08/18.
82. de la Sierra A, Banegas JR, Oliveras A, Gorostidi M, Segura J, de la Cruz JJ, et al. Clinical differences between resistant hypertensives and patients treated and controlled with three or less drugs. J Hypertens. 2012;30(6):1211–6. Epub 2012/04/25.
83. Papademetriou V, Doumas M, Faselis C, Tsioufis C, Douma S, Gkaliagkousi E, et al. Carotid baroreceptor stimulation for the treatment of resistant hypertension. Int J Hypertens. 2011;2011:964394. Epub 2011/08/09.
84. Doumas M, Faselis C, Papademetriou V. Renal sympathetic denervation in hypertension. Curr Opin Nephrol Hypertens. 2011;20(6):647–53. Epub 2011/09/03.
85. Schmieder RE, Redon J, Grassi G, Kjeldsen SE, Mancia G, Narkiewicz K, et al. ESH position paper: renal denervation - an interventional therapy of resistant hypertension. J Hypertens. 2012;30(5):837–41. Epub 2012/04/04.

86. Pickering TG, Davidson K, Gerin W, Schwartz JE. Masked hypertension. Hypertension. 2002;40(6):795–6. Epub 2002/12/07.

87. Stergiou GS, Salgami EV, Tzamouranis DG, Roussias LG. Masked hypertension assessed by ambulatory blood pressure versus home blood pressure monitoring: is it the same phenomenon? Am J Hypertens. 2005;18(6):772–8. Epub 2005/06/01.

88. Nasothimiou EG, Tzamouranis D, Roussias LG, Stergiou GS. Home versus ambulatory blood pressure monitoring in the diagnosis of clinic resistant and true resistant hypertension. J Hum Hypertens. 2012;26(12):696–700. Epub 2011/11/11.

89. Parati G, Ochoa JE, Bilo G. False versus true resistant hypertension. In: Mancia G, editor. Resistant hypertension: epidemiology, pathophysiology, diagnosis and treatment. Milan: Springer; 2013. p. 59–75.

90. Staessen JA, Thijs L, Fagard R, O'Brien ET, Clement D, de Leeuw PW, et al. Predicting cardiovascular risk using conventional vs ambulatory blood pressure in older patients with systolic hypertension. Systolic Hypertension in Europe Trial Investigators. JAMA. 1999;282(6):539–46. Epub 1999/08/18.

91. Kikuya M, Ohkubo T, Asayama K, Metoki H, Obara T, Saito S, et al. Ambulatory blood pressure and 10-year risk of cardiovascular and noncardiovascular mortality: the Ohasama study. Hypertension. 2005;45(2):240–5. Epub 2004/12/15.

92. Fagard RH, Celis H, Thijs L, Staessen JA, Clement DL, De Buyzere ML, et al. Daytime and nighttime blood pressure as predictors of death and cause-specific cardiovascular events in hypertension. Hypertension. 2008;51(1):55–61. Epub 2007/11/28.

93. Boggia J, Li Y, Thijs L, Hansen TW, Kikuya M, Bjorklund-Bodegard K, et al. Prognostic accuracy of day versus night ambulatory blood pressure: a cohort study. Lancet. 2007;370(9594):1219–29. Epub 2007/10/09.

94. Lacson Jr E, Lazarus JM. The association between blood pressure and mortality in ESRD-not different from the general population? Semin Dial. 2007;20(6):510–7. Epub 2007/11/10.

95. Mallion JM, Clerson P, Bobrie G, Genes N, Vaisse B, Chatellier G. Predictive factors for masked hypertension within a population of controlled hypertensives. J Hypertens. 2006;24(12):2365–70. Epub 2006/11/04.

96. Edmonds D, Foerster E, Groth H, Greminger P, Siegenthaler W, Vetter W. Does self-measurement of blood pressure improve patient compliance in hypertension? J Hypertens Suppl. 1985;3(1):S31–4. Epub 1985/04/01.

97. Agarwal R, Bills JE, Hecht TJ, Light RP. Role of home blood pressure monitoring in overcoming therapeutic inertia and improving hypertension control: a systematic review and meta-analysis. Hypertension. 2011;57(1):29–38. Epub 2010/12/01.

98. Logan AG, Dunai A, McIsaac WJ, Irvine MJ, Tisler A. Attitudes of primary care physicians and their patients about home blood pressure monitoring in Ontario. J Hypertens. 2008;26(3):446–52. Epub 2008/02/28.

99. Rothwell PM, Howard SC, Dolan E, O'Brien E, Dobson JE, Dahlof B, et al. Prognostic significance of visit-to-visit variability, maximum systolic blood pressure, and episodic hypertension. Lancet. 2010;375(9718):895–905. Epub 2010/03/17.

100. Kearney PM, Whelton M, Reynolds K, Muntner P, Whelton PK, He J. Global burden of hypertension: analysis of worldwide data. Lancet. 2005;365(9455):217–23. Epub 2005/01/18.

101. Kikuya M, Ohkubo T, Metoki H, Asayama K, Hara A, Obara T, et al. Day-by-day variability of blood pressure and heart rate at home as a novel predictor of prognosis: the Ohasama study. Hypertension. 2008;52(6):1045–50. Epub 2008/11/05.

102. Hashimoto T, Kikuya M, Ohkubo T, Satoh M, Metoki H, Inoue R, et al. Home blood pressure level, blood pressure variability, smoking, and stroke risk in Japanese men: the Ohasama study. Am J Hypertens. 2012;25(8):883–91. Epub 2012/06/08.

103. Johansson JK, Niiranen TJ, Puukka PJ, Jula AM. Prognostic value of the variability in home-measured blood pressure and heart rate: the Finn-Home Study. Hypertension. 2012;59(2):212–8. Epub 2012/01/05.

104. di Rienzo M, Grassi G, Pedotti A, Mancia G. Continuous vs intermittent blood pressure measurements in estimating 24-hour average blood pressure. Hypertension. 1983;5(2):264–9. Epub 1983/03/01.

105. Mancia G, Di Rienzo M, Parati G. Ambulatory blood pressure monitoring use in hypertension research and clinical practice. Hypertension. 1993;21(4):510–24. Epub 1993/04/01.
106. Mena L, Pintos S, Queipo NV, Aizpurua JA, Maestre G, Sulbaran T. A reliable index for the prognostic significance of blood pressure variability. J Hypertens. 2005;23(3):505–11. Epub 2005/02/18.
107. Matsui Y, Ishikawa J, Eguchi K, Shibasaki S, Shimada K, Kario K. Maximum value of home blood pressure: a novel indicator of target organ damage in hypertension. Hypertension. 2011;57(6):1087–93. Epub 2011/05/04.
108. Ushigome E, Fukui M, Hamaguchi M, Senmaru T, Sakabe K, Tanaka M, et al. The coefficient variation of home blood pressure is a novel factor associated with macroalbuminuria in type 2 diabetes mellitus. Hypertens Res. 2011;34(12):1271–5. Epub 2011/08/05.
109. Fukui M, Ushigome E, Tanaka M, Hamaguchi M, Tanaka T, Atsuta H, et al. Home blood pressure variability on one occasion is a novel factor associated with arterial stiffness in patients with type 2 diabetes. Hypertens Res. 2013;36(3):219–25. Epub 2012/10/26.
110. Hoshide S, Yano Y, Shimizu M, Eguchi K, Ishikawa J, Kario K. Is home blood pressure variability itself an interventional target beyond lowering mean home blood pressure during antihypertensive treatment? Hypertens Res. 2012;35(8):862–6. Epub 2012/04/06.
111. Nishimura M, Kato Y, Tanaka T, Todo R, Tone A, Yamada K, et al. Significance of estimating the glomerular filtration rate for the management of hypertension in type 2 diabetes with microalbuminuria. Hypertens Res. 2013;36(8):705–10. Epub 2013/04/05.
112. Schutte R, Thijs L, Liu YP, Asayama K, Jin Y, Odili A, et al. Within-subject blood pressure level--not variability--predicts fatal and nonfatal outcomes in a general population. Hypertension. 2012;60(5):1138–47. Epub 2012/10/17.
113. Ishikura K, Obara T, Kato T, Kikuya M, Shibamiya T, Shinki T, et al. Associations between day-by-day variability in blood pressure measured at home and antihypertensive drugs: the J-HOME-Morning study. Clin Exp Hypertens. 2012;34(4):297–304. Epub 2012/05/09.
114. Matsui Y, O'Rourke MF, Hoshide S, Ishikawa J, Shimada K, Kario K. Combined effect of angiotensin II receptor blocker and either a calcium channel blocker or diuretic on day-by-day variability of home blood pressure: the Japan Combined Treatment With Olmesartan and a Calcium-Channel Blocker Versus Olmesartan and Diuretics Randomized Efficacy Study. Hypertension. 2012;59(6):1132–8. Epub 2012/05/02.
115. Ushigome E, Fukui M, Hamaguchi M, Tanaka T, Atsuta H, Ohnishi M, et al. Beneficial effect of calcium channel blockers on home blood pressure variability in the morning in patients with type 2 diabetes. J Diabetes Investig. 2013;4(4):399–404. Epub 2014/05/21.
116. Pickering TG, Gerin W, Holland JK. Home blood pressure teletransmission for better diagnosis and treatment. Curr Hypertens Rep. 1999;1(6):489–94. Epub 2000/09/12.
117. Parati G, Omboni S. Role of home blood pressure telemonitoring in hypertension management: an update. Blood Press Monit. 2010;15(6):285–95. Epub 2010/11/19.
118. Rosenthal TC. The medical home: growing evidence to support a new approach to primary care. J Am Board Fam Med. 2008;21(5):427–40. Epub 2008/09/06.
119. Friedman RH, Kazis LE, Jette A, Smith MB, Stollerman J, Torgerson J, et al. A telecommunications system for monitoring and counseling patients with hypertension. Impact on medication adherence and blood pressure control. Am J Hypertens. 1996;9(4 Pt 1):285–92. Epub 1996/04/01.
120. Bosworth HB, Olsen MK, Gentry P, Orr M, Dudley T, McCant F, et al. Nurse administered telephone intervention for blood pressure control: a patient-tailored multifactorial intervention. Patient Educ Couns. 2005;57(1):5–14. Epub 2005/03/31.
121. Friedman RH. Automated telephone conversations to assess health behavior and deliver behavioral interventions. J Med Syst. 1998;22(2):95–102. Epub 1998/05/08.
122. Cottrell E, McMillan K, Chambers R. A cross-sectional survey and service evaluation of simple telehealth in primary care: what do patients think? BMJ Open. 2012;2(6), e001392. Epub 2012/11/30.
123. Parati G, Omboni S, Albini F, Piantoni L, Giuliano A, Revera M, et al. Home blood pressure telemonitoring improves hypertension control in general practice. The TeleBPCare study. J Hypertens. 2009;27(1):198–203. Epub 2009/01/17.

124. Parati G, Omboni S, Compare A, Grossi E, Callus E, Venco A, et al. Blood pressure control and treatment adherence in hypertensive patients with metabolic syndrome: protocol of a randomized controlled study based on home blood pressure telemonitoring vs. conventional management and assessment of psychological determinants of adherence (TELEBPMET Study). Trials. 2013;14:22. Epub 2013/01/25.
125. Omboni S, Gazzola T, Carabelli G, Parati G. Clinical usefulness and cost effectiveness of home blood pressure telemonitoring: meta-analysis of randomized controlled studies. J Hypertens. 2013;31(3):455–67. discussion 67-8. Epub 2013/01/10.
126. Omboni S, Guarda A. Impact of home blood pressure telemonitoring and blood pressure control: a meta-analysis of randomized controlled studies. Am J Hypertens. 2011;24(9):989–98. Epub 2011/06/10.
127. Ogedegbe G, Schoenthaler A. A systematic review of the effects of home blood pressure monitoring on medication adherence. J Clin Hypertens (Greenwich). 2006;8(3):174–80. Epub 2006/03/09.
128. Bobrie G, Postel-Vinay N, Delonca J, Corvol P, Investigators S. Self-measurement and self-titration in hypertension: a pilot telemedicine study. Am J Hypertens. 2007;20(12):1314–20. Epub 2007/12/01.
129. Carter BL, Bosworth HB, Green BB. The hypertension team: the role of the pharmacist, nurse, and teamwork in hypertension therapy. J Clin Hypertens (Greenwich). 2012;14(1):51–65. Epub 2012/01/13.
130. Chiu CW, Wong FK. Effects of 8 weeks sustained follow-up after a nurse consultation on hypertension: a randomised trial. Int J Nurs Stud. 2010;47(11):1374–82. Epub 2010/04/24.
131. Hebert PL, Sisk JE, Tuzzio L, Casabianca JM, Pogue VA, Wang JJ, et al. Nurse-led disease management for hypertension control in a diverse urban community: a randomized trial. J Gen Intern Med. 2012;27(6):630–9. Epub 2011/12/07.
132. Kim MT, Han HR, Hedlin H, Kim J, Song HJ, Kim KB, et al. Teletransmitted monitoring of blood pressure and bilingual nurse counseling-sustained improvements in blood pressure control during 12 months in hypertensive Korean Americans. J Clin Hypertens (Greenwich). 2011;13(8):605–12. Epub 2011/08/03.
133. Bosworth HB, Powers BJ, Olsen MK, McCant F, Grubber J, Smith V, et al. Home blood pressure management and improved blood pressure control: results from a randomized controlled trial. Arch Intern Med. 2011;171(13):1173–80. Epub 2011/07/13.
134. Magid DJ, Ho PM, Olson KL, Brand DW, Welch LK, Snow KE, et al. A multimodal blood pressure control intervention in 3 healthcare systems. Am J Manag Care. 2011;17(4):e96–103. Epub 2011/07/21.
135. Melnyk SD, Zullig LL, McCant F, Danus S, Oddone E, Bastian L, et al. Telemedicine cardiovascular risk reduction in veterans. Am Heart J. 2013;165(4):501–8. Epub 2013/03/30.
136. Zullig LL, Melnyk SD, Goldstein K, Shaw RJ, Bosworth HB. The role of home blood pressure telemonitoring in managing hypertensive populations. Curr Hypertens Rep. 2013;15(4):346–55. Epub 2013/04/30.
137. Zullig LL, Melnyk SD, Stechuchak KM, McCant F, Danus S, Oddone E, et al. The Cardiovascular Intervention Improvement Telemedicine Study (CITIES): rationale for a tailored behavioral and educational pharmacist-administered intervention for achieving cardiovascular disease risk reduction. Telemed J E Health. 2014;20(2):135–43. Epub 2013/12/07.
138. Omboni S, Sala E. The pharmacist and the management of arterial hypertension: the role of blood pressure monitoring and telemonitoring. Expert Rev Cardiovasc Ther. 2015;13(2):209–21. Epub 2015/01/13.
139. Harris IM, Baker E, Berry TM, Halloran MA, Lindauer K, Ragucci KR, et al. Developing a business-practice model for pharmacy services in ambulatory settings. Pharmacotherapy. 2008;28(2):285. Epub 2008/01/30.
140. Burke JM, Miller WA, Spencer AP, Crank CW, Adkins L, Bertch KE, et al. Clinical pharmacist competencies. Pharmacotherapy. 2008;28(6):806–15. Epub 2008/05/28.
141. Santschi V, Chiolero A, Burnand B, Colosimo AL, Paradis G. Impact of pharmacist care in the management of cardiovascular disease risk factors: a systematic review and meta-analysis of randomized trials. Arch Intern Med. 2011;171(16):1441–53. Epub 2011/09/14.

142. Carter BL, Bergus GR, Dawson JD, Farris KB, Doucette WR, Chrischilles EA, et al. A cluster randomized trial to evaluate physician/pharmacist collaboration to improve blood pressure control. J Clin Hypertens (Greenwich). 2008;10(4):260–71. Epub 2008/04/11.
143. McLean DL, McAlister FA, Johnson JA, King KM, Makowsky MJ, Jones CA, et al. A randomized trial of the effect of community pharmacist and nurse care on improving blood pressure management in patients with diabetes mellitus: study of cardiovascular risk intervention by pharmacists-hypertension (SCRIP-HTN). Arch Intern Med. 2008;168(21):2355–61. Epub 2008/11/26.
144. Wang V, Smith VA, Bosworth HB, Oddone EZ, Olsen MK, McCant F, et al. Economic evaluation of telephone self-management interventions for blood pressure control. Am Heart J. 2012;163(6):980–6. Epub 2012/06/20.
145. Reed SD, Li Y, Oddone EZ, Neary AM, Orr MM, Grubber JM, et al. Economic evaluation of home blood pressure monitoring with or without telephonic behavioral self-management in patients with hypertension. Am J Hypertens. 2010;23(2):142–8. Epub 2009/11/21.
146. Lovibond K, Jowett S, Barton P, Caulfield M, Heneghan C, Hobbs FD, et al. Cost-effectiveness of options for the diagnosis of high blood pressure in primary care: a modelling study. Lancet. 2011;378(9798):1219–30. Epub 2011/08/27.
147. Parati G, Bilo G. Home blood pressure measurements will or will not replace 24-hour ambulatory blood pressure measurement. Hypertension. 2009. Epub 2009/09/10.

Chapter 3
Activity Monitoring and the Effects of the Environment on Blood Pressure

George A. Mansoor

Introduction

Blood Pressure (BP), heart rate, and other cardiovascular parameters are not static biological variables. Multiple factors, internal and external to the human organism, affect human BP and heart rate variability. Important examples of these factors include the extent and nature of physical exercise and activity, the amount and quality of sleep, stress levels, the levels of anxiety and fear, anger, food consumption, hormones, and environmental factors such as temperature, noise, air pollutants and particulate matter, altitude, and latitude. This is a complex constantly changing set of inputs to cardiovascular variability. Untangling this lattice will not begin until good tools are developed that assess these factors reliably and then they can be related to cardiovascular parameter variability. Examples of such tools include electronic activity recording that has not only reached main street [1] with consumer-targeted activity devices, but have also provided significant insights into the relationship of activity both during awake hours and sleep hours to BP and its variability. Other tools are used to assess internal and external factors, but the ability to quantify many of these is rudimentary. In this chapter, we will review the expanding knowledge of activity and BP and other cardiovascular parameters and briefly review some of the other environmental influences on hemodynamic parameters.

G.A. Mansoor, M.Sc., M.B.B.S. (✉)
Mount Saint John Medical Center, St. Johns, Antigua and Barbuda
e-mail: gamansoor@gmail.com

© Springer International Publishing Switzerland 2016   45
W.B. White (ed.), *Blood Pressure Monitoring in Cardiovascular Medicine and Therapeutics*, Clinical Hypertension and Vascular Diseases,
DOI 10.1007/978-3-319-22771-9_3

Activity Monitoring and Cardiovascular Variability

Activity Monitoring: Methods and Limitations

It has long been appreciated that chronically sedentary lifestyles may play a role in the development of obesity and cardiovascular diseases. On a short-term basis, it was always recognized that physical activity is an important factor in the variability of heart rate and BP. Accurate monitoring of physical activities is a key step to understanding these relationships [2].

A pedometer is one type of motion sensor that tracks walking or running, hence the term also used is a step counter. The small highly portable units are attached to the waist belt. They are very location-specific and many do not function well if placed elsewhere as they detect vertical motion of the hips during walking. Recent models that do not require hip placement and take readings once held by the moving object or person have become available. Various algorithms in the software also deliver the amount of active time and calories burned. Pedometers are widely used in research and by health conscious individuals. Simple pedometers use a mechanical switch to count steps.

Accelerometers are pedometers that have micro-electro-mechanical systems; typically a cantilever beam with a piezo-electric crystal and an appropriate detection and recording apparatus. Acceleration deflects the device and generates a signal. Devices can be single, double, or triple axis in terms of the acceleration vector required. These devices can not only count steps, but also sense and quantify the force delivered. This allows more quantitative and precise data to be obtainable from triple axis devices; such data can be converted into calories or other pertinent health parameters. These are the type of devices most commonly used in cardiovascular research.

Data management by these devices can vary from use of an internal memory that can store 5–15 days of data with no download capability, to devices that can store multiple days and output the data to a computer, to devices that only detect the signal and beam data to a separate device such as a computer or phone.

It must be repeatedly appreciated that data collected by devices from different manufacturers are not interchangeable and that clinically important large differences have been observed in laboratory testing. There are three types of methods that have been in use in actigraphs to quantify activity; time above threshold (TAT), zero crossing mode (ZCM), and the newest format called digital integration. The TAT has a preset activity level as the threshold and activity is counted when this is exceeded. Each minute this process is repeated, a count is generated. The ZCM mode is similar to TAT except that the threshold is zero or close to it. Within each minute, counts are made and with each minute it is reset. With digital integration, acceleration signal is very frequently sampled (up to 40 times per second) and the signal is digitized and graphically analyzed to provide summary measures (e.g., total area under the curve) for that time. It should be realized that the TAT and ZCM modes are unable to determine the magnitude of any movement detected. Digital integration overcomes this limitation to some extent.

However, the sophistication and promise of such devices is exemplified by devices that not only have triple axis accelerometers, but also can sense skin temperature, a heat dissipation sensor, and skin impedance. These integrated multi-functionality devices may play major roles in research on the complex factors that affect cardiovascular reactivity.

Despite their promise, use of activity monitoring devices continues to have important limitations. First, each device and manufacturer uses their own units and algorithms to define activity amounts and intensities and various algorithms are used to infer inactivity, sleep, and its phases. Hence, as mentioned above, data generated by these devices are not interchangeable or linearly comparable to each other. Secondly, special attention must be paid to the number and location of devices used in a particular study. Special considerations may be needed when these devices are used to define various sleep parameters in different populations. In particular, these devices have poor ability to detect wakefulness during sleep periods [3]. This is not surprising since the actigraph detects movements while sleep may be associated with movement and complete inactivity may be an awake person and not a person who is asleep. We assume that reduced activity indicates sleep and that disturbed patterns of activity during sleep may reflect sleep disorders. These assumptions may be particularly untrue in some populations (e.g., elderly patients).

Physical Activity and Hemodynamic Parameters

There is a complex relationship between physical movements, BP, and heart rate. It is important to distinguish between short-term (e.g., minute by minute) activities and long-term (e.g., months or years) activities. Short-term physical activity is important to understand absolute BP levels, diurnal variations of BP, and overall BP variability.

Chronically higher activity levels are a key tool in the prevention of hypertension and vascular morbidity. Many cardiovascular society guidelines do recommend physical activity as a way to prevent hypertension. Ever since Paffenbarger made the initial observations [4], subsequent plethora of studies have confirmed this using a variety of experimental designs. What remains is a less than full understanding of the intensity and other characteristics of an exercise regimen that is optimal. We refer the reader to a recent update here [5]. Actigraphy has been recently applied to get around the limitations of self reporting of physical activity and confirms, in cross-sectional studies, that an inverse association is present between activity levels in general and vascular aging indices [6]. In this study, 432 relatively healthy participants between the ages of 30-60 years underwent ultrasonography and activity observations over 8 days. Data analysis revealed that the extent of physical activity was independently associated with carotid artery stiffness indices, but not intima media thickness.

Actigraphy and Sleep

One of the promises of activity monitoring has been the possibility of nonintrusively, in the patients' own environment, assess their sleep and its characteristics. Raw activity signals are subjected to various algorithms that define that period of interest as awake or asleep. Despite the promise of this methodology and its usefulness in defining "sleep," there remains a search for its optimal use.

Use in Ambulatory BP Monitoring

The use of actigraphy to refine the definition of awake and asleep periods during ambulatory BP monitoring is largely restricted to research purposes. Some ambulatory BP monitors have a built-in activity monitor to allow simultaneous acquisition of activity data. This work has been extended to the use of activity to relate sleep characteristics to the BP profile from day to night (dipping or non-dipping). The hypothesis is that poor sleep quality may directly or indirectly cause persistent elevation of BP. Sherwood et al. [7] recently evaluated whether sleep quality may play a role in the more prevalent non-dipping BP profile in African Americans. In 128 participants, triplicate 24-h BP monitoring studies, actigraphy, sleep interviews, and self-report of sleep and fractionated catecholamines were measured about one week apart on a regular weekday. Regression analyses suggested that body mass index, sleep quality, and sleep period reduction in sympathetic nervous system activity were likely independent factors in systolic BP dipping. Ethnicity was not a significant factor once these three factors were in the model.

Similarly, Agarwal and colleagues (8) studied the relationships of activity to ambulatory BP and dipping in 103 veterans ranging 18–90 years, with chronic kidney disease. Activity was monitored with actigraphy for 6–7 days and then an ambulatory BP monitoring study was done with simultaneous actigraphy. This set of evaluations was repeated about 1 month later. Patients who were morbidly obese, with an eGFR of 15 mL/min/$1.73m^2$ with uncontrolled hypertension, or who had been hospitalized within the prior 2 months were excluded. The results showed that in patients who normally sleep well, the use of an ambulatory BP monitor causes them to spend less time in bed and be less asleep during that time and there was reduced sleep efficiency. These results suggest that the wearing and repeated inflation deflation of an ambulatory monitor may alter sleep and cause more patients to have non-dipping BP. However, these data may only be true in elderly males and studies in other populations are needed. Sleep itself, when altered by any factor, may affect awake–sleep BP variability. Similar results were obtained by Hinderliter et al. [9] in their study of 115 untreated adults with untreated hypertension. These patients underwent study in triplicate with ambulatory BP monitoring and an actigraph monitor about a week apart. BP averages were relatively stable. Systolic dipping variability was greater in subjects with higher awake BP. In addition, day-to-day variations in dipping were related to variations in the fragmentation index. Again actigraphy-determined sleep parameters suggest that sleep quality affects BP variability.

Activity Monitoring and Neurological Disorders

There is an attraction to the idea that actigraphy and motion monitoring systems may quantify disorders in which abnormal or reduced movements predominate (e.g., Parkinsons or restless legs syndrome or stroke). In the monitoring of stroke patients, there are small studies that have described activity levels of paretic limbs over time. It is not yet known how stroke location and size affect the actigraphic output. In stroke patients, it is likely that 2–4 devices should be worn on all limbs to provide adequate information on movement or activity.

In the case of Parkinson's Disease, there are not only tremors but these patients frequently have gait and sleep disorders. Actigraphy can be useful to quantify over-all changes in activity levels, either as a reflection of the natural history or to assess the effects of drug therapy [10].

Activity Monitoring and Sleep Apnea

A large number of studies continue to be conducted in the area of sleep medicine. The small, battery-efficient, and automated analysis aspects of actigraphy seem to vastly outweigh the labor-intensive polysomnography sleep studies typically required for sleep apnea diagnosis. However, it has become clear that actigraphy may be complementary to polysomnography, a technique that remains the gold standard for diagnosis of sleep apnea. Lack of standardization of data capture and analysis continues to pose significant hurdles in the understanding of the perfor-mance in sleep disorders (e.g., apnea). It has been suggested [11] that one advanta-geous use may be as an extension to a diagnostic polysomnograph. When utilized for 9 days or more after a full polysomnograph, it can provide valuable information on naps taken during the daytime. In situations where PSG is not available, actigra-phy may provide a high level assessment of activity levels during day and night, but it will not provide the detailed assessment of sleep stages.

Sadeh [3] recently reviewed the role and validity of actigraphy in sleep disorders and has articulated a limited role and highlights the low specificity of actigraphy in detecting wakefulness during sleep periods. It was also suggested that where actig-raphy is used complementary assessment methods be considered.

Seasonal Effects, Temperature and BP, and Heart Rate

Multiple clinical studies show that office, home, and ambulatory BPs are higher in winter months than in the summer months [12]. Studies of season, temperature, and latitude and their effects on hemodynamic parameters have been consistent in showing an association between colder temperatures and increases in BP. The effect has an onset within days and recurs with each cold period.

Such variations in BP across seasons can be of a clinically meaningful magnitude, especially in the elderly, and have implications for cardiovascular risk, and also the conduct and interpretation of clinical trials especially ones that are conducted over a substantial portion of the year. Despite these observations, the complex changes in a number of climatic (sunlight and ultraviolet light) and behavioral factors (physical activity, dietary changes in food and alcohol and sleep quality) with seasons require directed study to unravel their effects independently.

Several physiological perturbations have been observed during temperature changes in the laboratory setting that may explain this phenomenon. Studies in the laboratory have shown that a reduction in environmental temperatures was associated with an increase in BP and less so in heart rate. Furthermore, acutely skin vasoconstriction and elevations of catecholamines with significant drops in temperature are reported suggesting a causal link [13, 14].

In a recent longitudinal study [15] that explored the association of temperature and BP, 1831 hypertensive patients were followed up for 3 years with measurement not only of BP, but also ambient temperatures. In this study, BP showed an inverse association with ambient temperature and explained clinically important percentages of BP variability. Interestingly, the use of the antihypertensive medication, benazepril, attenuated the level of the change though the inverse association remained.

Further insight into this complex relationship was obtained in the REGARDS study [16] that suggested that it is likely that the observed variations of BP with season are mostly mediated via temperature changes (REGARDS). In this cross-sectional study of >26,000 participants over the age of 45, minimum and maximum temperatures and previous week temperatures at various self-reported geographical residencies, as well as clinical and demographic data, were analyzed using multivariable models. This study shows that the effect of temperature on SBP was consistent across race, age, stroke risk region, education, and other factors.

Environmental Noise and Cardiovascular System

Increasingly, there is considerable environmental noise that is present not just during the day time periods but also at night. The source of the noise is road traffic, airplanes, and various industrial sources. Using noise maps in large cities has shown that about 20% of the population was exposed to excessive levels of noise due to traffic [17]. It is likely that this finding is similar in most large cities.

Chronic exposure to traffic, railway, or aircraft noise may not be just a nuisance. Studies have suggested that as road noise increases, the prevalence of hypertension also increases. Similarly, there are some but not all studies suggesting that road noise predisposes persons to myocardial infarction and stroke. Further work is needed to clarify the strength of the association of noise with these cardiovascular complications.

Brief and long-term exposure to noise may not only raise BP, but also be associated with the development of hypertension.

In human studies, increases in norepinephrine have been observed with repetitive noise exposure. In other types of noise exposure, there are observed increases in epinephrine [18].

Night time noise due to aircraft even when not loud enough to wake patients can be associated with disrupted sleep and also impaired endothelial function. In the HYENA study, night noise but not day noise was associated with BP increases [18].

Particulate Matter and Cardiovascular Risk

Particulate matter air pollution refers to particulate matter that is <2.5 μm in diameter. Problematic in understanding the effects of particulate matter is the fact that it is always present with other particulates and with several gases. Inhalation of fine particulate matter does induce an inflammatory reaction with release of cytokines. Similarly, there is an increase in endothelin activity as well as a shift towards dominance of the sympathetic nervous system [19, 20, 21]. With these changes also observed is an increase in atherosclerotic burden. Long considered an interesting topic by cardiovascular disease experts, it has not received patient level consideration by physicians and instead considered more of a societal issue.

Recently, using double blind randomized studies in relatively healthy young volunteers, fine particulate matter and not ozone was suggested to be the main factor increasing diastolic BP and possibly reducing brachial artery flow-mediated dilation.

Summary and Conclusions

In this chapter I focused on some of the variables that influence cardiovascular variability and in particular BP and heart rate. These include activity, temperature, noise, and atmospheric particulate matter. Chronic physical activity such as exercise has an important effect to reduce cardiovascular complications. Day-to-day activity using actigraphy is an important factor in understanding short-term changes in BP and heart rate and in defining sleep versus awake periods for the analysis of 24-h ambulatory BP monitoring. Indeed, actigraphy has become a mass-marketed consumer gadget that may allow individuals to monitor their own daily levels of activity. Other novel uses of actigraphy include supplementing polysomnography for sleep studies and also in a variety of neurological or other disorders. There seems little doubt that colder temperatures are associated with somewhat higher BP and heart rate. What is needed is a better understanding of whether the effects are due to temperature alone or due to other factors that change during the seasons. Environmental noise has come to full attention as an important factor in cardiovascular risk. Potential mechanisms are being elucidated that are known to link to worse cardiovascular outcomes. Regulations should be able to keep exposure below critical thresholds. Lastly, the effects of air pollution and, in particular, fine particulate matter are now well-recognized by many cardiovascular groups as being adverse on cardiovascular disease. Studies suggest that there is a direct effect of fine particulate matter to raise BP and also to increase sympathetic nervous system activity. It is likely that further refinements will be made to these factors influencing BP variability.

References

1. http://well.blogs.nytimes.com/2013/06/12/how-accurate-are-fitness-monitors/
2. Tryon WW. The ambulatory measurement of physical activity. In: Luiselli JK, Reed DD, editors. Behavioral sport psychology, evidence based approaches to performance enhancement. New York: Springer; 2011.
3. Sadeh A. The role and validity of actigraphy in sleep medicine: An update. Sleep Med Rev. 2011;259–267.
4. Paffenbarger Jr RS, Thomas MC, Wing AL. Chronic disease in former college students. VIII. Characteristics in youth predisposing to hypertension in later years. Am J Epidemiol. 1968;88:25–32.
5. Diaz KM, Shimbo D. Physical Activity and the Prevention of Hypertension. Curr Hypertens Rep. 2013;15:659–68.
6. Kozakova M, Palombo C, Mhamdi L, Konrad T, Nilsson P, Staehr PB, Paterni M, et al. Habitual physical activity and vascular aging in a young to middle-age population at low cardiovascular risk. Stroke. 2007;38(9):2549–55.
7. Sherwood A, Routledge FS, Wohlgemuth WK, Hinderliter AL, Kuhn CM, Blumenthal JA. BP Dipping: Ethnicity, sleep quality and sympathetic nervous system activity. Am J Hypertens. 2011;24(9):982–8.
8. Agarwal R, Light RP. Physical activity and hemodynamic reactivity in chronic kidney disease. Clin J Am Soc Nephrol. 2008;3(6):1660–8.
9. Hinderliter AL, Routledge FS, Blumenthal JA, Koch G, Hussey M, Wohlgemuth WK, et al. Reproducibility of BP dipping: Relation to day to day variability in sleep quality. Am J Hypertens. 2013;7(6):423–39.
10. Pan W, Song Y, Kwak S, Yoshida S, Yamamoto Y. Quantitative evaluation of the use of actigraphy for neurological and psychiatric disorders. Behav Neurol. 2014;4:1–6.
11. De Weerd AW. Actigraphy, the alternative way? Front Psychiatry. 2014;155:1–3.
12. Barnett AG, Sans S, Salomaa V, Kuulasmaa K, Dobson AJ, WHO MONICA Project. The effect of temperature on systolic BP. Blood Press Monit. 2007;12(3):195–203.
13. Babisch W. Stress hormones in the research on cardiovascular effects of noise. Noise Health. 2003;5(18):1–11.
14. Munzel T, Gori T, Babisch W, Basner M. Cardiovascular effects of environmental noise exposure. Eur Heart J. 2014;35:829–36.
15. Chen Q, Wang J, Tian J, et al. Association between Ambient Temperature and BP and BP Regulators: 1831 Hypertensive Patients Followed Up for Three Years. PLoS One. 2013;8(12):e84522.
16. Kent ST, Howard G, Crosson WL, Prineas RJ, McClure LA. The association of remotely-sensed outdoor temperature with BP levels in REGARDS: a cross-sectional study of a large, national cohort of African-American and white participants. Environ Health. 2011;10(1):7.

17. Stansfeld S, Crombie R. Cardiovascular effects of environmental noise: Research in the United Kingdom. Noise Health. 2011;13(52):229–33.
18. Jarup L, Babisch W, Houthuijs D, HYENA Study Team, et al. Hypertension and exposure to noise near airports: the HYENA study. Environ Health Perspect. 2008;116(3):329–33.
19. Newby DE, Mannucci PM, Tell GS, ESC Working Group on Thrombosis, European Association for Cardiovascular Prevention and Rehabilitation, ESC Heart Failure Association, et al. Expert position paper on air pollution and cardiovascular disease. Eur Heart J. 2015;36(2):83–93.
20. Brook RD, Rajagopalan S, Pope 3rd CA, American Heart Association Council on Epidemiology and Prevention, Council on the Kidney in Cardiovascular Disease, and Council on Nutrition, Physical Activity and Metabolism, et al. Particulate matter air pollution and cardiovascular disease: An update to the scientific statement from the American Heart Association. Circulation. 2010;121(21):2331–78.
21. Brook RD, Urch B, Dvonch T, et al. Insights into the mechanisms and mediators of the effects of air pollution exposure on BP and vascular function in healthy humans. Hypertension. 2009;54(3):659–67.

Chapter 4
Ambulatory Monitoring of Blood Pressure: An Overview of Devices, Analyses, and Clinical Utility

William B. White and Vanessa Barber

Introduction

Ambulatory blood pressure monitoring (ABPM) has been available for more than 40 years, and despite substantial evidence that this diagnostic tool provides a more precise picture of BP status in individual persons, in most countries, clinic BP measurements remain the primary method used for hypertension screening, diagnosis, and management. Ambulatory blood pressure (ABP) monitors have become increasingly popular in clinical practice. The numerous benefits include the avoidance of potential blood pressure measurement errors such as observer bias and terminal digit preference and provision of more comprehensive information on blood pressure behavior than is possible with office or home blood pressure measurement [1].

Blood pressure varies reproducibly over a 24-h cycle with a number of well-recognized patterns. Most patients are "dippers;" these individuals are characterized by at least a 10 % decline in nocturnal blood pressure compared to their awake blood pressure [2]. Some patients may have an exaggerated drop in nocturnal pressures of >20 % and have been referred to as "extreme" dippers. Kario et al. demonstrated that extreme dippers in an older Japanese population were more likely to have ischemic lesions on magnetic resonance imaging compared to dippers; however, these data have not been reproduced in other populations [3]. Approximately 10–30 % of patients are "non-dippers," in whom the blood pressure decline is blunted or absent during sleep [4, 5]. This may be the result of various types of autonomic dysfunction

W.B. White, M.D. (✉)
Calhoun Cardiology Center, University of Connecticut School of Medicine,
263 Farmington Avenue, Farmington, CT 06030-3940, USA
e-mail: wwhite@uchc.edu

V. Barber
Clinical Research Center, University of Connecticut School of Medicine, CT, USA

© Springer International Publishing Switzerland 2016
W.B. White (ed.), *Blood Pressure Monitoring in Cardiovascular Medicine and Therapeutics*, Clinical Hypertension and Vascular Diseases,
DOI 10.1007/978-3-319-22771-9_4

or certain causes of secondary hypertension and the loss of nocturnal BP decline is also a risk factor for target organ damage [6]. Multiple studies, in hypertensives as well as normotensives (NTs), have consistently shown that target organ damage is more likely in non-dippers than dippers [7]. Additionally, nocturnal BP is an independent, powerful indicator of cardiovascular disease [2]. A small proportion of patients exhibit an "inverse" dipping pattern [8]. Here, the nocturnal blood pressures do not fall during sleep and, in some cases, may actually be higher than the daytime readings. Other 24-h blood pressure patterns that have been observed resulting from the advent of ABP include "white coat" hypertension (WCH) or the "white coat effect" [9]. In these patients, medical care environment blood pressures are substantially higher than ambulatory awake blood pressure averages. There are also some individuals who may present with "masked hypertension," where ABP is elevated but office blood pressure is normal. This phenomenon may, in part, be the result of factors not present in the physician's office (e.g., smoking cigarettes, mental stress, or physical activity). Liu et al. reported that people with masked hypertension are as likely to have left ventricular hypertrophy (LVH) and carotid artery intimal-medial thickening as those patients with definite hypertension [10]. More recently, a 10-year follow-up of the Ohasama study showed that the cardiovascular mortality and stroke rates were significantly higher in masked hypertensives as compared with normotensives (relative hazard ratio = 2.1) [11]. Another pattern identified by ABP that has been linked to increased incidence of stroke in hypertensive patients is the "morning surge," which is a marked rise in BP during the early morning awakening hours [12].

Most research has shown that isolated clinic blood pressure values do not accurately estimate a patient's overall hypertension burden since they represent only one or two points in time on a patient's 24-h blood pressure profile. ABP monitors overcome this problem by obtaining multiple readings over the 24-h period and capturing the blood pressure variability. Numerous studies have also shown that clinic blood pressures are inferior in predicting hypertensive target end-organ damage, as well as long-term cardiovascular outcomes, compared with ambulatory BP averages. This chapter will focus on the various types of ABPM devices and their validation and discuss their clinical application in managing patients with hypertension.

ABPM Devices: Auscultatory and Oscillometric

Ambulatory BP monitors are automated and programmable devices that detect blood pressure either by the auscultatory method or the oscillometric route. Some devices have the option of using both techniques. Each method has its own advantages and limitations. The auscultatory devices employ the use of a microphone to detect Korotkoff sounds. Unfortunately, these devices are also sensitive to external artifact noise, which may limit their accuracy. They may also be less precise in the obese upper extremity. In some devices, these limitations have been overcome by synchronizing the Korotkoff sounds with the R-wave of the electrocardiogram (electrocardiographic gating) [13]. The oscillometric technique, which is utilized in the majority of present-day monitors, detects the initial and maximal arterial vibrations or the mean arterial blood pressure and is less affected by external artifacts. The systolic and diastolic blood pressure values used in this technique are actually computed via set algorithms. Hence, the more sensitive the algorithm, the more accurate the device. Extreme blood pressure values increase the likelihood of error with the oscillometric devices [14]. Modern ABP recorders are compact, lightweight monitors that can be programmed to take blood pressure readings at various intervals (e.g., every 15 min during the day and every 30 min at night). In most devices, the bleed rates of deflation of the cuff and maximal inflation pressures can be programmed; some devices also have a patient-initiated event button (to monitor symptoms). Most devices have algorithms to screen out most erroneous readings and will perform a repeat of the blood pressure measurement within 1–2 min. Prior to initiation and again at the termination of a 24-h monitoring study, the ABP device may be calibrated against either an aneroid or a mercury-column sphygmomanometer to verify that the systolic blood pressure and diastolic blood pressure agree within about 5 mmHg. It is most practical that the cuff be fitted to the nondominant arm. If there is a large discordance between arms in BP measurement, it is recommended to apply the cuff to the higher value arm if the difference in systolic BP is greater than 10 mmHg [12, 15]. Patients should be educated regarding the use of the ABPM at device hookup. Most experts recommend that a written set of instructions be given for at-home reference along with verbal counseling [12]. For example, the patient needs to be aware that when the actual readings are being measured, the arm should be held motionless to avoid artifact and repetitive readings [16]. Excessive heavy physical activity during measurements should be discouraged, as it usually interferes with the accuracy of the measurements. A diary that records wake-up and sleep times, time of medication administration, meals, and any occurrence of symptoms should be maintained.

Ambulatory BP monitoring should be performed on a routine working day rather than a nonworking day or on the weekend to obtain the most representative blood pressure values. A study conducted by Devereux et al. demonstrated that daytime (work) blood pressures were a more sensitive determinant of left ventricular mass index compared to daytime values taken at home [17]. The clinical advantages of ABPM studies are many and the disadvantages are few (Table 4.1). Ambulatory BP monitoring eliminates observer error as well as the white coat effect, and it allows for a more comprehensive assessment of antihypertensive therapy. In addition, ABP is a superior prognostic indicator for hypertensive target end-organ damage as compared to clinic blood pressures. The potential limitations of ABP devices include poor technical results in patients with rapid atrial fibrillation or in those patients with very obese or large, muscular upper arms that exceed a mid-bicep circumference of 44 cm. Imprecise data may also be recorded in patients with weak pulses or an auscultatory gap. The devices are usually well-tolerated by patients, although occasionally there may be bruising or petechiae at the upper or distal arm, particularly in the elderly or patients on anticoagulation therapies. Some subjects may experience a lack of sleep at night or poor sleep quality because of the repeated cuff inflations.

Table 4.1 Advantages and disadvantages of ambulatory blood pressure monitoring compared to clinic blood pressures

Advantages	Disadvantages
Elimination of observer bias/error	Cost
Elimination of the white coat effect	Time commitment on behalf of
More comprehensive assessment of antihypertensive	Patient
therapy	Disturbed sleep
Superior prognostic indicator	Cuff discomfort
Calculation of blood pressure loads	May be inaccurate in atrial fibrillation
Evaluation of dipping/non-dipping status	
Ability to better assess blood pressure variability	
More reproducible over time	

Validation of ABP Monitors

The Association for the Advancement of Medical Instrumentation (AAMI) has long recognized the importance of evaluation of the accuracy of ABP monitors. A protocol was first developed in 1987 for the assessment of device accuracy and reliability [18]. The AAMI protocol was followed by a more complex method of independent validation from the British Hypertension Society (BHS) in 1990 [19]. Although the protocols differed, their aim was to establish minimum accuracy standards for these devices in order for them to be considered reliable clinical tools. Since then, both protocols have been revised [20, 21]. In addition to clinical testing, the protocols include recommendations such as labeling information, details for environmental performance, as well as stability and safety requirements.

In an updated version in 1992, the AAMI [20] advised that blood pressure should be measured at the onset and conclusion of the validation study in three positions (supine, seated, and standing) and the difference between the ABPM vs. the reference standard should not be more than 5 mmHg with a standard deviation of 8 mmHg. Additionally, the disparity between the ABPM and the reference sphygmomanometer should be assessed in 20 subjects at the beginning and at the end of a 24-h blood pressure study. This difference should not exceed 5 mmHg in at least 75 % of the readings. For reliability testing, three different instruments should be assessed in a minimum of ten subjects for a total of thirty 24-h ABP studies. It is recommended that a minimum of 75 readings in each of the 24-h studies be obtained, with 15-min intervals during the awake period and 30-min intervals during sleep. The number of satisfactory readings (i.e., no error codes) should exceed 80 % of the total number of readings programmed for the day.

The BHS protocol is a more complex validation protocol that has the grading system outlined in Table 4.2. The BHS protocol calls for multiple phases of validation: (1) before use device validation, (2) in-use (field) assessment, (3) after-use device calibration, (4) static device calibration where the device is rechecked after 1 month of usage, and (5) report of evaluation. Each phase has its passing criteria [21].

Table 4.2 British Hypertension Society Grading Criteria

Absolute difference between standard and test device (mmHg)			
Grade	≤5 (%)	≤10 (%)	≤15 (%)
A	60	85	95
B	50	75	90
C	40	65	85
D		Worse than C	

Grades are derived from percentages of readings within 5, 10, and 15 mmHg. To achieve a grade, all three percentages must be equal to or greater than the tabulated values

From ref. [21]

In 2002, the Working Group on Blood Pressure Monitoring of the European Society of Hypertension approved a new protocol—the European Society of Hypertension International Protocol (ESH_IP) [22]. The main purpose of this protocol was to simplify the previous protocols without compromising their integrity. Briefly, this protocol consists of the following steps:

1. Observer training and assessment.
2. Familiarization session.
3. Validation measurements (done in two phases, with 15 patients required in the first phase and 33 in the second).
4. Analysis after each phase.
5. Reporting of results.

This protocol uses "pass" or "fail" for grading the devices as opposed to the A–D classification of the BHS protocol. One of the other differences from the BHS protocol is the exclusion of the pre-validation phases (phases 1–3 in the previous list), thereby considerably reducing time and labor. Also, the specifications regarding observer training reduce errors in the actual measurement of blood pressures and resolve major differences between individual observers. A reduced sample size, a refinement in the range of test blood pressure, and a two-phase system of evaluation will decrease the time and cost required for validation by using fewer total subjects and eliminating extremely inaccurate devices in an initial phase of testing. The international protocol has also been criticized for certain differences from prior protocols [23]. First, the protocol does not specify a range of arm circumference over which the device must be tested. Arm circumference is known to affect the accuracy of blood pressure measurement. Second, the protocol does not specify the maximum number of subjects that can be excluded. Some experts have brought up concerns that this might give the manufacturers excessive control over data reporting. In 2010, the ESH-IP was revised with more stringent validation specifications [24]. These specifications include forms with standardized options for responses in the place of open-ended responses, an age restriction of ≥25 years, and more stringent pass levels [25]. The 2002 ESH-PI1 and 2010 ESH-PI2 have been the most frequently used validation protocols primarily due to their ease of use compared to the AAMI and BHS guidelines [15, 26].

Hodgkinson et al. conducted a systematic review of validation studies using the AAMI, BHS, ESH-IP1, ISO, and ESH-IP2 protocols and found that the less complicated ESH-IP generated fewer major protocol deviations than the AAMI and BHS [27]. Ultimately, Hodgkinson et al. recommended the ESH-IP2 protocol citing its "simplicity of method and greater accuracy requirement" [27].

Analysis of ABPM Data

Upon completion of the 24-h ABP recording, the data are downloaded and analyzed statistically to calculate blood pressure averages (i.e., 24-h, awake or daytime, and sleep or nighttime) as well as variations on the blood pressure load. The American Society of Hypertension as well as other expert groups have proposed limits of normal blood pressure and blood pressure loads as depicted in Table 4.3 [28].

Descriptive Blood Pressure Data from ABPM

Data are generally reported separately for the 24-h, daytime, and nighttime periods. These averages should be accompanied by the standard deviations as a simple indicator of blood pressure variability. A study by Kikuya et al. found an association between increased cardiovascular mortality risk and daytime SBP variability [29]. Some studies have indicated that there is a significant relationship between blood pressure variability and target end-organ damage [30], especially with beat-to-beat intra-arterial data. Frattola et al. conducted a study on 73 essential hypertensives that underwent intra-arterial blood pressure monitoring at the initiation of the study [31]. Subsequently, echocardiography was performed to assess left ventricular mass

Table 4.3 Suggested upper limits of normal average ambulatory blood pressure and load

Blood pressure measure	Probably normal	Borderline	Probably abnormal
Systolic average			
Awake	<135	135–140	>140
Asleep	<120	120–125	>125
24-h	<130	130–135	>135
Diastolic average			
Awake	<85	85–90	>90
Asleep	<75	75–80	>80
24-h	<80	80–85	>85
Awake	<15	15–30	>30
Asleep	<15	15–30	>30
Awake	<15	15–30	>30
Asleep	<15	15–30	>30

From ref. [28]

on subjects at the onset and at the conclusion of the study 7 years later. The standard deviations were obtained, and the average blood pressure variability for the group was calculated as 10.8 mmHg. The authors observed that end-organ damage was significantly higher in patients who had a greater than average blood pressure variability (for the group as a whole) given that the 24-h mean arterial pressure was similar in both groups. Unfortunately, 24-h blood pressure monitoring was not conducted at the end of the study to confirm if the same level of blood pressure variability persisted.

Blood Pressure Loads

The blood pressure load is calculated as the proportion of blood pressures >135/85 mmHg during the awake period and >120/75 mmHg during the sleep hours. White et al. was one of the first groups to introduce the concept of blood pressure loads [32]. They conducted a study in 30 previously untreated hypertensives and observed that the blood pressure load was a sensitive predictor of indices of hypertensive cardiac involvement. The results demonstrated that when the systolic or diastolic blood pressure loads were less than 30 %, the likelihood of LVH was negligible. However, with a systolic blood pressure load exceeding 50 %, the incidence of LVH approached 90 %, and with the diastolic blood pressure load more than 40 %, LVH occurred in 70 % of the subjects [33]. Similar results were obtained when Mule et al. studied 130 patients with mild to moderate hypertension [34]. Subjects with a higher systolic blood pressure load, adjusted for average 24-h SBP, were found to have increased relative myocardial wall thickness and total peripheral vascular resistance as well as increased prevalence of hypertensive retinopathy. These studies suggest that blood pressure load is an independent predictor of hypertensive target organ damage and adverse cardiovascular risk profile. However, this parameter has fallen out of favor in recent years since 'load' is not a continuous variable and has no means to differentiate moderate versus severely hypertensive individuals.

White Coat Hypertension (WCH) and the White Coat Effect (WCE)

White coat hypertension (also called isolated clinic hypertension) is diagnosed when the untreated patient's 24-h blood pressure is within normal limits, but blood pressure in the clinic is persistently elevated (Fig. 4.1), with clinic BP measurements ≥140/90 mmHg, 24-h ABPM <130/80 mmHg, awake ABPM <135/85 mmHg, and nocturnal ABPM <120/70 mmHg [35]. The prevalence of WCH is reported to be 10 to 20 % of patients with untreated Stage 1 hypertension [36]. Originally thought to be a benign condition, recent WCH studies have found evidence that CV risk in individuals with WCH is between that of normotensives and sustained hypertensives. A meta-analysis by Cuspidi et al. in 2014 showed that people with WCH had

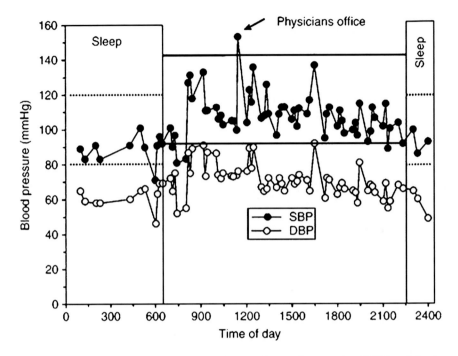

Fig. 4.1 *Plot* showing 24-h pressure curve depicting white coat hypertension (WCH) and dipping status. The patient's blood pressure in the physician's office is 153/76 mmHg. The daytime ambulatory average is normal at 108/71 ± 13/9 mmHg. The subject has WCH with a 45/5 mmHg rise in blood pressure in the physician's office. The patient also has a normal drop in nocturnal pressures, with a night time average of 90/60 ± 7/6 mmHg

increased left ventricular mass index, decreased mitral E/A ratio, and greater left atrial diameter compared to a matched group of normotensive individuals [37]. A key utility of ambulatory BP monitoring in clinical practice is its ability to identify WCH, thereby preventing excessive drug therapy [12, 15]. Nevertheless, patients with WCH do need close observation with ABP performed every 2–3 years to determine whether a more sustained hypertensive pattern has developed [38]. The white coat effect (WCE) is defined as an additional presser response in patients with established and treated hypertension, which causes an overestimation of true blood pressure when measured in the clinic setting (Fig. 4.2). White coat effect parameters are typically defined as: treated patients with hypertension where the office BP is ≥140/90 mmHg, 24-h ABPM <130/80 mmHg, daytime ABPM <135/85 mmHg, and nocturnal ABPM <120/70 mmHg [12].

Masked Hypertension

Masked hypertension ("white coat normotension" or "reverse white coat hypertension") is an entity that has been closely studied during the past decade.

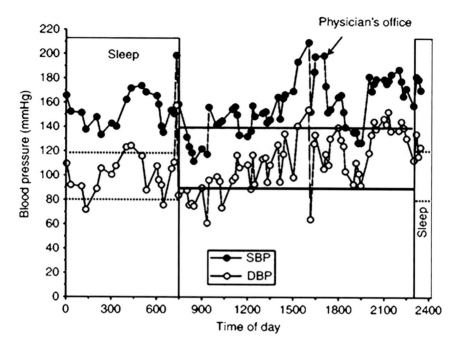

Fig. 4.2 *Plot* showing 24-h blood pressure curve depicting white coat effect and non-dipper status. The patient is hypertensive with a daytime average of 158/110±21/23 mmHg. The nighttime blood pressure does not drop significantly (157/105±15/16 mmHg). The patient, in addition to his hypertension, has a significant white coat effect in which the blood pressure is 216/98 mmHg in the physician's office

Masked hypertension is diagnosed when an individual has a normal office (or clinic) blood pressure and an elevated ABP in those patients either not currently being treated for hypertension or on therapy which is not controlling the BP during a 24-h period. The parameters for this condition are typically: untreated patients with office BP <140/90 mmHg, 24-h ABP ≥130/80 mmHg, daytime ABP ≥135/85 mmHg, and/or nighttime ABP ≥120/70 mmHg [35]. Patients with normal office BP in conjunction with stressful occupations, kidney disease, obstructive sleep apnea, LVH, target organ damage, familial history of hypertension, and increased blood pressure during exercise should be considered for ambulatory BP assessment to confirm or deny a diagnosis of masked hypertension [12]. Masked hypertension, which occurs in 10–15 % of normotensive people, is associated with an increased risk of target organ damage as well as cardiovascular mortality [10].

Dipping/Non-dipping/Extreme Dipping

Blood pressure normally has a circadian pattern in which blood pressure drops during sleep and is higher during the awake hours of the day. This pattern is referred to as "dipping" (Fig. 4.1). The dipping status can be determined by evaluating awake and sleep blood pressures and calculating differences between the two averages. The percentage "dip" is then determined by dividing this difference by the awake average. The degree of decline in blood pressure varies from person to person, but a general consensus is that 10–20 % drop in blood pressure during sleep is "normal" [39]. The patient who has *less* than a 10 % drop in blood pressure at night is referred to as a "nondipper" (Fig. 4.2).

Reporting of Ambulatory BP Data for Medical Records

Using all of the above-referenced values, an informative report can be generated indicating the status of the patient's blood pressure. The reports should include demographics, all medications taken during the study, the number of accurate readings obtained, the awake/sleep times, and any symptoms that were experienced. The clinical report could also graphically depict blood pressures and heart rates over a 24 h period as shown in Figs. 4.1, 4.2, and 4.3.

Reproducibility of ABPM

The majority of clinical trials conducted to evaluate ABP reproducibility confirm both superior short-term (<1 year) [40, 41] and long-term (>1 year) [42–44] reproducibility of ABPM as compared to clinical blood pressure measurement. One

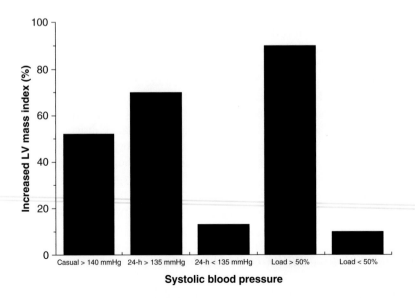

Fig. 4.3 Bars show percentage of increased left ventricular (LV) mass in subjects with elevated systolic blood pressures (both clinical and ambulatory) and systolic blood pressure loads (From ref. [45])

substudy from the Systolic Hypertension in Europe (SYST-EUR) trial evaluated 112 patients who were randomized to receive placebo [42]. Clinical and ABPM readings done at baseline were repeated after 1 month in 51 subjects and a full year in 112 subjects. The results indicated that differences in 24-h ambulatory systolic blood pressure (2.4 ± 10.7 mmHg [$p < 0.05$]) were far less than for clinical systolic blood pressure (6.6 ± 15.9 mmHg [$p < 0.001$]) taken at 1 year (Fig. 4.4). Another large-scale trial that also observed better reproducibility for ABP monitoring than clinical blood pressure was the Hypertension and Ambulatory Recording Study (HARVEST), in which 508 subjects were evaluated [43]. Ambulatory BP monitoring was conducted at baseline and 3 months later in the untreated state. A very modest difference in the two sequential ABPMs for the group as a whole was observed (0.4/0.7 mmHg).

Studies evaluating the reproducibility of the circadian rhythm have not had such promising results. For example, in a study by Mochizuki et al., it was found that there was limited reproducibility of the circadian rhythm [45]. In that study, 253 untreated essential hypertensives were monitored for 48 h. In these 2 days, 16 % of dippers "converted" into non-dippers and 13 % of non-dippers "converted" into dippers (Fig. 4.5). The authors suggested that 48-h ABP monitors be performed to assess the circadian blood pressure profile of an individual [46]. Although this will not solve the problem entirely, it should decrease the likelihood of error.

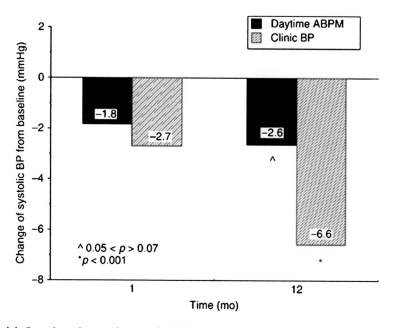

Fig. 4.4 *Bars* show the superior reproducibility of ambulatory blood pressure (ABP) vs. clinic/office blood pressure from the SYST-EUR trial ($n = 112$). Blood pressures were measured 1 and 12 months after baseline measurements (From ref. [42])

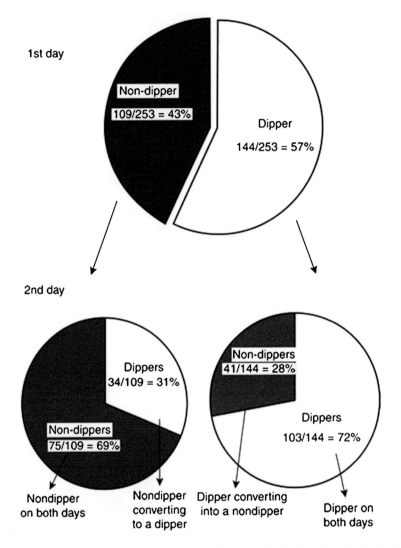

Fig. 4.5 Illustration of the limited reproducibility of the circadian rhythm (i.e., the dipping/non-dipping status) with ambulatory blood pressure monitoring studies conducted over 48 h in 253 subjects (From ref. [45])

Indications for ABPM

ABPM has been recognized as an important clinical tool by a number of expert medical groups and societies. In the US, the Joint National Committee (JNC VII) recommended ABP monitoring for a number of clinical situations (Table 4.4) [39].

The 2014 ESH practice guidelines for ambulatory blood pressure monitoring report that ABPM should be extended to not only to WCH, but also to suspected

Table 4.4 Primary indications for ambulatory blood pressure monitoring

Suspected white coat hypertension
Apparent drug resistance
Hypotensive symptoms with antihypertensive medications
Episodic hypertension
Autonomic dysfunction
Suspected white coat effect
Suspected masked hypertension, particularly in treated patients

cases of nocturnal hypertension, dipping, to assess 24 h BP, masked controlled and uncontrolled hypertension , and daytime hypertension [47]. These guidelines also highlighted that ABP analysis could be used in any patient who is hypertensive with presence of target organ damage, diabetics, and those who have a family history of CVD [47]. Recently, the National Institute for Health and Clinical Excellence (NICE) updated their guidelines for the management of hypertension to include ABPM as a confirmatory test in patients with an office blood pressure $\geq 140/90$ mmHg, citing ABPM's cost-effectiveness and greater accuracy over HBPM [48]. A 2014 systematic review found that hypertension is inaccurately diagnosed at an exceedingly higher rate when office BP measurements are solely used; they found that studies that required confirmatory testing had better accuracy in diagnosis and concluded that ABPM should be employed as a confirmatory test in instances for which office BP is elevated [49].

White Coat Hypertension

WCH, a well-recognized clinical entity since 1983 [9], is a result of the presser response that patients experience when entering a medical environment. These patients have normal blood pressure outside of the doctor's office during activities of regular daily life. The prevalence has been estimated to be approximately 20 % in untreated borderline and stage I hypertensives [50]. The prognostic significance of this diagnosis has been the subject of considerable debate over the past three decades. Multiple prospective as well as cross-sectional studies have been performed looking at this issue, a large majority of which have shown no significant difference in long-term cardiovascular outcomes in people with WCH versus those with normotension. In one of the initial long-term studies, Verdecchia et al. prospectively followed 1187 subjects from the PIUMA registry for up to 7.5 years [51]. In their study, WCH was defined as an ambulatory daytime blood pressure of <131/86 mmHg for women and <136/87 mmHg for men, and the clinic blood pressure was >140/90 mmHg. No difference was initially observed between the WCH and normotensive groups, although follow-up of this database was later conducted with the use of a larger number ($n = 1500$) of patients [52]. The WCH patients were stratified into two subgroups. The first subgroup had a more restrictive and conservative definition of WCH (daytime ABP <130/80 mmHg), whereas the second group had more liberal limits for ABP (daytime ABP <131/86 mmHg for women and <136/87 mmHg for men). Cardiovascular morbid events in the first group were similar to the normal BP controls, but event rates in the more liberally defined group were significantly higher than the normotensive population. In the HARVEST trial, 722 hypertensive patients were evaluated using a more restrictive threshold to define WCH [53]. There was a significantly higher left ventricular mass index in the population with WCH (threshold <130/80 mmHg) when compared with the normo- tensive population (Fig. 4.6). The PAMELA study also showed that patients with WCH have cardiac morphological and functional indices that seem to be intermedi- ate between normals and sustained hypertensives [54]. Given the results of these rather large trials, WCH might be considered a prehypertensive state in some patients. Thus, close monitoring and follow-up is required, and at some point the institution of therapy may be needed. Careful follow-up is necessary even in the 6–8 % of true WCH patients with daytime ABP <130/80 mmHg.

Therapeutic Interventions

Accurate blood pressure measurement is the key step in formulating an effective treatment plan for hypertensive patients. ABPM can be used to assess the need for and effectiveness of both initial and additional antihypertensive therapy. To illus- trate this benefit, Staessen et al. conducted a randomized controlled trial evaluating 419 untreated hypertensive patients over a course of approx. 6 months [55]. The

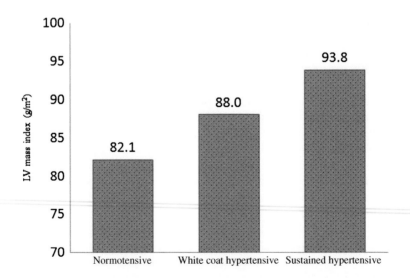

Fig. 4.6 *Bars* show the left ventricular mass in three categories of patients (*n* = 722): normoten- sives, those with white coat hypertension (threshold <130/80 mmHg), and sustained hypertensives (HARVEST trial) (From ref. [53])

Ambulatory Blood Pressure Monitoring and Treatment of Hypertension (APTH) trial randomized patients to an ABP arm vs. a clinical blood pressure arm.

Drug treatment was adjusted in a stepwise fashion based on daytime ABP readings vs. the average of three clinical measurements. At the end of the study, it was shown that more subjects in the ABP group discontinued antihypertensive drug therapy. Furthermore, fewer subjects in the ABP group had progressed to receive multiple antihypertensive drugs (Fig. 4.7). There were no significant differences in the final blood pressure, left ventricular mass, or reported symptoms between groups. Therefore, ABP monitors can complement conventional approaches in determining optimal medication dosage and frequency of dosing.

Resistant Hypertension

Resistant hypertension has been defined as the failure to achieve goal blood pressure despite strict adherence to near-maximal doses of an appropriate 3- or 4-drug therapy regimen that includes a diuretic [39]. Ambulatory BP monitors have proven useful in the evaluation of those patients who do not appear to be responding to therapy or for those on complicated medication regimens. With data derived from an ABPM, one can ascertain if and at what time additional therapy is needed or if it is needed at all. Mezzetti et al. evaluated 27 subjects with resistant hypertension by ABPM [56]. They observed that more than 50 % of the subjects showed a large white coat effect and were actually normotensive (<135/85 mmHg) on their current

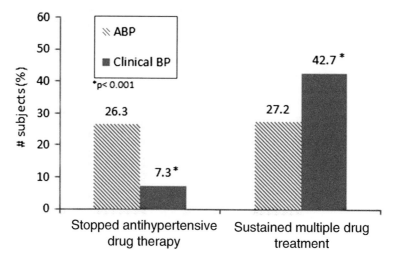

Fig. 4.7 *Bars* depict the percentage of subjects (*n*=419) who stopped antihypertensive therapy and those who sustained multiple-drug therapy with the medication regimen being controlled either by ambulatory blood pressure monitoring results or by clinical measurements (APTH trial) (From ref. [55])

medication regimens. Later, Muxfeldt et al. conducted a cross-sectional study in 286 resistant hypertensives and divided them based on their ABP into a true resistant group (56.3 %) and a white coat resistant group (43.7 %) [57]. The former group was found to have a significantly increased prevalence of both LVH and nephropathy. In a 5-year follow-up study, Pierdomenico et al. found that the cardiovascular event rate was much lower in false resistant patients than true resistant hypertensives (1.2 vs. 4.1 events per 100 patient–year) [58]. Finally, Redon et al. conducted a study in 86 refractory hypertensives over 49 months [59]. These patients were divided into tertiles of average diastolic blood pressure from the ABPM. The office blood pressures were not different among the three groups. It was found that subjects in the highest tertile group (diastolic blood pressure > 97 mmHg) had greater progression of hypertensive end-organ damage compared to the lower two tertile groups. Thus, ABPM was capable of identifying high-, medium-, and low-risk patients with refractory hypertension that was not apparent by office blood pressure measurements alone.

Type of Therapy/Chronotherapeutics

It has been well-documented that a majority of cardiovascular events occur in the morning hours because of a number of inciting hemodynamic, hormonal, and hematological factors. Gosse et al. established in 181 patients that the arising blood pressure correlated with left ventricular mass better than did the office blood pressures [60]. Hence, the higher the early morning blood pressure, the greater the left ventricular mass. The rise in post-awakening morning blood pressure can be obtained best by a 24-h ABP monitoring study. More recently, a prospective study performed in older hypertensives showed a higher incidence of stroke (relative risk=2.7; p=0.04) in subjects with a morning blood pressure surge after matching for age and 24-h blood pressures [61]. These studies stress the importance of identifying vulnerable subjects and targeting antihypertensive therapy to avoid morning surges of blood pressure.

Orthostatic Hypotension/Autonomic Dysfunction

Individuals with autonomic dysfunction (e.g., diabetics) or orthostatic hypotension tend to lose the normal circadian variation in blood pressure and may even demonstrate an inverse dipping phenomenon (Fig. 4.8).

The Ohasama, Japan, study clearly demonstrated in 1542 subjects that patients with inverse dipping had a significantly worse cardiovascular outcome as compared to the other patient groups (Fig. 4.9) [8]. Generally, there is also considerable variability of blood pressure noted in the inverse-dipping patient population. Patients with inverse dipping may benefit from short-acting medications that can be taken at bedtime to reduce the nighttime blood pressure average. In addition, some complicated patients with idiopathic orthostatic hypotension may be severely hypertensive

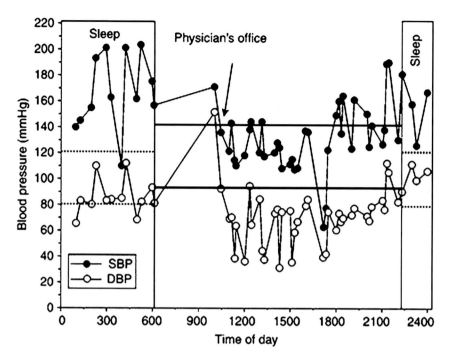

Fig. 4.8 *Plot* showing a 24-h blood pressure curve depicting autonomic dysfunction and inverse dipping. There is significant variability of blood pressure, as seen by the standard deviation. The awake blood pressure average is $132/71 \pm 26/23$ mmHg, and the sleep average is $164/89 \pm 28/15$ mmHg. The sleep averages are higher than awake averages, indicating an inverse dipping pattern

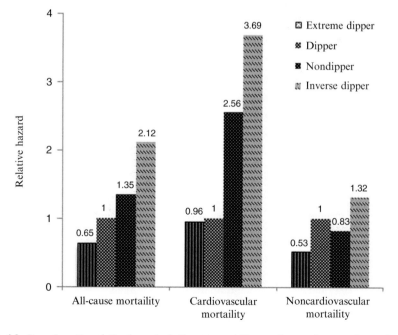

Fig. 4.9 *Bars* show the relative hazard of all-cause mortality, cardiovascular mortality, and noncardiovascular mortality in four subsets of patients ($n = 1542$): the extreme dipper, the dipper, the non-dipper, and the inverse dipper (From ref. [8])

in the supine position and markedly hypotensive in the upright position. Medication regimens can be tailored individually for these patients by using the detailed blood pressure information obtained via a 24-h ABPM.

Other indications for an ABPM study include evaluation of symptoms and episodic hypertension. With the help of a patient-initiated event button, the physician can determine if the symptoms correlate with either a severely hypertensive (in the case of pheochromocytoma) or hypotensive period (in the case of excessive medication or autonomic dysfunction).

Cost-Effectiveness of ABPM

ABPM studies generally cost $150–400 in the United States. In 2002, a national insurance policy was created by the Centers for Medicare and Medicaid Services to cover 24-h ABPM for "suspected white coat hypertension." The International Classification of Diseases (ICD)-9 code for this diagnosis is somewhat elusive, since it is under a different category than the hypertension codes (transient increases in blood pressure, hypertension nonconfirmed, 796.2). Many private insurance carriers have followed the lead of Medicare and also cover some of the cost of an ambulatory blood pressure monitoring study. Kent et al. looked at ABPM claims submitted between 2007 and 2010 and found that claims that used code 796.2 (International Classification of Diseases, Ninth Revision, diagnosis code) were reimbursed 93.8 % of the time [62].

However, there has been some controversy regarding the cost-effectiveness of ABPM. Moser argued that if 24-h ABPM were to be performed on just 3–5 million of persons with hypertension in the United States, it would add an additional $600 million to $1.75 billion per year to the cost of management [63]. However, the APTH trial [55] performed a cost–benefit analysis of ABPM vs. clinical blood pressure monitoring. They observed that the cost of medication was less for the ABP arm compared to patients who were solely evaluated by office blood pressures ($3390 vs. $4188 per 100 patients per month of therapy). Additionally, the ABP arm required fewer office visits for close blood pressure monitoring, thereby reducing physician fees. The authors concluded that the potential savings in the ABP group were offset by the cost of the study, rendering it equally cost-effective but therapeutically more beneficial. Ambulatory BP guidelines published by the ESH in 2014 suggested that pharmacies equipped with ABP monitors could place these on patients with doctor's referrals reducing the individual financial burden of such monitors on physicians and expanding the availability of such services [47]. In 1994, Yarows et al. from Michigan also conducted a cost-effective study in clinical practice [64]. They followed two sets of patients: the treatment group that had documented hypertension on an ABPM and was given appropriate antihypertensive therapy ($n = 192$) and a diagnostic group that was documented to be hypertensive in the physician's office and was off all antihypertensive therapy ($n = 131$). The diagnostic group had a 24-h ABPM conducted, and the prevalence of WCH in this group was determined to be 34 % (using a 24-h mean diastolic pressure of 85 mmHg) [65].

The authors ascertained the average yearly cost of antihypertensive medications for the 192 hypertensive subjects to be $578.40 (range $94.90–$4361.75). They concluded that in the diagnostic group, the fee for the ABPM ($188) would be offset by the savings for 1 year of antihypertensive therapy (if no medications were used for the WCH patients). In a cost-effectiveness analysis, Krakoff used the most up-to-date information on the prevalence of WCH, probability of WCH transitioning to a sustained hypertension, and the costs of medical care and testing [66]. His analysis predicted savings of 3–14 % in healthcare costs for hypertension when ABP monitoring was routinely used as a diagnostic tool. The annual cost savings calculated for secondary screening using ABPM was also less than 10 % of treatment costs, based on the current reimbursement rates. Hopefully, these types of important analyses [66, 67] will convince the payers as well as clinicians that ambulatory blood pressure monitoring has matured into a useful tool for both the diagnosis and management of many patients with hypertension.

References

1. Prisant LM. Ambulatory blood pressure monitoring in the diagnosis of hypertension. Cardiol Clin. 1995;13(4):479–90.
2. Snyder F, Hobson JA, Morrison DF, Goldfrank F. Changes in respiration, heart rate, and systolic blood pressure in human sleep. J Appl Physiol. 1964;19:417–22.
3. Kario K, Matsuo T, Kobayashi H, Imiya M, Matsuo M, Shimada K. Nocturnal fall of blood pressure and silent cerebrovascular damage in elderly hypertensive patients. Advanced silent cerebrovascular damage in extreme dippers. Hypertension. 1996;27(1):130–5.
4. Pickering TG. The clinical significance of diurnal blood pressure variations. Dippers and non-dippers. Circulation. 1990;81(2):700–2.
5. O'Brien E, Sheridan J, O'Malley K. Dippers and non-dippers. Lancet. 1988;2(8607):397.
6. Hany S, Baumgart P, Battig B, Walger P, Vetter W, Vetter H. Diagnostic aspects of 24-hour blood pressure determination. Schweiz Rundsch Med Prax. 1987;76(17):450–4.
7. Shimada K, Kawamoto A, Matsubayashi K, Nishinaga M, Kimura S, Ozawa T. Diurnal blood pressure variations and silent cerebrovascular damage in elderly patients with hypertension. J Hypertens. 1992;10(8):875–8.
8. Ohkubo T, Imai Y, Tsuji I, et al. Relation between nocturnal decline in blood pres- sure and mortality. The Ohasama Study. Am J Hypertens. 1997;10(11):1201–7.
9. Mancia G, Bertinieri G, Grassi G, et al. Effects of blood-pressure measurement by the doctor on patient's blood pressure and heart rate. Lancet. 1983;2(8352):695–8.
10. Liu JE, Roman MJ, Pini R, Schwartz JE, Pickering TG, Devereux RB. Cardiac and arterial target organ damage in adults with elevated ambulatory and normal office blood pressure. Ann Intern Med. 1999;131(8):564–72.
11. Ohkubo T, Kikuya M, Metoki H, et al. Prognosis of "masked" hypertension and "white-coat" hypertension detected by 24-h ambulatory blood pressure monitoring 10-year follow-up from the Ohasama study. J Am Coll Cardiol. 2005;46(3):508–15.
12. Head GA, McGarth BP, Mihailidou AS, Nelson MR, Schlaich MP, Stowasser M, Mangoni AA, Cowley D, Brown MA, Ruta LA, Wilson A. Ambulatory blood pressure monitoring in Australia: 2011 consensus position statement. J Hypertens. 2012;30:253–66.
13. White WB, Schulman P, McCabe EJ, Nardone MB. Clinical validation of the accutracker, a novel ambulatory blood pressure monitor using R-wave gating for Korotkoff sounds. J Clin Hypertens. 1987;3(4):500–9.

14. Anwar YA, Giacco S, McCabe EJ, Tendler BE, White WB. Evaluation of the efficacy of the Omron HEM-737 IntelliSense device for use on adults according to the recommendations of the Association for the Advancement of Medical Instrumentation. Blood Press Monit. 1998; 3(4):261–5.
15. O'Brien E, et al. European Society of Hypertension Position Paper on Ambulatory Blood Pressure Monitoring. J Hypertens. 2013;31:1731–68.
16. White WB, Lund-Johansen P, Omvik P. Assessment of four ambulatory blood pressure monitors and measurements by clinicians vs intraarterial blood pressure at rest and during exercise. Am J Cardiol. 1990;65(1):60–6.
17. Devereux RB, Pickering TG, Harshfield GA, et al. Left ventricular hypertrophy in patients with hypertension: importance of blood pressure response to regularly recurring stress. Circulation. 1983;68(3):470–6.
18. Association for the Advancement of Medical Instrumentation, A.V. American National Standard for Electronic or Automated Sphygmomanometers, in ANSI/AAMI SP10-1987. Arlington: AAMI.
19. O'Brien E, Petrie J, Littler W, et al. The British Hypertension Society protocol for the evaluation of automated and semi-automated blood pressure measuring devices with special reference to ambulatory systems. J Hypertens. 1990;8(7):607–19.
20. White WB, Berson AS, Robbins C, et al. National standard for measurement of resting and ambulatory blood pressures with automated sphygmomanometers. Hypertension. 1993;21(4):504–9.
21. O'Brien E, Petrie J, Littler W, et al. An outline of the revised British Hypertension Society protocol for the evaluation of blood pressure measuring devices. J Hypertens. 1993;11(6):677–9.
22. O'Brien E, Pickering T, Asmar R, et al. Working Group on Blood Pressure Monitoring of the European Society of Hypertension International Protocol for validation of blood pressure measuring devices in adults. Blood Press Monit. 2002;7(1):3–17.
23. Campbell NR, McKay DW. Do we need another protocol for assessing the validity of blood pressure measuring devices? Blood Press Monit. 2002;7(1):1–2.
24. O'Brien E, Atkins N, Stergiou G, Karpettas N, Parati G, Asmar R, Working Group on Blood Pressure Monitoring of the European Society of Hypertension, et al. European Society of Hypertension International Protocol revision 2010 for the validation of blood pressure measuring devices in adults. Blood Press Monit. 2010;15:23–38.
25. O'Brien E, et al. European Society of Hypertension International Protocol revision 2010 for the validation of blood pressure measuring devices. Blood Press Monit. 2010;15(1):23–38.
26. Stergiou GS, Karpettas N, Atkins N, O'Brien E. Impact of applying the more stringent validation criteria of the revised European Society of Hypertension International Protocol 2010 on earlier validation studies. Blood Press Monit. 2011;16:67–73.
27. Hodgkinson JA, Sheppard JP, Heneghan C, Martin U, Mant J, Roberts N, Mcmanus RJ. Accuracy of ambulatory blood pressure monitors: a systematic review of validation studies. J Hypertens. 2013;31:239–50.
28. Pickering T. Recommendations for the use of home (self) and ambulatory blood pressure monitoring. American Society of Hypertension Ad Hoc Panel. Am J Hypertens. 1996;9(1):1–11.
29. Kikuya M, Hozawa A, Ohokubo T, Tsuji I, Michimata M, Matsubara M, et al. Prognostic significance of blood pressure and heart rate variabilities: the Ohasama study. Hypertension. 2000;36.
30. Parati G, Pomidossi G, Albini F, Malaspina D, Mancia G. Relationship of 24-hour blood pressure mean and variability to severity of target-organ damage in hypertension. J Hypertens. 1987;5(1):93–8.
31. Frattola A, Parati G, Cuspidi C, Albini F, Mancia G. Prognostic value of 24-hour blood pressure variability. J Hypertens. 1993;11(10):1133–7.
32. White WB, Dey HM, Schulman P. Assessment of the daily blood pressure load as a determinant of cardiac function in patients with mild-to-moderate hypertension. Am Heart J. 1989; 118(4):782–95.
33. White WB. Accuracy and analysis of ambulatory blood pressure monitoring data. Clin Cardiol. 1992;15(5 Suppl 2):II10–3.

34. Mule G, Nardi E, Andronico G, et al. Relationships between 24 h blood pressure load and target organ damage in patients with mild-to-moderate essential hypertension. Blood Press Monit. 2001;6(3):115–23.
35. Gorostidi M, Vinyoles E, Banegas JR, Sierra A. Prevalence of white-coat and masked hypertension in national and international registries. Hypertens Res. 2015;38:1–7.
36. Sipahioglu NT, Sipahioglu F. A closer look at white-coat hypertension. World J Methodol. 2014;4(3):144–50.
37. Cuspidi C, Rescaldani M, Tadic M, Sala C, Grassi G, Mancia G. White-coat hypertension, as defined by ambulatory blood pressure monitoring, and subclinical cardiac organ damage: a meta-analysis. J Hypertens. 2014;32:24–32.
38. Mancia G, De Backer G, Dominiczak A, Cifkova R, Fargard R, Germano G, et al. Management of Arterial Hypertension of the European Society of Hypertension; European Society of Cardiology: the Task Force for the Management of Arterial Hypertension (ESH) and of the European Society of Cardiology (ESC). J Hypertens. 2007;25.
39. Chobanian AV, Bakris GL, Black HR, et al. The Seventh Report of the Joint National Committee on Prevention, Detection, Evaluation, and Treatment of High Blood Pressure: the JNC 7 report. JAMA. 2003;289(19):2560–72.
40. James GD, Pickering TG, Yee LS, Harshfield GA, Riva S, Laragh JH. The reproducibility of average ambulatory, home, and clinic pressures. Hypertension. 1988;11(6 Pt 1):545–9.
41. Fotherby MD, Potter JF. Reproducibility of ambulatory and clinic blood pressure measurements in elderly hypertensive subjects. J Hypertens. 1993;11(5):573–9.
42. Staessen JA, Thijs L, Clement D, et al. Ambulatory pressure decreases on longterm placebo treatment in older patients with isolated systolic hypertension. J Hypertens. 1994;12(9): 1035–9.
43. Palatini P, Mormino P, Canali C, et al. Factors affecting ambulatory blood pressure reproducibility. Results of the HARVEST Trial. Hypertension and Ambulatory Recording Venetia Study. Hypertension. 1994;23(2):211–6.
44. Mansoor GA, McCabe EJ, White WB. Long-term reproducibility of ambulatory blood pressure. J Hypertens. 1994;12(6):703–8.
45. Mochizuki Y, Okutani M, Donfeng Y, et al. Limited reproducibility of circadian variation in blood pressure dippers and nondippers. Am J Hypertens. 1998;11(4 Pt 1):403–9.
46. Tamura K, Mukaiyama S, Halberg F. Clinical significance of ABPM monitoring for 48h rather than 24h. Statistician. 1990;39:301–6.
47. Parati F, et al. European Society of Hypertension practice guidelines for ambulatory blood pressure monitoring. J Hypertens. 2014;32(7):1359–66.
48. Krause T, Lovibond K, Caulfield M, McCormack T, Williams B. Management of hypertension: summary of NICE guidance. BMJ. 2011;343.
49. Piper MA, Evans CV, Burda BU, Margolis KL, O'Connor E, Whitlock EP. Diagnostic and predictive accuracy of blood pressure screening methods with consideration of rescreening intervals: an updated systematic review for the U.S. Preventative Services Task Force. Ann Intern Med. 2014;162(3):192–204. doi:10.7326/M14-1539.
50. Pickering TG, James GD, Boddie C, Harshfield GA, Blank S, Laragh JH. How common is white coat hypertension? JAMA. 1988;259(2):225–8.
51. Verdecchia P, Porcellati C, Schillaci G, et al. Ambulatory blood pressure. An independent predictor of prognosis in essential hypertension. Hypertension. 1994;24(6):793–801.
52. Verdecchia P, Schillaci G, Borgioni C, Ciucci A, Porcellati C. White-coat hypertension. Lancet. 1996;348(9039):1444–6.
53. Palatini P, Mormino P, Santonastaso M, et al. Target-organ damage in stage I hypertensive subjects with white coat and sustained hypertension: results from the HARVEST study. Hypertension. 1998;31(1):57–63.
54. Sega R, Trocino G, Lanzarotti A, et al. Alterations of cardiac structure in patients with isolated office, ambulatory, or home hypertension: data from the general population (Pressione Arteriose Monitorate E Loro Associazioni (PAMELA) Study). Circulation. 2001;104(12): 1385–92.

55. Staessen JA, Byttebier G, Buntinx F, Celis H, O'Brien ET, Fagard R. Antihypertensive treatment based on conventional or ambulatory blood pressure measurement. A randomized controlled trial. Ambulatory Blood Pressure Monitoring and Treatment of Hypertension Investigators. JAMA. 1997;278(13):1065–72.
56. Mezzetti A, Pierdomenico SD, Costantini F, et al. White-coat resistant hypertension. Am J Hypertens. 1997;10(11):1302–7.
57. Muxfeldt ES, Bloch KV, Nogueira AR, Salles GF. Twenty-four hour ambulatory blood pressure monitoring pattern of resistant hypertension. Blood Press Monit. 2003;8(5):181–5.
58. Pierdomenico SD, Lapenna D, Bucci A, et al. Cardiovascular outcome in treated hypertensive patients with responder, masked, false resistant, and true resistant hypertension. Am J Hypertens. 2005;18(11):1422–8.
59. Redon J, Campos C, Narciso ML, Rodicio JL, Pascual JM, Ruilope LM. Prognostic value of ambulatory blood pressure monitoring in refractory hypertension: a prospective study. Hypertension. 1998;31(2):712–8.
60. Gosse P, Ansoborlo P, Lemetayer P, Clementy J. Left ventricular mass is better correlated with arising blood pressure than with office or occasional blood pressure. Am J Hypertens. 1997; 10(5 Pt 1):505–10.
61. Kario K, Pickering TG, Umeda Y, et al. Morning surge in blood pressure as a predictor of silent and clinical cerebrovascular disease in elderly hypertensives: a prospective study. Circulation. 2003;107(10):1401–6.
62. Kent ST, Shimbo D, Huang L, Diaz KM, Viera AJ, Kilgore M, Oparil S, Muntner P. Rates, amounts, and determinants of ambulatory blood pressure monitor claim reimbursement among Medicare beneficiaries. Am Soc Hypertens. 2014;8(12):898–908.
63. Moser M. Hypertension can be treated effectively without increasing the cost of care. J Hum Hypertens. 1996;10 Suppl 2:533–58.
64. Yarows SA, Khoury S, Sowers JR. Cost effectiveness of 24-hour ambulatory blood pressure monitoring in evaluation and treatment of essential hypertension. Am J Hypertens. 1994; 7(5):464–8.
65. Khoury S, Yarows SA, O'Brien TK, Sowers JR. Ambulatory blood pressure monitoring in a nonacademic setting. Effects of age and sex. Am J Hypertens. 1992;5(9):616–23.
66. Krakoff LR. Cost-effectiveness of ambulatory blood pressure: a reanalysis. Hypertension. 2006;47(1):29–34.
67. Pessanha P, Viana M, Ferreira P, Bertoquini S, Polonia J. Diagnostic value and cost-benefit analysis of 24 hours ambulatory blood pressure monitoring in primary care in Portugal. BMC Cardiovascular Disord. 2013;13:57.

Chapter 5
Validation and Reliability Testing of Blood Pressure Monitors

Neil Atkins and Eoin O'Brien

Introduction

Though the importance of checking the accuracy of blood pressure measurement techniques was recognised when it was introduced in the early years of the twentieth century [1], it was largely ignored until the 1980s, when observational concerns about the London School of Hygiene sphygmomanometer, developed to remove measurement bias in scientific studies, led to a validation which proved its inaccuracy [2]. Similar concerns were later demonstrated that another device, also developed as a gold standard for research—the Hawksley Random Zero Sphygmomanometer, was also inaccurate [3]. At that time, there was no standardised protocol for the evaluation of blood pressure measuring devices. Obvious discrepancies between clinic measurements and automatic measurements in the early years of electronic devices led to validation studies using ad-hoc protocols [4–6], but with the dawn of electronic measurement and the advent of 24-h ambulatory blood pressure measurement (ABPM), the need for a standardised protocol became compelling [7].

N. Atkins
Medaval Ltd., 28-32 Upper Pembroke Street, Dublin 2, Ireland

E. O'Brien, M.D. (✉)
The Conway Institute, University College Dublin, Dublin, Ireland
e-mail: proeobrien@icloud.com

© Springer International Publishing Switzerland 2016
W.B. White (ed.), *Blood Pressure Monitoring in Cardiovascular Medicine and Therapeutics*, Clinical Hypertension and Vascular Diseases,
DOI 10.1007/978-3-319-22771-9_5

Validation Protocols

AAMI/ISO Standards

Standardised protocols for the validation of the accuracy of blood pressure monitors were first introduced in 1987 when the Association for the Advancement of Medical Instrumentation (AAMI) published a standard for electronic and aneroid sphygmomanometers that included a protocol for the evaluation of device accuracy [8]. This protocol required the mean systolic and diastolic measurements of three measurements on the test devices to be compared against simultaneous measurements recorded using standard mercury sphygmomanometer on each of 85 subjects. If the mean difference, from the 85 subjects, was no more than 5 mmHg and the standard deviation was no more than 8 mmHg, then the device was deemed accurate.

The protocol was revised in 1992 (published 1993 and amended 1996) [9, 10]. In this revision, the accuracy was based on the differences of all 255 measurements. This effectively made the standard deviation requirements more stringent. The option of using the test and control measurements sequentially was also introduced.

The AAMI standard was revised again in 2002 (published 2003), 2007, 2009 and 2013 [11–14]. The 2002 revision introduced a second passing criterion based on the mean measurements from 85 subjects, but standard deviations based on the mean pressure ensure that the average error in at least 85 % of the subjects is at most 10 mmHg. Since 2007, the AAMI standard has been adopted by the International Standards Organization (ISO).

BHS Protocols

In 1990, the British Hypertension Society (BHS) published a protocol devoted solely to the validation of devices in the clinical setting [15]. While basing sample requirements on the rationale of the 1987 AAMI protocol, it was also based on evidence from validations carried out for Which? consumer magazine [5, 6] and from research into the comparison of simultaneous and sequential measurements both in the same arm and in opposite arms [16]. It consisted of five phases—observer training, before-use inter-device variability, in-use (field) assessment, after-use inter-device variability and device validation. The protocol recommended sequential same-arm comparisons in order to remove bias due to insufficient inflation or deflation by the test device. Passing requirements were based on the percentage of measurements falling within 5 mmHg, 10 mmHg and 15 mmHg of the control device and with A and B pass grades and C and D fail grades.

The BHS protocol was revised in 1993 [17]. This revision introduced a period of device usage prior to validation, so that validation was not performed on brand new devices. It also consisted of five phases—before-use device calibration, in-use (field) assessment, after-use device calibration, static device validation and report of evaluation. It was the first time a calibration procedure for sphygmomanometers was defined carefully with a specific procedure and pressures. Recruitment requirements were tightly defined over five ranges for both systolic and diastolic pressures (<90, 90–129, 130–160, 161–180 and >180 mmHg for SBP and <60, 60–79, 80–100, 101–110 and >110 mmHg for DBP). The criteria for analysing sequential-measurement differences and the passing criteria were amended and the report required separate analysis of performance in low, medium and high pressure ranges. Descriptions of follow-up validations, for devices that achieved an A or B grade, in special circumstances, namely pregnant women, elderly subjects, paediatric subjects and during exercise, were included.

Importantly, the 1993 BHS protocol included an appendix describing the methodology for observer training that was based on previous work [18] and a video method of recording was introduced [19].

International Protocols of the ESH

In 2002, the Working Group on Blood Pressure Monitoring of the ESH published a protocol, updated from the BHS protocol, named the International Protocol (ESH-IP) [20]. The Working Group had the advantage of being able to examine and analyse the data from 19 validation studies performed according to the earlier protocols at the Blood Pressure Unit in Dublin [21]. While a large number of BP measuring devices were evaluated according to one or both of the AAMI and BHS protocols, experience demonstrated that the conditions demanded for validation were extremely difficult to fulfil because of the large number of individuals that needed to be recruited and the ranges of BP required [22]. Recruitment in very high ranges of pressure became increasingly difficult due to advances in treatment and, as adults in the low, normal and hypotensive ranges were not to be referred to hypertension centres, these also became very difficult to recruit. These factors made validation studies difficult to perform and very costly, with the result that fewer centres were prepared to undertake them. Technological improvements, both in reliability (time to failure), device size and device use, also meant that the in-use phase, as described, was insufficient to highlight device failure [22].

The main change in this protocol was the reduction in the number of subjects required to 33, 11 of whom had to be recruited from three SBP and three DBP ranges. This was based on the re-analysis of data gathered from validations studies using the BHS protocol. The ABCD grading system, used in the BHS protocol, was abandoned, as it had effectively been a Pass (AB)—Fail (CD) system anyway, but the pass requirements introduced a subject-based requirement to ensure that errors were distributed by chance, rather than by subject, which had been defined as a weakness of earlier protocols by Gerin et al. [23]. The validation procedure was confined to adults over the age of 30 years. A procedure of stopping, after 45 subjects, in the case of "hopeless" devices was introduced. Validation in special groups, as defined in the BHS 1993 protocol, was not defined.

In 2010, the ESH International Protocol was revised [24], based on the evidence and experience acquired from 104 validation studies conducted using the 2002 protocol [25]. The main purpose of this revision was to require more stringent accuracy requirements. The accuracy requirements of both the BHS and ESH protocols had been a compromise of technological ability and problems, such as terminal digit preference, in the use of manual sphygmomanometers [26]. Advances in technology therefore demanded that these be revised. Experience with the 2002 ESH-IP showed that, in many studies, recruitment pressures were not reflected in the distribution of control measurements and, therefore, measures were included to ensure that these were not statistically significantly different. The early termination of the study for "hopeless" devices was removed, as no study availed of this; the age requirement was changed to 25 years and a small relaxation in recruitment requirements was coupled with the introduction of minimum overall SBP and DBP ranges. Strict reporting requirements were also introduced in order to minimise the number of protocol violations that had been an on-going problem.

A review assessed the impact the more stringent criteria of the revised ESH International Protocol 2010 would have had on the previous studies that had used the ESH International Protocol 2002. If the devices validated according to the earlier protocol [20] had been validated according to the 2010 revision of the ESH International Protocol [24], the failure rate would have increased markedly from 17 to 42 % [27].

Protocol Use

In an analysis of validations carried out prior to the publication of the revised ESH-IP protocol in 2010 [24], it was noted that, in relation to the 2002 ESH-IP protocol [20], there was "an impressive increase in the publication of validation studies conducted using this protocol", while "the use of the BHS [17] and the AAMI [10–12] protocols remained rather static" [25]. Since 2007, more than twice as many validations were carried out using this protocol than the other protocols put together (Table 5.1 and Fig. 5.1).

In its introduction, the 2002 ESH-IP protocol included the sentence "It is anticipated that the relative ease of performance of the International Protocol will encourage manufacturers to submit blood pressure measuring devices for validation in order to obtain the minimum approval necessary for a device to be used in clinical medicine, and that, in time, most devices on the market will be assessed according to the protocol for basic accuracy". The figures demonstrate that while the goal of having "most devices on the market" validated has still some way to go, the protocol did encourage manufacturers to submit devices for validation.

The analysis demonstrates the importance of practicality in the development of protocols. Protocols that are difficult and onerous to complete are less attractive both to centres and to manufacturers. Furthermore, they are rarely carried out correctly. Ideal evaluation is therefore best achieved, and perhaps can only be achieved, by a set of simple validations rather than by a single complex one.

Table 5.1 Number of validation studies according to the ESH-IP, the BHS, and the AAMI protocol reported per year starting from 2000 (2 years before the ESH-IP publication) until June 2009. *Adapted from Stergiou* et al. [25]

Year	BHS (only)	BHS + AAMI	AAMI (only)	BHS (all)	AAMI (all)	ESH-IP	Total
2000	2 (20 %)	4 (40 %)	0 (0 %)	6 (60 %)	4 (40 %)	—	10
2001	1 (8 %)	5 (42 %)	1 (8 %)	6 (50 %)	6 (50 %)	—	12
2002	4 (29 %)	3 (21 %)	1 (7 %)	7 (50 %)	4 (29 %)	3 (21 %)	14
2003	2 (13 %)	0 (0 %)	6 (38 %)	2 (13 %)	6 (38 %)	8 (50 %)	16
2004	1 (6 %)	5 (29 %)	1 (6 %)	7 (41 %)	6 (35 %)	4 (24 %)	17
2005	2 (12 %)	4 (24 %)	0 (0 %)	6 (35 %)	4 (24 %)	7 (41 %)	17
2006	4 (13 %)	5 (17 %)	1 (3 %)	9 (30 %)	6 (20 %)	15 (50 %)	30
2007	1 (3 %)	2 (6 %)	3 (9 %)	3 (9 %)	5 (16 %)	24 (75 %)	32
2008	3 (9 %)	2 (6 %)	1 (3 %)	6 (17 %)	4 (11 %)	25 (71 %)	35
2009[a]	4 (14 %)	3 (10 %)	0 (0 %)	8 (28 %)	3 (10 %)	18 (62 %)	29
2002–2009[a]	21 (11 %)	24 (13 %)	13 (7 %)	48 (25 %)	38 (20 %)	104 (55 %)	190

AAMI Association for the Advancement of Medical Instrumentation, *BHS* British Hypertension Society, *ESH-IP* European Society of Hypertension International Protocol
[a]Until 15/06/2009

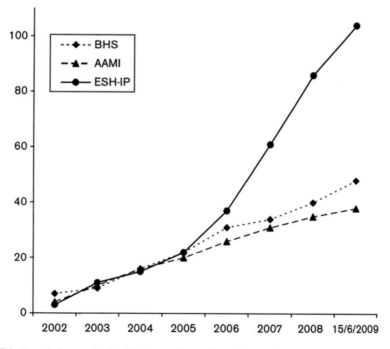

Fig. 5.1 Cumulative graph of validation studies performed according to the European Society of Hypertension International Protocol (ESH-IP) compared with the British Hypertension Society (BHS) and Association for the Advancement of Medical Instrumentation (AAMI) protocols from 2002 (publication of ESH-IP) until June 2009. *Reproduced from Stergiou et al.* [25] *with permission from the authors*

Differences Between Protocols

At present, the ESH-IP validation protocol is the most widely used, followed by the AAMI/ANSI/ISO standard. There are some substantial differences between these validation procedures, as described below and shown in Table 5.2. A detailed comparison has also been made by Ng [28]. Nevertheless, they both have a common objective, namely the standardisation of validation procedures to establish minimum standards of accuracy and performance, and to facilitate comparison of one device with another. With the substantial data available, it is perhaps timely that a common protocol be developed that will become a world standard.

Passing Requirements

The AAMI/ISO standard requires two criteria to be fulfilled. In Criterion 1, the mean error of at least 255 measurements must be at most 5 mmHg with a standard deviation of at most 8 mmHg. In Criterion 2, the mean error of the mean measurements from at least 85 subjects must be at most 5 mmHg and the standard deviation at most a value to ensure that the mean error on at least 85 % of subjects is within 10 mmHg. (By extension, this definition also means that the expected number of subjects with average errors within the more commonly accepted error of 5 mmHg is around 50 %.) A table, showing the acceptable standard deviations for ranges of mean errors, is provided. For ABPM devices, similar criteria must also be applied to a further raised-heartrates test.

The ESH-IP protocol provides two sets of cut-off points. The primary set is for at least 73/99 measurement errors to be within 5 mmHg, at least 87/99 to be within 10 mmHg and at least 96/99 to be within 15 mmHg. The secondary set is for at least 65/99 measurement errors to be within 5 mmHg, at least 81/99 to be within 10 mmHg and at least 95/99 to be within 15 mmHg. Devices must fulfil at least two of the primary set and all of the secondary set. In addition, in at least 24/33 subjects, the errors in at least two of the three measurements recorded must be no more than 5 mmHg and there can be no more than 3/33 subjects with errors over 5 mmHg in all three measurements.

Methodology

The AAMI/ANSI/ISO standard allows simultaneous same-arm comparisons if the test device inflates to at least 20 mmHg above SBP and deflates to at least 20 mmHg below DBP at a rate of between 2 and 3 mmHg/s. Otherwise, sequential same-arm comparisons or simultaneous opposite-arm comparisons must be used. The ESH-IP protocol stipulates sequential same-arm comparisons in all circumstances.

Table 5.2 Comparison of ESH-IP 2010 [24] and AAMI/ANSI/ISO 81060-2:2013 [14] requirements for noninvasive validation of blood pressure devices

Protocol provision			ESH-IP 2010	AAMI/ANSI/ISO 81060-2:2013	
Sample demographics					
Sample size			33	85+	
Age			≥25 years	Adult and adolescent	>12 years
				Adult, adolescent, and children	35 subjects 3–12 years and
					50+ subjects >25 years
Sex			≥10 Male and ≥10 Female	≥30 % Male and ≥30 % Female	
Arm circumference	1 cuff		No requirements	≥40 % upper ½, ≥40 % lower ½,	
				≥20 % upper ¼, ≥20 % lower ¼	
	n cuffs, n > 1			≥1/2n subjects/cuff	
Methodology					
Sequential same arm			7 alternating measurements (4 observer, 3 test device)	7 alternating measurements (4 observer, 3 test device)	
			Control measurement is the nearer on the preceding and succeeding mean observer measurements to test measurement	Control measurement is average of 4 values (preceding and succeeding measurements of each observer)	
				Exclude measurement if observer measurements differ by >12 mmHg SBP or >8 mmHg DBP from other 2 measurements. (Max. 10 % of subjects; exclude subject if >10 %)	
Simultaneous same arm			Not permitted	Test device: Inflates ≥SBP+20 mmHg, deflates ≤DBP−20 mmHg, deflation rate 2 mmHg/s to 3 mmHg/s	
				3 Pairs of measurements	
				Control measurement is mean observer measurement	
				Exclude subject if observer measurements differ by >12 mmHg SBP or >8 mmHg DBP	

(continued)

Table 5.2 (continued)

Protocol provision	ESH-IP 2010	AAMI/ANSI/ISO 81060-2:2013
Simultaneous opposite arm	Not permitted	3 Pairs of measurements with test device on left arm +3 pairs with test device on right arm
		Control measurement is mean observer measurement with lateral arm difference adjustment
		Exclude subject if observer measurements on same arm differ by >12 mmHg SBP or >8 mmHg DBP of if lateral difference >15 mmHg SBP or >10 mmHg DBP

Recruitment blood pressure

SBP	90–100 mmHg[a]	10–12	≥1
	101–129 mmHg	10–12	Initial pressures are recorded on each subject but they are not used in any calculations. Blood pressure distribution requirements are based on the reference control measurements only
	130–160 mmHg	10–12	
	161–169 mmHg	10–12	
	170–180 mmHg[a]		≥1
DBP	40–50 mmHg[a]	10–12	≥1
	51–79 mmHg	10–12	
	80–100 mmHg	10–12	
	101–119 mmHg	10–12	
	120–130 mmHg[a]		≥1

Control BP distribution

SBP	≤100 mmHg	22/99–44/99	Max. difference ≤19/99 ≥5 % (13/255)
	101–129 mmHg		≤75 % (191/255)
	130–139 mmHg	22/99–44/99	
	140–159 mmHg		≥20 % (51/255)
	160 mmHg		
	>160 mmHg	22/99–44/99	≥5 % (13/255)

DBP				
≤60 mmHg	22/99–44/99	Max. difference ≤19/99		≥5 %
61–79 mmHg				≤75 %
80–84 mmHg	22/99–44/99			
85–99 mmHg				≥20 %
100 mmHg				
>100 mmHg	22/99–44/99			≥5 %

Passing requirements (SBP and DBP)

ESH-IP

Part 1 based on individual measurement errors

No. of errors	≤5 mmHg	≤10 mmHg	≤15 mmHg
≥2 of	≥73/99	≥87/99	≥96/99
All of	≥65/99	≥81/99	≥95/99

Part 2 based on measurement errors per subject

No. of subjects	≥2/3 errors	0/3 errors
	≤5 mmHg	≤5 mmHg
Both	≥24/33	≤3/33

81060-2:2013

Criterion 1 based on individual measurement errors

For comparison with ESH-IP, expected error rates within bands are shown when the mean error is 5 mmHg ±8 mmHg

	≤5 mmHg	≤10 mmHg	≤15 mmHg
Mean error (255 measurements)			
5 mmHg	39.3 %	70.1 %	88.5 %

Max. SD			
8 mmHg			

Criterion 2 based on mean subject errors such that, using the normal distribution, the probability of a mean subject error being within 10 mmHg is ≥0.85. Selected examples shown

Probability of mean subject error within bands, based on normal distribution

Sample mean error and SD combinations that satisfy criteria

Mean error (85 subject mean BPs)	Max. SD	≤5 mmHg	≤10 mmHg	≤15 mmHg
0 mmHg	6.95 mmHg	0.528	0.850	0.969
1 mmHg	6.87 mmHg	0.529	0.850	0.969
2 mmHg	6.65 mmHg	0.528	0.850	0.969
3 mmHg	6.25 mmHg	0.525	0.850	0.971
4 mmHg	5.64 mmHg	0.515	0.850	0.974
5 mmHg	4.79 mmHg	0.482	0.851	0.982

Special circumstances — No requirements

Exercise — Supplementary study using 35 subjects

[a] Maximum of four instances in total with SBP<90 mmHg, SBP>180 mmHg, DBP<40 mmHg or DBP>130 mmHg

Recruitment Requirements

For Criterion 1, the AAMI/ISO standard requires 255 measurements to be recorded in at least 85 subjects, with at most three measurements per subject. For Criterion 2, 85 subjects with at least three measurements per subject are required. This number of measurements per subject is doubled if the simultaneous opposite-arm methodology is used, with each arm being used for half the control and test measurements. For ABPM devices, a further 35 subjects are required for a validation with raised heartrates following exercise.

The ESH-IP protocol requires three measurements to be recorded in each of 33 subjects. However, strict requirements generally necessitate several more subjects to be recruited in order for these to be satisfied.

Pressure-Range Requirements

The ESH-IP protocol requires between 10 and 12 subjects with SBP in the ranges <130, 130–160 and >160 mmHg; between 10 and 12 subjects with DBP in the ranges <80, 80–100 and >100 mmHg; a total of at most for subjects with pressures outside the "ideal" range of 90–180 mmHg for SBP and 40–130 mmHg for DBP and minimum ranges of 100–170 mmHg for SBP and 50–120 mmHg for DBP. In addition, the 99 control measurements must not be statistically different from the ideal 33 measurements in each range; that is each range must contain 22 and 44 measurements and the difference between the range with the highest count and that with the lowest count cannot exceed 19.

The AAMI/ISO standard requires at least 5 % (13 measurements, requiring at least five subjects) of reference systolic blood pressures have to be at least 160 mmHg, at least 20 % (51 measurements, requiring at least 17 subjects) at least 140 mmHg and at least 5 % at most 100 mmHg. Similarly, at least 5 % of reference diastolic blood pressures have to be at least 100 mmHg, at least 20 % at least 85 mmHg and at least 5 % at most 60 mmHg.

Age Distribution Requirements

The ESH-IP protocol requires all subjects to be at least 25 years of age. The AAMI/ISO standard defines two types of studies based on age. The first is for an adult/adolescent population defined simply as on persons over the age of 12. The alternative population is a combined adult/paediatric population where 35 subjects must be between the ages of 3 and 12; the remainder (minimum 50) must be over the age of 12.

Sex Distribution Requirements

Both the ESH-IP protocol and the AAMI/ISO standard are at ad idem requiring a minimum of 30 % (stated as 10/33 in the ESH-IP protocol) male and 30 % female subjects.

Arm Circumference and Cuff Requirements

The ESH-IP protocol does not specify requirements for arm circumference distribution. The appropriate cuff, as defined by the manufacturer for the respective arm circumference, must be used.

In the AAMI/ISO standard, where the device has a single cuff, at least 40 % (minimum 34) of arm circumferences must be in the upper half of the cuff range with 20 % (minimum 17) in the uppermost quarter of the cuff range and at least 40 % must be in the lower half of the cuff range with 20 % in the lowest quarter of the cuff range. Where "n" cuffs are supplied ($n > 1$), each must be tested in at least $1/2n$ subjects.

Intra-subject Blood Pressure Variability

In the AAMI/ANSI/ISO standard, comparisons, where control determinations differ by more than 12 mmHg SBP or 8 mmHg DBP, are excluded. Where simultaneous comparisons are used, all measurements from the relevant subjects are excluded. Where sequential same-arm comparisons are used, a single pair of measurements can be excluded in up to 10 % of subjects, with extra subjects being added to make up the 255 measurements. Where simultaneous opposite-arm comparisons are used, subjects are also excluded if their lateral difference is more than 15 mmHg SBP or 10 mmHg DBP.

No determinations are excluded using the ESH-IP protocol. Allowance for high variability, based on the analysis of data from previous studies, is included in the passing criteria.

Control Pressures

In both the AAMI/ISO standard and the ESH-IP protocol, the mean observer pressures, where they differ by no more than 4 mmHg, are used as control measurements and are retaken if they differ by more than 4 mmHg.

In the ESH-IP protocol, the nearer control measurement (of those taken either side of the test measurement) to the test measurement is used.

In the AAMI/ISO standard, the control measurement used is dependent on the method used. For simultaneous same arm comparisons, there is just one control measurement. For sequential same-arm comparisons, the mean of the control measurements taken either side of the test measurement is used. For simultaneous opposite-arm comparisons, the control measurements are used but, in calculating the errors, a lateral difference (the mean left-arm control measurement subtracted from the mean right-arm control measurements) is added to the left arm measurements.

Validation in Special Groups

The AAMI/ISO protocol describes procedures for supplementary validations where a device is intended to be used in an exercise stress-testing environment, in neonatal and infant populations or in pregnant (including pre-eclamptic) patient populations.

Sphygmomanometers have been validated in pregnancy (including normotensive pregnancy, non-proteinuric hypertension in pregnancy and pre-eclampsia), children, children and adolescence, the elderly, the obese, Black women, in the supine position, before, during and after haemodialysis, in end-stage renal disease, and in Parkinson's disease [29].

Where a device is intended for use in a specific population, it should be validated in that population. Devices intended for clinical use should be validated in at least three special-group populations. Validation protocols should provide clear instructions on validation in these groups.

Validation in subjects with arrhythmias continues to be elusive and research is needed to establish a reliable and effective method to solve this ongoing problem.

Device Equivalence

Manufacturers of blood pressure measuring devices that have been previously validated successfully for accuracy may make modifications to a device, which do not affect its measurement accuracy and should not require further validation [30]. These "modifications" tend to fall into three categories: (1) Manufacturers provide a "family" of devices around the same measuring technology, differing only in the "extras" provided; (2) Manufacturers produce a device in different languages; (3) OEM manufacturers provide devices to several OBL manufacturers using the same measuring technology.

Equivalence is a scientific comparison of an applicant device against a device which has undergone, and passed, a formal validation. All features are compared. Critical features, upon which measurement is dependent, should not differ and include: the algorithm for oscillometric measurements, the algorithm for auscultatory measurements, artefact and error detection, microphones, the pressure transducer, the cuff and bladder, the inflation mechanism and the deflation mechanism.

Differences are permitted in items not critical to blood pressure measurement, which include: the model name and number, the device casing, the display layout, any carrying or mounting facilities, software other than the pressure detection algorithm, memory capacity and the number of stored measurements, printing facilities, communication facilities and power supply.

Manufacturers are obliged to provide sufficient evidence to prove equivalence.

Since the procedure was first described in 2006, there have been regularity changes that have had an impact on how the procedure must be performed. In particular, IEC 80601-2-30:2009 requires that all devices include rated pressure ranges and technical alarm conditions (measurements outside the rated range that are deemed technical errors). This ruling does not affect algorithms relating to the detection of blood pressure, but it does impact how the detected pressures are treated, as those that outside the rated range must be treated as error readings. Therefore, it is essential that these conditions are considered in equivalence checks.

It is necessary to record that some equivalence procedures performed by the dabl Educational Trust have recently approved devices in which there may have been differences in pressure transducers and/or cuffs, [29] whereas it is an essential requirement of the equivalence process that the transducers or cuffs are themselves proved to be equivalent.

Validation Quality

In a critical review of 69 studies carried out using the ESH-IP 2002 protocol [20], 23 (33.3 %) were found to have protocol violations, with eight (11.6 %) of these having major violations [25]. Given that ease of compliance was a major consideration in the design of this protocol, it is reasonable to hypothesise that validations according to other protocols contain at least the same rate of violations. Indeed, it is not hard to find validations according to AAMI/ISO protocols not showing Criterion 2 results. Validations according to the BHS protocol rarely carry out the first three phases and recruitment violations are common.

This raises serious questions about the quality of peer review of validation studies. In theory, these reviews should be straightforward, essentially ensuring that the studies follow a checklist of requirements. The approval of devices where the protocol has not been followed or where there is inadequate detail is incorrect. Where details are omitted, it is not possible to know whether this was inadvertent or deliberate. This leads to further problems if the papers are not recognised subsequently as sufficient evidence of accuracy.

One of the difficulties in ensuring compliance is the concept that "minor violations" are acceptable. For instance, in the ESH-IP 2010 protocol, a fifth subject outside the ideal range or a maximum or minimum pressure requirement being shy of the mark. The problem is that protocols already include the statistically allowable deviations and, while in certain circumstances, minor violations might not affect the results, in others they will. Therefore, they are often "justified by the results". The corollary of this is that the violation will only be corrected if they cannot be "justified by the results". This, of course, is simply a form of bias.

The ESH-IP 2010 protocol [24] provides for strict requirements and reporting. Many of the studies have carried out using the dabl Educational Trust ESH-IP 2010 Online Service [29], which guarantees protocol adherence. Future protocols should provide a strict report format or checklist and, perhaps, this should be supplied along with papers when being sent for peer review.

Validation Centres

In 2010, Turner highlighted a major weakness of the current validation process, namely reliance on peer-reviewed publications alone without formal certification of the centres performing validation studies, as is common practice with other measurement systems [31]. He called for formal accreditation of laboratories. The process would be overseen by independent agencies, such as the United Kingdom Accreditation Service, a not-for-profit organisation funded by accredited laboratories, which is answerable to the International Bureau of Weights and Measures in Paris, France, the peak laboratory in the international measurement framework of cooperating national and commercial laboratories that provide reference standards and traceable calibration for all scientific, industrial and trade measurements worldwide.

In 2010, O'Brien and Stergiou, in an article entitled 'Who will bell the cat?' noted that "This process of accreditation is complex and presumably costly. The technicians, nurses and doctors involved in validation must receive specialised training; the test measurement system must be calibrated traceably, according to an international standard [32]; the laboratory must be shown to operate a quality system conforming to international standards [33] and accredited laboratories would be required to participate in inter-laboratory comparisons." These authors went on: "The process detailed by Turner raises important questions that need to be considered carefully. Will the proposed accreditation process lead to more BP measuring devices being validated or could it have the effect of making the accreditation of validation laboratories so unworkable and expensive as to be counter-productive? How can the process be implemented taking into consideration the fact that BP device validation studies have previously been considered akin to research projects that have been conducted on a voluntary basis? How much will the proposed process add to the cost of device validation and who will pay?" [22].

The BHS has established a system for training and for accrediting laboratories for device validation by ensuring that certain minimum criteria apply [34].

The issues raised by Turner need to be considered and integrated into the device validation procedure. A creditable accreditation procedure is fundamental to ensuring confidence in the quality of validation studies. Ideally, there should be no direct links between validation centres and manufacturers. Direct employment of investigators by manufacturers introduces an unhealthy relationship whereby investigators may be reluctant to fail a device, or to allow the results of failures to be published, for fear of loss of future business.

Manufacturers requiring validation on a device should approach an independent authority who would allocate the validation to an accredited centre that would remain blind to the manufacturer until the study was completed. If a device was already on the market, the independent authority would always publish the results. If the device was validated prior to release, the manufacturers would be provided with the results first and, in the event the device failed, be provided with the opportunity to fix the problem and to have it validated again prior to release. Manufacturers who endeavour to produce only high-quality validated devices should not be penalised by the publication of failed validations when they do not supply those devices for use.

Practical Aspects of Validation

Blinding Process

It is critical that, in all validations, observers are blinded to each-other's readings. A method of blinding was described in relation to observer training in the 1990 BHS protocol [15], the 1993 BHS protocol [17] and the 2002 ESH-IP [20]. These descriptions, with accompanying diagrams, show the importance of separating observers by means of partitions. The descriptions in these papers refer to observer training; an adaptation of the method, for use during the validation procedure, is described in the appendix at the foot of this chapter.

The Sphygmocorder

Though the sphygmocorder was first described 20 years ago [35] and has had a number of updated descriptions incorporating changes in technology [36, 37], it never gained any popularity in device validation. The most recent version has undergone several modifications and is currently being subjected to rigorous testing. With endorsement from organisations, such as the IEEE [38], it is hoped that its use will eventually become the norm in sphygmomanometer validation.

The fundamental principal behind the sphygmocorder is the ability to record both the audio and barometric parameters during a blood pressure measurement, which enables replaying as often as required, a facility that is particularly useful with low Korotkov sounds, especially between K4 and K5. As the records can be reassessed, by independent arbitrators, bias can be effectively removed. The requirement to retake measurements due to observer differences is also removed.

Both audio and barometric waveforms can be shown visually together, thereby greatly assisting accurate measurement. The technique also ensures a complete and comprehensive record of the study.

The setting required for a study using the sphygmocorder is far simpler. As the sphygmocorder effectively replaces the observers, there is no need for the observers to be present at the time of the recording and there is no need for separate booths. In the pneumatic system, the sphygmocorder replaces all of the mercury manometers with the air-hose connected appropriately. In the auscultatory system, the diaphragm section, containing a microphone, is connected to the sphygmomanometer and headphones replace the stethoscope headsets.

Observers can review the measurements later, replaying them, as required, to ensure they are recorded accurately. Where observers differ, an independent arbitrator can also assess the measurements. Other features are also possible, such as randomising the recordings so that measurements from the same subject are separated from each other and including a random sample of the measurements twice, to reduce bias and to provide reliability and consistency checks.

The use of the sphygmocorder minimises observer error, which subsequently minimises the consideration of this error in the passing criteria which become more stringent as a consequence. This in turn can ensure that devices are validated eventually to the highest standards possible.

Manufacturer Compliance

While many manufacturers prioritise device validation in the development of new devices, there are several who make no effort at all in this regard. Regularity requirements ensuring the safety of a device can be assumed by consumers to include their validity. Validation is an expensive process adding to the cost of development and therefore on the cost of a device to consumers.

Even the term "manufacturer" is confusing and can refer to sole manufacturers, contract manufacturers, original design manufacturers, original equipment manufacturers, regulatory manufacturers, own brand labellers and even distributers. The confusion is compounded by the use of device brands and trademarks that are often difficult to distinguish from manufacturers. Own brand labellers frequently source devices from different original equipment manufacturers. Indeed, the actual maker of a device does not always appear in any of the manuals and the role of the manufacturer shown may be no more than to source devices and provide the makers with labelling decal details.

Many of these devices are sold without any validations and may have labels familiar to the target consumers and with which the consumers assume quality. It is therefore important that a manufacturer grading system is developed. This is desirable for consumers so that they are provided with evidence-based information on the devices they are considering to purchase. It is also important for compliant manufacturers that their brands are associated with approved devices.

Consumer Awareness

Availability of Information at Present

It is now expected that all information is provided on-line. It is the first and, for most, the only place consumers seek information. While other sources, such a professional recommendation, also play a factor, consumers are fully aware that these are more limited. However, on-line information also brings with it the issue of volume and dispersion.

Sites, such as www.dableducational.org [29], provide information on the accuracy of hundreds of blood pressure devices. However, information on the devices themselves must be sought elsewhere. Manufacturers provide this information, but the quality varies considerably. On-line retail sources provide pricing information, some also with details on the devices. Naturally much of this information is provided with an advertising agenda, rather than from a purely objective perspective.

While professional organisations can afford to research possible options, it is difficult, particularly for home consumers, and the amount of information can be more bewildering than informative. It is likely that many give up on this process entirely and simply seek advice from the local outlet, where the concept of whether or not a device is validated is unlikely to have penetrated.

Where a consumer seeks information about a device that has not been validated, there is no trigger to alert the consumer. There are hundreds non-validated devices available and consumers can easily spend considerable time researching devices, particularly in non-English sites, without ever coming across accuracy or validation requirements.

Requirements for On-line Information

For on-line information to be successful, and useful, there must be a single site, which provides comprehensive information on devices currently available. This must include information on the validity of each device, in particular it should state when a device has not been validated independently—this is not available anywhere at present.

The information should include a set of device features and an ability to compare a number of selected devices. The countries where the devices are available should also be provided. At the very least, consumers should be able to compare a device on sale at their local supplier on an independent site and check its validity.

Full manufacturer details for each device should be provided along with statistics, for each manufacturer, that provides information to the user on the number and percentage of its devices that are validated.

The site should be provided in languages other than English and should be written in simple sentences. This not only makes it easier to understand by all readers, but also makes it more suitable for accurate translation by on-line translation services.

Apps

Apps can provide a facility for accessing information in a manner more suitable for mobile phones. Other features can be added, such as scanning a bar code to access the information. However, there are two major drawbacks with apps. The first is that separate versions have to be written for each operating system and the second is that there are so many apps available users have become very selective in downloading only those apps that they expect to use regularly. Given that BP monitor purchase decisions are irregular events, it is unlikely that users will want to download an app. Therefore, a well-written mobile-friendly website is probably the most effective approach.

Increasing Awareness

The accuracy of blood pressure devices (and many other medical devices), which was once the responsibility of hospitals and health care professionals, is now a matter of considerable concern for home users of measuring devices and presents challenges to the medical community that have not yet been acknowledged.

There are several consumer factors to consider. Concerns of health issues in general can vary from obsession to obliviousness. Knowledge of diagnosed illnesses can range from minimal to total trust in a practitioner. Access to on-line information can range from none to efficient and, the ability to use the information supplied can vary considerably. The ability to understand information presented, both medical and technological, can be influenced by the language used and the understanding of terminology. Age and mental ability correlate strongly with all of these and, of course, location, education and financial circumstances can be confounding factors.

The quality of the information itself can be difficult to assess. Misinformation and advertising can often mislead. Different regulatory and organisational approval markings are not always clear as to what exactly is approved. Even the best scientific validation studies have an element of chance and are not always correct.

One simple method of increasing awareness is to establish a single mark of approval, showing that a device has been validated to an agreed standard that is acceptable to the main standard organisations and hypertension societies. This mark of approval can then be advertised, not only on the web but also in clinics, pharmacies and any outlet selling blood pressure monitors and on the media, particularly, for instance, on World Hypertension Day. Regardless of the complexity and diversity of the consumers, devices and information, the fundamental message of whether or not a device has been proven to be accurate can be conveyed with a simple universal mark of approval.

Device Reliability

Validation invariably occurs at the beginning of a new line of production. None of the current protocols makes any reference to reliability; in other words, for how long the device is expected to work. In essence, the validation applies indefinitely. For monitors used in the home, this is perhaps not unreasonable, as their frequency of use is likely to be low in comparison to failure tests such as required by IEC 60601-1 [39].

Technological advances tend towards disposability and devices are no longer serviced and are destined to a short shelf life, being discontinued after a relatively short time and usually without notice to consumers.

Devices used in clinic settings however, especially ABPM monitors, are often used for well over a decade. However, these generally require regular return for maintenance and calibration, which provides protection against loss of accuracy. Moreover, devices that are supplied for long periods may undergo difficulties in the acquisition of certain electronic parts that are no longer produced and alternative replacements may require software changes. Such changes are effectively device changes that are not always publicised by manufacturers. This issue was identified as far back as the 1993 BHS protocol: "When manufacturers incorporate modifications into externally identical or indistinguishable versions of a device, this should be indicated clearly by a specific device number and full details concerning how the device differs from earlier versions should be provided. In particular, the probable effect of all such modifications on the performance and accuracy of the device should be stated. Updated and modified devices must be subjected to full independent validation" [17]. Without data, it is difficult to justify or eliminate the need for re-validation or to determine when such a re-evaluation should occur.

However, it is reasonable to impose a limit on a device for equivalence purposes. Firstly, it is likely that the family of devices based on a particular technology is developed within a short time-frame, either together or in the immediate aftermath of a successful validation. Secondly, it is unlikely that the same technologies are used in new devices developed after a number of years. Thirdly, the incorporation of new technologies should be encouraged and manufacturers should not use older technologies merely to enable a device to be validated by equivalence. Nevertheless, there is a special case where devices are identical except for the branding and it clearly does not make sense to approve a device under one brand but not under another. It therefore seems reasonable to allow a device to be available for equivalence for 4 years from the date of approval of a full validation, except in the case where the applicant device is identical to the validated device, where there would be no limit.

Protocol Harmonisation

Ng identifies differences between the ISO [13] and ESH-IP [24] protocols in reference devices and methods, sample size, blood pressure levels and distribution, arm circumference and cuff sizes, procedures for recording and pairing measurements, criteria for excluding/handling subjects with high BP fluctuations, accuracy criteria and statistical methods and provisions for special populations and circumstances that need to be resolved in order to develop a harmonised protocol [28]. He also notes that provisions for monitors that require patient-specific calibration, as required by many of the newer measurement techniques, are not catered for at all in any protocol and provides reasoned analysis showing how aspects from both protocols could form the basis for harmonisation.

At present, both the differences in the protocols and in their recognition make it difficult and unnecessarily expensive for manufacturers to achieve compliance. Fundamentally, the aim of all the protocols is identical. They all include some compromise in order to balance an unworkable ideal and a practical solution.

Back in the 1980s and 1990s, there was little data available. Indeed, the concept of standard validation protocols was revolutionary. Therefore, the idea of two protocols with different but statistically valid approaches was, scientifically, the correct and best approach. However, the concept of reconciliation was always the intention [40]. Yet, more ideas needed to be tested. The BHS protocol essentially evolved into the ESH-IP protocols and the AAMI standards also evolved. While, on one hand, they appear to have become more divergent in these changes, in reality they have complemented each other refining different compromises. The very fact that they have evolved, based on data and reports on studies that have used them, is a recognition that they are not perfect.

There is also now substantial data available to test protocols and upon which to generate models for Monte-Carlo simulation of new protocols [41]. It is time, therefore, for the experts behind each of the protocols to use the substantial experience, knowledge and data gained to develop a joint protocol that will not only serve the validation of blood pressure monitors, but a basis upon which protocols for the validation of other medical devices can be based.

The Future

Despite improvements in technology, the standard method of blood pressure measurement has essentially changed little in over a century. The vast majority of devices require a cuff to occlude either a brachial or radial artery. Non-occlusive methods of measuring blood pressure, such as pulse wave velocity [42], applanation tonometry [43], and photoplethysmography [44], have been described for some time. With the drive to develop new wearable devices, it is inevitable that new technologies for blood pressure measurement will also be developed.

One of the challenges in the future will be the development of a suitable "gold standard". The current auscultation method is flawed, but has become the reference standard for diagnosis and treatment. As technologies improve and as more is learnt about the reasons for differences between central aortic pressure and brachial pressure, the use of this method as a reference will become harder to justify. Even with algorithms to modify results from new technologies to align with current reference methods, there will come a time when it will be clear that this will not be correct.

Conclusion

The validation of blood pressure monitors has come a long way since the inception of standard protocols in the late 1980s. The information gained has provided a platform upon which a unified protocol can now be developed at a time where technological development is at a stage to allow passing criteria to be based on medical considerations only. Such a protocol can also serve as a template upon which protocols for the validation of other medical devices can also be based.

It is also incumbent on the medical profession to ensure that this information is provided to all consumers, from home users to hospital procurement decision makers, and also to providers. It is essential to increase awareness of the importance of using validated devices and to provide an easily identifiable means of checking whether or not a device is validated to a recognised standard.

Blood pressure monitoring at home or using ABPM is now accepted as mandatory for the diagnosis and treatment of hypertension. Remote expert assessment and self-regulation of treatment may become more commonplace in order to optimise efficacy, to minimise side-effects, and to reduce the effect of geographic location on the access to quality management of hypertension.

Underpinning all of this is the need for accurate measurement. All stakeholders, manufacturers, suppliers, medical professionals, validation investigators, regulatory authorities and consumers must appreciate the importance of accurate devices and the need for a methodology that is practical and robust to ensure that accuracy. As we enter an age of measurement of many cardiovascular parameters, the time has surely come to consolidate experience, knowledge and technology to make the most important haemodynamic measurement—blood pressure—accurate and reliable, thereby not only benefitting the millions of patients world-wide who suffer from hypertension, but also establishing a process for the evaluation of other measuring technologies.

Appendix: Observer Blinding During Validation Procedure

This appendix provides a generalised description of the observer blinding procedure required during validation. It is an adaptation of the method described for observer training in the 1990 BHS protocol [15], the 1993 BHS protocol [17] and the 2002 ESH-IP [20].

Observer Isolation

The observers and supervisor are seated at a bench fitted with partitions so that each is isolated from each other in a "booth". It must not be possible for an observer to have any indication of any blood pressure measurement other than by viewing his/her mercury column and listening with his/her own headset.

Booth Contents

The only objects in the observer booths are a mercury column (or other reference device), a stethoscope headset, two pens (one spare) and prepared forms to write down the observed measurements.

The supervisor booth will have space for both the supervisor and the subject. It will contain a mercury column (or other reference device), a full stethoscope, cuffs, an inflation bulb, the test device, two pens (one spare) and prepared forms.

The Pneumatic System

For sequential same-arm measurements and simultaneous opposite-arm measurements, all of the mercury columns and inflation bulb and a facility to connect a cuff are appropriate to the subject. This will not be a cuff supplied with the test device.

For simultaneous same-arm measurements, all of the mercury columns are connected to the device pneumatic system. The cuff used will be the appropriate cuff for the subject as supplied with the test device.

The system must be closed, and regardless of whether inflation and deflation are controlled by a bulb or by the test device, the system must be calibrated to test for air leaks and for stability.

The Auscultatory System

All of the stethoscope headsets must be connected to the one diaphragm. The lengths of tubing to each of the observer headsets must be the same. The system must be tested to ensure that Korotkov sounds are audible clearly on each headset.

Subject Forms

For the ESH-IP, supervisors must use the Subject Form as published. A similar form should be prepared, containing spaces for all subject details required, including observer measurements, for validations carried out according to the AAMI/ANSI/ISO standard.

Observer forms must contain a space for the subject number, spaces for the measurements and possible repeat measurements. For example, for the ESH-IP protocol, observers will record measurements A, 1, 3, 5 and 7; for the AAMI/ANSI/ISO standard with simultaneous same-arm measurements, observers will record an entry measurement and measurements 1, 2 and 3.

Procedure for Each Subject

After each observer reading, the supervisor checks the observers' readings and, if they differ by at most 4 mmHg for both SBP and DBP, the supervisor simply states "OK" and continues. If not, the supervisor simply states "Repeat measurement n", *n* being the number of the respective measurement. If there are three consecutive repeat measurement or mmm repeat measurements on the same subject, the supervisor simply states "OK" but the subject is excluded.

When the all measurements have been completed on the subject, the supervisor collects the forms and enters the observer measurements on the supervisor form. The forms are stapled together, in the order of Supervisor, Observer 1 and Observer 2. After entry into a computer, they are stored as evidence.

References

1. O'Brien E, Fitzgerald D. The history of indirect blood pressure measurement. In: O'Brien E, O'Malley K, Birkenhager WH, Reid JL, editors. Blood pressure measurement. Handbook of hypertension. Amsterdam: Elsevier; 1991. p. 1–54.
2. Fitzgerald D, O'Callaghan W, O'Malley K, O'Brien E. Inaccuracy of the London School of Hygiene Sphygmomanometer. Br Med J. 1982;284:18–9.
3. O'Brien E, Mee F, Atkins N, O'Malley K. Inaccuracy of the Hawksley random-zero sphygmomanometer. Lancet. 1990;336:1465–8.
4. Fitzgerald D, O'Callaghan WG, McQuaid R, O'Malley K, O'Brien E. Accuracy and reliability of two ambulatory blood pressure recorders: Remler M 2000 and cardiodyne sphygmology. Br Heart J. 1982;48:572–9.
5. O'Brien E, Mee F, Atkins N, O'Malley K. Keep blood pressure Down. WHICH? Magazine. August 1989. p. 372–5.
6. O'Brien E, Mee F, Atkins N, O'Malley K. Inaccuracy of seven popular sphygmomanometers for home-measurement of blood pressure. J Hypertens. 1990;8:621–34.
7. O'Brien E, O'Malley K, Sheridan J. The need for a standardized protocol for validating noninvasive ambulatory blood pressure measuring devices. J Hypertens. 1989;7 (suppl 3):S19–20.
8. American National Standards Institute, Association for the Advancement of Medical Instrumentation. ANSI/AAMI SP10-1987, Electronic or automated sphygmomanometers. Arlington: AAMI; 1987.
9. American National Standards Institute, Association for the Advancement of Medical Instrumentation. ANSI/AAMI SP10-1992, electronic or automated sphygmomanometers. Arlington: AAMI; 1993.
10. American National Standards Institute, ANSI/AAMI SP10-1992/A1, Association for the Advancement of Medical Instrumentation. American National Standard. Electronic or automated sphygmomanometers. Arlington: AAMI; 1996.
11. American National Standards Institute, Association for the Advancement of Medical Instrumentation. ANSI/AAMI SP10-2002 & SP10-2002/A1, Manual, electronic or automated sphygmomanometers. Arlington: AAMI; 2003.
12. Association for the Advancement of Medical Instrumentation, American National Standards Institute, International Organization for Standardization. AAMI/ANSI/ISO 81060-1:2007/(R)2013, Non-invasive sphygmomanometers—Part 1: Requirements and test methods for non-automated measurement type. Geneva: AAMI; 2007.

13. American National Standards Institute, Association for the Advancement of Medical Instrumentation, International Electrotechnical Commission. ANSI/AAMI/IEC 80601-2-30:2009 & A1:2013, Medical electrical equipment—Part 2-30: Particular requirements for basic safety and essential performance of automated type non-invasive sphygmomanometers and Amendment 1. Geneva: IEC Central Office; 2009.

14. Association for the Advancement of Medical Instrumentation, American National Standards Institute, International Organization for Standardization. AAMI/ANSI/ISO 81060-2:2013, non-invasive sphygmomanometers—Part 2: Clinical investigation of automated measurement type. Geneva: AAMI; 2013.

15. O'Brien E, Petrie L, Littler WA, et al. British Hypertension Protocol: Evaluation of automated and semi-automated blood pressure measuring devices with special reference to ambulatory systems. J Hypertens. 1990;8:607–19.

16. Atkins N, O'Brien E, Mee F, O'Malley K. The relative accuracy of simultaneous same arm, simultaneous opposite arm and sequential same arm measurements in the validation of automated blood pressure measuring devices. J Hum Hypertens. 1990;4:647–9.

17. O'Brien E, Petrie J, Littler WA, et al. The British Hypertension Society Protocol for the evaluation of blood pressure measuring devices. J Hypertens. 1993;11 (suppl 2):S43–63.

18. O'Brien E, Mee F, Atkins N, O'Malley K, Tan S. Training and assessment of observers for blood pressure measurement in hypertension research. J Hum Hypertens. 1991;5:7–10.

19. Jamieson M, Petrie J, O'Brien E, Padfield P, Littler WA, De Swiet M. Blood Pressure Measurement. London: Video for the British Hypertension Society, distributed by British Medical Journal Publications; 1989.

20. O'Brien E, Pickering T, Asmar R, on behalf of the Working Group on Blood Pressure Monitoring of the European Society of Hypertension, et al. International protocol for validation of blood pressure measuring devices in adults. Blood Press Monit. 2002;7:3–17.

21. O'Brien E, Atkins N. Validation and reliability of blood pressure monitors. In: White W, editor. Blood pressure monitoring in cardiovascular medicine and therapeutics. Totowa: Humana; 2007. p. 97–132.

22. O'Brien E, Stergiou G. Who will bell the cat? A call for a new approach for validating blood pressure measuring devices. J Hypertens. 2010;28:2378–81.

23. Gerin W, Schwartz AR, Schwartz JE, et al. Limitations of current validation protocols for home blood pressure monitors for individual patients. Blood Press Monit. 2002;7:313–8.

24. O'Brien E, Atkins N, Stergiou G, on behalf of the Working Group on Blood Pressure Monitoring of the European Society of Hypertension, et al. European Society of Hypertension International Protocol for the validation of blood pressure measuring devices in adults: 2010 revision. Blood Press Monit. 2010;15:23–38.

25. Stergiou G, Karpettas N, Atkins N, O'Brien E. European Society of Hypertension International Protocol for the validation of blood pressure monitors: A critical review of its application and rationale for revision. Blood Press Monit. 2010;15:39–48.

26. Keary L, Atkins N, O'Brien E. Terminal digit preference and heaping in blood pressure measurement. J Hum Hypertens. 1998;12:787–8.

27. Stergiou GS, Karpettas N, Atkins N, O'Brien E. Impact of applying the more stringent validation criteria of the revised European Society of Hypertension International Protocol 2010 on earlier validation studies. Blood Press Monit. 2011;16:67–73.

28. Ng KG. Clinical validation protocols for noninvasive blood pressure monitors and their recognition by regulatory authorities and professional organizations: rationale and considerations for a single unified protocol or standard. Blood Press Monit. 2013;18(5):282–9. doi:10.1097/MBP.0b013e3283624b3b.

29. dabl Educational Trust [Internet]. Dublin: dabl Educational Trust; 2006 [Updated 2015 Feb 19; Cited 2015 Mar 9] Available from: www.dableducational.org.

30. Atkins N, O'Brien E. The dabl®Educational Trust device equivalence procedure. Blood Press Monit. 2007;12:245–9.

31. Turner MJ. Can we trust automatic sphygmomanometer validations? J Hypertens. 2010; 28:2353–6.

32. International Organization for Standardization, International Electrotechnical Commission. ISO/IEC 17025:2005, General requirements for the competence of testing and calibration laboratories. Geneva, Switzerland: ISO; 2005.

33. International Organization for Standardization, International Electrotechnical Commission. ISO/IEC 9001:2008, Quality management systems—requirements. Geneva, Switzerland: ISO; 2008.

34. Caulfield M, Heagerty T, Ian Wilkinson I, et al on behalf of the BHS Strategic Review Group. British Hypertension Society Strategic Review 2010-2016 [Internet]. Leicester, UK: BHS; 2009. 20 p. [Cited 2015 Mar 19] Available from: www.bhsoc.org/pdfs/BHS%20Strategic%20 Review%202009.pdf.

35. O'Brien E, Atkins N, Mee F, Coyle D, Syed S. A new audio-visual technique for recording blood pressure in research: the Sphygmocorder. J Hypertens. 1995;13:1734–7.

36. Atkins N, O'Brien E, Wesseling KH, Guelen I. Increasing observer objectivity with audio-visual technology: the Sphygmocorder. Blood Press Monit. 1997;2:269–72.

37. Lee J, Park D, Oh H, Kim I, Shen D, Chee Y. Digital recording system of sphygmomanometry. Blood Press Monit. 2009;14(2):77–81. doi:10.1097/MBP.0b013e3283262f45.

38. IEEE Xplore Digital Library. P1708/D02, Aug 2013—IEEE Draft Standard for Wearable Cuffless Blood Pressure Measuring Devices [Internet]. New York: Institute of Electrical and Electronics Engineers [Cited 2015 Mar 12] Available from: http://ieeexplore.ieee.org/xpl/ login.jsp?tp=&arnumber=6626346&url=http%3A%2F%2Fieeexplore.ieee.org%2FielD%2F 6626344%2F6626345%2F06626346

39. International Electrotechnical Commission. IEC 60601-1, Medical electrical equipment— Part 1: General requirements for basic safety and essential performance. 3rd ed. Geneva, Switzerland: IEC Central Office; 2005.

40. O'Brien E, Atkins N. A comparison of the BHS and AAMI protocols for validating blood pressure measuring devices: can the two be reconciled? J Hypertens. 1994;12:1089–94.

41. Metropolis N, Ulam S. The Monte Carlo method. J Am Stat Assoc. 1949;44:335–41. doi:10.2307/2280232.

42. Lu W, Li H, Tao S, et al. Research on the main elements influencing blood pressure measurement by pulse wave velocity. Front Med Biol Eng. 1992;4(3):189–99.

43. Siebenhofer A, Kemp C, Sutton A, Williams B. The reproducibility of central aortic blood pressure measurements in healthy subjects using applanation tonometry and sphygmocardiography. J Hum Hypertens. 1999;13(9):625–9.

44. Laurent C, Jönsson B, Vegfors M, Lindberg LG. Non-invasive measurement of systolic blood pressure on the arm utilizing photoplethysmography: development of the methodology. Med Biol Eng Comput. 2005;43:131–5.

Part II
Concepts in the Circadian Variation of Cardiovascular Disease

Chapter 6
Circadian and Cyclic Environmental Determinants of Blood Pressure Patterning and Implications for Therapeutic Interventions

Michael H. Smolensky, Francesco Portaluppi, and Ramón C. Hermida

Abbreviations

ABPM	Ambulatory blood pressure monitoring
ACE	Angiotensin converting enzyme
ACEIs	Angiotensin converting enzyme inhibitor medications
ACTH	Adrenocorticotropic hormone
ANG II	Angiotensin II
ANP	Atrial natriuretic peptide
ANS	Autonomic nervous system
ARBs	Angiotensin receptor blocker medications
AT1 receptor	Angiotensin type-1 receptor
BP	Blood pressure
BTCT	Bedtime chronotherapy: full dose of one or more hypertension medications ingested at bedtime
CCBs	Calcium-channel blocker medications
cGMP	Cyclic guanosine monophosphate
CGRP	Calcitonin gene-related peptide
Cl	Chloride

M.H. Smolensky, Ph.D. (✉)
Department of Biomedical Engineering, Cockrell School of Engineering, The University of Texas at Austin, 107 W. Dean Keaton St., Austin, TX 78712-0238, USA
e-mail: michael.smolensky@utexas.edu
URL: http://msmolensky@austin.rr.com

F. Portaluppi, M.D., Ph.D.
Hypertension Center, S. Anna University Hospital, University of Ferrara, Ferrara, Italy

R.C. Hermida, Ph.D.
Bioengineering and Chronobiology Laboratories, Atlantic Research Center for Information and Communication Technologies (AtlantTIC), University of Vigo, Vigo, Spain

© Springer International Publishing Switzerland 2016
W.B. White (ed.), *Blood Pressure Monitoring in Cardiovascular Medicine and Therapeutics*, Clinical Hypertension and Vascular Diseases,
DOI 10.1007/978-3-319-22771-9_6

CMTT	Conventional morning time therapy: full dose of one or more hypertension medications ingested upon morning awakening
CO	Cardiac output
CRH	Corticotropin-releasing hormone
CV	Cardiovascular
DBP	Diastolic blood pressure
EEG	Electroencephalography
ET-1	Endothelin 1
FMD	Brachial artery flow-mediated endothelium-dependent vasodilatation
GFR	Glomerular filtration rate
h	Hour
HOPE	Heart outcomes prevention evaluation trial
HPAA	Hypothalamic–pituitary–adrenal axis
HPTA	Hypothalamic–pituitary–thyroid axis
HR	Hazard ratio
ipRGC	Intrinsic photoreceptive retinal ganglion cells
K	Potassium
MAPEC trial	Monitorización Ambulatoria para Predicción de Eventos Cardiovasculares (English: Ambulatory blood pressure monitoring for prediction of cardiovascular events)
min	Minutes
MTCT	Morning-time conventional therapy
Na	Sodium
NO	Nitric oxide
NREM	Non-rapid eye movement sleep
PRA	Plasma renin activity
RAAS	Renin–angiotensin–aldosterone system
REM	Rapid eye movement sleep
SBP	Systolic blood pressure
SCN	Suprachiasmatic nuclei
s	Seconds
SNS	Sympathetic nervous system
TPR	Vascular total peripheral resistance
TRH	Thyrotropin-releasing hormone
TSH	Thyroid stimulating hormone
Ultradian	Oscillations with period less than 20 h

Introduction

The systolic and diastolic blood pressure (SBP/DBP) 24 h pattern typical of diurnally active normotensive and uncomplicated hypertensive persons is characterized by: (1) striking morning-time BP rise, (2) two daytime peaks—the first 2–3 h after awakening and the second early evening, (3) small mid-afternoon nadir, and (4) 10–20 % decline during sleep relative to the daytime mean, with greater nyctohemeral variation in SBP than DBP [1]. Such BP temporal variation also is substantiated, although often of diminished amplitude, in recumbent normotensive and hypertensive individuals [2, 3] and males and females with fixed heart rate [4]. The importance of cyclic 24 h environmental factors, such as temperature and noise, plus behavioral factors, such as food, liquid, salt, and stimulant consumption, posture, mental stress, and physical activity, is well established [5–9]; nonetheless, there is substantial evidence that various biological rhythms also play a critical role (Table 6.1). This chapter addresses the contribution of innate circadian determinants

Table 6.1 Contribution of exogenous environmental 24 h cycles and innate circadian rhythms to the typical nyctohemeral blood pressure pattern of most normotensive and uncomplicated hypertensive persons

Exogenous day–night cycles
• Light: bright daytime/dark nighttime
• Sound: noisy daytime/quiet nighttime
• Posture: erect daytime/supine nighttime
• Physical activity and exertion: high daytime/low or nil nighttime
• Arousal, mental, and emotional stress: high daytime/nil nighttime
• Eating behavior: primarily daytime/none or nil nighttime
• Salt and water consumption: primarily daytime/none or nil nighttime
• Caffeine and other stimulant consumption: daytime/none or nil nighttime
Endogenous circadian rhythms
• Plasma melatonin concentration: nil or none daytime/elevated nighttime
• SNS[a]: dominant daytime/suppressed, except during REM sleep, nighttime
• Vagal tone: reduced daytime/dominant nighttime
• Plasma active noradrenaline and adrenaline concentration: elevation before morning awakening and peaking late morning or afternoon/nighttime trough
• Vasoconstriction: predominates daytime/vasodilatation predominates nighttime
• Vascular TPR[a]: increased markedly on morning awakening/decreased early in nighttime sleep, but increased there after during sleep
• α_2 and β_2-adrenergic receptors: up-regulated morning/normal or down-regulated afternoon and nighttime
• Baroreflex response: up-regulated morning/down-regulated nighttime
• HR[a] and CO[a]: elevated during morning and daytime/reduced during nighttime sleep
• Peripheral capillary and arteriovenous-anastomoses blood flow: enhanced before and on nighttime sleep onset/reduced on morning-time sleep offset
• Plasma cortisol: highest in morning/lowest or nil nighttime
• RAAS[a]: activated during middle to late nighttime sleep span/down-regulated late evening and early sleep
• PRA[a] and ACE activity[a] and Ang II[a], and aldosterone concentration: significantly elevated late sleep and morning/reduced evening and early sleep
• GFR[a] and NA[a], K[a], Cl[a], and H_2O[a] diuresis: elevated daytime, peaking in afternoon/depressed nighttime
• ANP[a] and CGRP[a] plasma concentrations: highest during nighttime sleep/lowest afternoon or early evening

(continued)

Table 6.1 (continued)

• Plasma NO[a] concentration: lowest on morning awakening/highest early evening
• Plasma ET-1[a] concentration: first peak on morning awakening and second peak 12 h later/lowest early evening
• BP[a] regulating-natriuresis mechanism: down-regulated daytime/up-regulated nighttime

[a]*SNS* sympathetic nervous system, *TPR* total peripheral resistance, *HR* heart rate, *CO* cardiac output, *RAAS* renin–angiotensin–aldosterone system, *ACE* angiotensin converting enzyme, *GFR* glomerular filtration rate, *ANG II* angiotensin II, *Na* sodium, *K* potassium, *Cl* chloride, *H₂O*water, *ANP* atrial natriuretic peptide, *CGRP* calcitonin gene-related peptide, *NO* nitric oxide, *ET-1* endothelin 1, *BP* blood pressure

to the BP day/night pattern of diurnally active normotensive and uncomplicated hypertensive human beings through presentation of a broad array of relevant research findings as well as recently completed circadian rhythm-based hypertension-treatment outcomes trials.

Overview of Biological Time-Keeping

Master and Peripheral Circadian Clocks

Given the subject matter, a brief introduction to the mechanisms of biological time-keeping is central to appreciating the materials subsequentially presented. Circadian rhythms in pressor and all other biological processes are generated and orchestrated by a self-oscillating master brain clock, the suprachiasmatic nuclei (SCN) of the hypothalamus [10, 11]. The clock mechanism in the SCN and peripheral oscillators is similar; it consists of a network of transcriptional–translational feedback loops that drive rhythmic, i.e., ~24 h, expression patterns of the core clock components—clock genes such as *Clock*, *Bmal*, *Per*, and *Cry*—whose protein products generate and regulate cellular circadian rhythms of all tissues, organs, and systems. Because the inherited period of the SCN and peripheral oscillators differs somewhat from exactly 24.0 h, external time cues are required to synchronize it for efficient functioning. The primary environmental time cue is the 24 h light/day cycle. Environmental time information in the form of the onset (sunset) and offset (sunrise) of darkness is sensed by intrinsic non-rod/non-cone ganglion cells (ipRGC) of the retinae and conveyed via the retinohypothalamic neural pathway first to the SCN and thereafter via the paraventricular nucleus, hindbrain, spinal cord, and superior cervical ganglion pathways to β- and α-receptors within the pineal gland to initiate melatonin synthesis [12]. Accordingly, the period of the SCN and subservient peripheral clocks, and the circadian rhythms they drive, is synchronized, i.e., set and reset from one day to the next, to 24.0 h, and additionally, the phasing (peak and trough) of these circadian oscillators and the rhythms they generate is correctly timed to support optimal biological efficiency during daytime wakefulness and activity and rest and repair during nighttime sleep.

Pineal Gland and Melatonin

The short-half-life molecule melatonin, the so-called hormone of darkness, plays a central role in biological time-keeping. Its synthesis and circulation take place only during the nighttime dark span; thus, in humans plasma and tissue melatonin concentration peaks during nocturnal sleep, while it is essentially undetectable during the daytime [12]. Normal daytime and artificial nighttime light, especially of the blue spectrum, inhibits melatonin synthesis. The period and phasing of the melatonin synthesis circadian rhythm of the pinealocytes are synchronized to external time by the onset, duration, and cessation of environmental darkness, and the circulation of melatonin, in turn, synchronizes the period and phasing of the other 24 h bodily rhythms [10].

The melatonin 24 h rhythm, itself, appears to play a role in the observed BP day/ night variation via its direct effects on the arterial wall [13], cardiomyocytes [14], baroreflex set point [15], and sympathetic nervous system (SNS) through modulation in the adrenal medulla of the catecholamine synthesis circadian rhythm [16]. Moreover, bedtime melatonin supplementation reduces human BP, particularly sleep-time BP [15, 17]. Such observations are consistent with the contention that the BP day/night variation is endogenous in origin, even though it is often masked by the more dominant external influences [18], especially those of physical and mental activity [19] as clearly demonstrated by studies of rotating shift workers [20].

Wake/Sleep Circadian Rhythm

The wake/sleep cycle, the most evident circadian rhythm of life, is an important endogenous determinant of the BP nyctohemeral variation. The wake/sleep cycle, which is controlled by a multitude of basic sensory, motor, autonomic, endocrine, and cerebral 24 h rhythms [21], derives from the alternating-in-time dominance of mutually inhibitory actions of arousal/activating systems—cholinergic, serotonergic, and histaminergic nuclear groups of the rostral pons, midbrain, and posterior hypothalamus, and cholinergic neurons of the basal forebrain—and hypnogenic/deactivating systems— those of the medial preoptic-anterior hypothalamic region and adjacent basal forebrain, medial thalamus, and medulla plus the pineal gland via melatonergic mechanisms. Circadian change in autonomic nervous system (ANS) tone plays an essential mechanistic role, and it also mediates the impact of the sleep and wake states on cardiac and vascular 24 h rhythms [22]. Melatonin, serotonin, arginine vasopressin, vasoactive intestinal peptide, somatotropin, insulin, and steroid hormones and their biologically active metabolites are associated with nighttime sleep induction, while corticotropin-releasing hormone (CRH), adrenocorticotropic hormone (ACTH), thyro-tropin-releasing hormone (TRH), endogenous opioids, and prostaglandin E_2 are associ-ated with morning arousal [23]. The nyctohemeral alteration of these constituents is surely reflected in the phasic oscillations of cardiovascular (CV) function and status.

Most biologically active substances, e.g., hormones, peptides, and neurotransmitters, among others, exhibit significant circadian variability that is superimposed on feedback control systems. Secretion of these substances is typically episodic, i.e., as high fre-quency pulses, and "gated" by mechanisms directly coupled to sleep or the pacemaker SCN clock [24]. Thus, it is not surprising that BP also exhibits short period (ultradian) oscillations in association with sleep staging [25]. BP is lowest during deepest (stages 3/4) sleep and highest, although not to the level when fully awake, during less deep (stages 1/2 and REM) sleep. Sleep-time BP ultradian oscillations also may be mediated through temporal patterns of respiration [26]. After sleep onset and during light NREM sleep, breathing tends to be periodic with only sporadic occurrence of central apneas. Oscillations in breathing occur every 20–30 s in association with synchronous fluctua-tions in cortical EEG activity, BP, heart rate, and oxygen saturation. During deep NREM sleep, breathing is more regular and BP and heart rate decline. During REM sleep, breathing and heart rate are more erratic with irregularly expressed central apneas or hypopneas lasting 20–30 s that typically coincide with bursts of REM and BP spikes as great as 30–40 mmHg, often beyond the threshold of normotension [25, 26].

In part, the BP nocturnal decline is the consequence of blood volume redistribu-tion associated with the normal late night decrease of core and brain temperature that gates sleep onset [27, 28]. The core body temperature circadian rhythm, gov-erned by the SCN master clock, peaks in the late afternoon/early evening, descends slightly ~20:00 h and more markedly ~35 min before sleep onset, attains its nadir 1–2 h before morning arousal when sleep tends to be deepest, and rises thereafter [28]. The late evening and sleep-time body temperature fall results from activation of physiologic heat loss mechanisms mediated by reduced SNS outflow, and aug-mented by recumbency, that increases peripheral vasodilatation by 30–40 % just before sleep commences and as much as 80 % during sleep [27]. This results in enhanced capillary blood flow to the proximal (trunk and limb) skin and especially the arteriovenous-anastomoses of the distal glabrous (hand, fingers, feet, toes, ear) skin, the latter thought to be mediated, at least in part, by the melatonin circadian rhythm [27, 28]. The circadian rhythm-dependent change in peripheral blood flow plus associated fluid shift to extracellular compartments result in sleep-time reduc-tion of plasma volume, as documented in non-human primate studies [29].

BP rises markedly in the morning upon awakening, although the morning rise usually commences beforehand in association with the high prevalence of less deep stages and, additionally, the redistribution of blood volume from the distal and proximal skin to the central arterial circulation mediated by the SCN-orchestrated circadian rise in core body temperature related to the physiology of morning arousal [27, 28, 30]. Deep sleep density, which is greatest during the first part of the night, is correlated with BP rapid decline. REM sleep and brief episodes of arousal, gener-ally in response to external stimuli, are more common during the last half of the sleep span and trigger spurts of BP elevations. When 24 h-recorded intra-arterial BP data of a large group of normal subjects were individually aligned to the exact time of waking, it became evident that the BP morning rise commences some hours before the termination of sleep. Thus, it is highly implausible that the BP morning rise results from morning arousal, alone [31].

Neural, Neuroendocrine, and Endocrine Systems

Autonomic Nervous System

SNS tone dominates during the daytime wake span, while vagal tone dominates during the nighttime sleep span [32–34]. Plasma norepinephrine and epinephrine plus urinary catecholamine concentrations are greatest during the initial span of diurnal activity, i.e., morning to early afternoon, when SBP and DBP attain near peak or peak values and lowest during nocturnal sleep when SBP and DBP are least [35, 36]. The temporal relationship between the 24 h alteration in plasma dopamine and norepinephrine/epinephrine concentrations is strong, suggesting dopaminergic modulation of the circadian rhythm of SNS activity [36, 37]. In human beings, catecholamine sulfates are biologically inactive, and in normotensive recumbent persons the circadian pattern is opposite that of biologically active free catecholamines [38]: plasma noradrenaline and adrenaline sulphates rise to peak levels early during the nighttime sleep span, and plasma-free noradrenaline and adrenaline rapidly increase before morning awakening.

Environmental cycles, especially the one of light and darkness, in conjunction with the activity/sleep circadian rhythm, significantly influence catecholamine concentration [39]. The day/night change in plasma norepinephrine and metabolite 3-methoxy-4-hydroxyphenylglycol, but not epinephrine, is strongly affected by activity, arousal, posture, and food consumption [36, 39, 40]. Nonetheless, nocturnal decline in norepinephrine is observed even in sleep-deprived individuals, suggesting the inherent 24 h variation in norepinephrine secretion is controlled by an endogenous circadian clock [41].

The ANS nyctohemeral variation, together with the day-night pattern in physical activity, mental and emotional stress, and posture, plays a prominent role in the BP 24 h profile of both normotensive and uncomplicated hypertension [4–9]. In most normotensive subjects the sleep-time heart rate decreases by 18 beats/min, cardiac output by 29 %, stroke volume by 7 %, and vascular total peripheral resistance (TPR) although declining early in sleep increases by 22 % compared to average daytime values [42]. Comparable changes are observed in uncomplicated essential dipper hypertensive subjects [43].

Renin–Angiotensin–Aldosterone System

The renin–angiotensin–aldosterone system (RAAS) modulates BP through various mechanisms—body sodium (Na) and water (H_2O), SNS, and vasomotor tone balance. Renal blood flow reduction induces renal juxtaglomerular cells to release the enzyme renin. Liver-derived angiotensinogen is converted by renin to angiotensin I, which in turn is converted by lung tissue-derived angiotensin-converting (ACE) enzyme to angiotensin II (ANG II). ANG II elevates BP by signaling aldosterone release from the adrenal cortex, which acts to increase renal Na and H_2O reabsorption, stimulate SNS activity, and initiate blood vessel vasoconstriction.

Circadian rhythms of prorenin, plasma renin activity (PRA) and serum ACE activity, plasma ANG II and aldosterone concentration, plus tissue angiotensin type-1 (AT1) receptor expression contribute strongly to the BP day/night oscillation in both normotensive and uncomplicated hypertensive conditions, and for some of the variables even under conditions of long-term recumbence [6, 44–51]. The RAAS activates during the night, i.e., mid-sleep span, with highest and lowest PRA and ANG II concentration found in the morning and late evening, i.e., at the commencement of the wake and sleep span, respectively. However, this temporal patterning persists in the absence of the wake/sleep cycle, i.e., in sleep-deprived subjects, although generally with reduced amplitude [52]. Some investigators have failed to detect PRA circadian patterning [53–55], finding instead an ultradian periodicity of ~100 min strongly correlated with sleep staging—PRA declining during REM sleep and peaking during deep and light sleep transitions. SNS and dopaminergic mechanisms appear to be important modulators of the PRA, ANG II, and aldosterone circadian rhythms [56]. The PRA circadian rhythm determines the magnitude of response to external challenge, explaining why the exercise-induced PRA response is markedly greater in the afternoon at 16:00 h than middle of the night at 04:00 h [57]. Plasma aldosterone 24 h variation is predominantly regulated by the ACTH circadian rhythm that peaks between the middle and late portion of sleep [24]; although, during the wake span aldosterone is modulated mainly by the renin-angiotensin system [58].

ACE circadian rhythmicity has been demonstrated in both healthy normotensive and uncomplicated essential hypertensive individuals studied under a controlled meal-time and activity/rest routine. Two Italian studies [48, 49] reported a late afternoon rather than the expected morning peak, while a third Japanese study reported a late nighttime sleep/early daytime activity peak (06:00–09:00 h) [50], both in normotensive and essential hypertensive subjects. Inconsistency in the circadian time of peak ACE activity between studies could represent differences during the 24 h in meal composition and liquid consumption and their timings, subject activity and posture patterning, and blood sampling paradigm. Moreover, in the two Italian studies [48, 49], absence of the early morning peak in ACE activity might be indicative of a circadian rhythm of ACE turnover: during sleep when ANG II generation is maximum, ACE consumption is maximum, and circulating ACE level is reduced, and during the daytime when ANG II generation is minimal, ACE consumption is minimal, and circulating ACE level is elevated. Finally, it is of interest that circadian rhythmicity in SCN AT1-receptor expression has been demonstrated in laboratory animals with peak expression early during the nocturnal activity span and lowest expression during the middle to late rest span [51]. This finding implicates central clock modulation of the BP 24 h variation [51] and further suggests the possibility of AT1-expression circadian rhythmicity in other tissues.

Hypothalamic–Pituitary–Adrenal Axis

Adrenocortical hormones, in general, mediate electrolyte, extracellular fluid, and plasma volume balance through effects on epithelial, smooth muscle, and cardiac cells [59]. They and their active metabolites also modulate energy and other processes of adipose, liver, kidney, and vascular tissue; they also play a role in atherogenesis, vascular homeostasis, and vascular remodeling following intra-vascular injury or ischemia [60, 61]. Additionally, they are involved in the elevated vascular risk induced by long-term stress [62]. Several studies suggest the late sleep/morning-time marked rise in glucocorticoids may up-regulate at the commencement of the diurnal activity span both α_2 and β_2-adrenergic receptor expression in heart, blood vessel, and other tissues, which may explain the greater morning-time effects of certain adrenergic agonist and antagonist agents as well as marked SNS-driven increase in morning heart rate and BP [63–65].

The master SCN oscillator drives the ACTH circadian rhythm, and this along with circadian SCN-mediated SNS activity gives rise to cortisol 24 h periodicity [24]; plasma ACTH concentration peaks during the latter span of sleep, and cortisol adrenocortical synthesis and circulation is highest just prior to or upon waking and lowest early during sleep [24]. The sensitivity of the adrenal cortex to both endogenously produced and exogenously administered ACTH, itself, is circadian-time dependent [24], explaining in part the enhanced secretion of cortisol in response to stressful stimuli in the morning [66]. The ACTH and ACTH-dependent 24 h oscillation of cortisol contributes to the nyctohemeral variation in cardiac output and SBP, but without effect upon blood vessel peripheral resistance [59, 67]. The BP 24 h pattern is disrupted, especially BP sleep-time decline, in Cushing's syndrome and also Addison's disease, in which the adrenocortical-derived circadian rhythms of cortisol and aldosterone are abnormal or absent, thereby implicating the significance of hypothalamic–pituitary–adrenal axis (HPAA) periodicity in the BP day/night variation under normal conditions [56, 68].

Hypothalamic–Pituitary–Thyroid Axis

Plasma thyroid stimulation hormone (TSH) concentration exhibits circadian variation, rising during the afternoon and peaking after midnight [24]. The hypothalamic–pituitary-thyroid axis (HPTA) exerts effects on the CV system at multiple levels, including direct positive inotropic and cronotropic actions on the myocardium plus stimulation of tissue metabolic rate and positive modulation of the agonistic sensitivity of heart tissue ß-adrenergic receptors [69]. Surprisingly, there have been few studies of the exact role of the HPTA nyctohemeral cycle on BP day/night variation. Evidence of its effects is based on clinical observations of persons with abnormal thyroid states—increased vascular resistance, often depressed systolic function, left ventricular diastolic dysfunction at rest, systolic and diastolic dysfunction on effort, endothelial dysfunction, arterial wall thickness, atherosclerotic injury [69–71], plus altered BP regulation and 24 h non-dipping patterning [72].

Opioid, Vasoactive peptide, and Endothelial Factors

Opioid Factors

Various opioid peptides and receptors are present in the central nervous system and peripheral neural elements, some of which exert CV system effects. In normotensive and spontaneously hypertensive rats, both free and cryptic metenkephalin heart tissue concentration exhibits circadian rhythmicity [73]. In humans, plasma ß-endorphins (but not metenkephalin) also are circadian rhythmic [74], as is the binding of ligand to opiate receptors [75]. Involvement of both the sympathetic and parasympathetic nervous systems in the actions of these peptides on CV function is established; although little is known to date about underlying mechanisms in humans. In man, endogenous opioids modulate central nervous system BP control, particularly its nocturnal decline [76]. ∂-Opioid receptors, in particular, are suspected of playing a role in BP nocturnal decline through suppression of the SNS and HPAA [77, 78] and the phase (peak and trough) relationships of the respective circadian rhythms.

Vasoactive Peptide Elements

Both atrial natriuretic peptide (ANP) and calcitonin gene-related peptide (CGRP) are circadian rhythmic [79, 80], and both exert regulatory control of the 24 h BP pattern. ANP, a 28 amino acid polypeptide, suppresses PRA, ANG II, aldosterone, and catecholamine concentrations; increases Na excretion and plasma and urinary cGMP levels; and shifts the renal pressure-natriuresis mechanism so Na balance during sleep can take place at lower arterial pressures. ANP is principally involved in short-term electrolyte balance and BP control, while the RAAS primarily exerts long-term BP control [81]. Thus, ANP acts to reduce vascular TPR and as a consequence arterial BP. Peak ANP concentration occurs between 23:00 and 04:00 h and coincides approximately with the nadir of the PRA and aldosterone circadian rhythms of diurnally active normotensive and essential hypertensive persons, with the ANP peak-to-trough 24 h variation that is independent of posture amounting to ~10 pmol/L [79, 81, 82]. Blunting of the nocturnal BP decline, e.g., in chronic renal and congestive heart failure patients, is paralleled by concomitant alteration of the ANP circadian rhythm, both before and after treatment [83–85].

CGRP is a 37 amino-acid peptide involved in various metabolic and behavioral functions [86]. CGRP-containing fibers exist throughout the CV system, particularly within the coronary arteries, sinoatrial and atrioventricular nodes, and papillary heart muscle fibers [87]. CGRP blood levels are most likely representative of peptide spillover from nerve terminals that promote vasodilatation. A circadian rhythm in plasma CGRP has been demonstrated in both normotension and uncomplicated hypertension [80, 88, 89]. The RAAS modulates plasma CGRP secretion, either directly through vasopressor effect on peripheral blood vessels or indirectly through neurohumoral mechanisms that modulate vascular tone and thus BP [90–92]. Intravenous CGRP infusion in pharmacological doses decreases mean BP and increases heart rate in humans [93, 94]. CGRP also plays a role in response to postural and vasomotor changes; plasma CGRP levels rapidly rise, as do those of norepinephrine and aldosterone, in healthy subjects after assuming an upright position or following low-dose ANG II infusion [91].

Endothelial Factors

Circadian rhythms of the endothelial vasodilator and vasoconstrictor factors of nitric oxide (NO) and endothelin 1 (ET-1) modulate vascular tone and BP. In diurnally active healthy individuals, vasodilator NO concentration is lowest around the transition between the sleep and wake span and highest 12 h later [95–97]. Accordingly, brachial artery flow-mediated endothelium-dependent vasodilatation (FMD) is least in the early morning and most elevated in the late afternoon and evening. The FMD circadian rhythm is substantiated in both men and pre-menopausal women, although based on the results of a single investigation not in menopausal women [98]. The vasoconstrictor ET-1 exhibits 12 h variability, with two peaks of equal magnitude, one in the morning at the beginning of the wake span and the other early evening [97].

Renal Hemodynamics

Circadian rhythms with afternoon to early evening peak times of renal blood flow, glomerular filtration rate (GFR), urine volume, and urinary excretions of Na, potassium (K), and chloride (Cl) are well-known and persist independent of meal timings, activity level, sleep, and posture [99, 100]. Renal blood flow, vascular resistance, and GFR decline at night, although the decrease of urine flow observed in non-elderly persons is much more pronounced than expected, suggesting circadian rhythmicity with nighttime peak of tubular reabsorption perhaps mediated by intrarenal ANG II and also vasopressin, whose circadian rhythm also peaks during sleep [101–103]. Significant correlation is detectable at night between BP and Na and K excretion when the balance between Na-retaining and Na-sparing mechanisms favors natriuresis. However, the correlation is masked during waking by dominating Na-retaining factors [100]. The circadian rhythm of renal Na and K handling appears to be driven by the circadian rhythm of aldosterone. Dopamine and the renal kallikrein–kinin system also play a role in the daily variation of H_2O and Na handling, as suggested by the close timing of the peak and trough among the circadian rhythms of urinary dopamine, Na, kinin, kallikrein, and H_2O excretion [104, 105]. The circadian rhythm of ANP that peaks early during sleep also modulates the urinary Na excretion 24 h rhythm [106]. Urinary excretion of kinin, kallikrein, and prostaglandin E is circadian rhythmic, being highest in the afternoon and lowest overnight, both in recumbent and non-recumbent healthy volunteers [105, 107]. The day/night alteration of urinary kallikrein and plasma aldosterone concentration is strongly and positively correlated, suggesting the circadian rhythm of aldosterone drives the circadian rhythm of urinary kallikrein excretion.

Circadian BP Profile of Different Hypertensive Conditions

Pathologic and other disturbances of the ANS, renal hemodynamics, and vasoactive neurohumoral, peptide, opioid, and endothelial circadian rhythms that play a role in the regulation of blood volume and central and peripheral vascular tone are clearly involved in the genesis of altered BP 24 h patterning. As reviewed elsewhere [23], attenuated or reversed nocturnal decline in BP is common in many medical conditions, for example: orthostatic autonomic failure, Shy–Drager syndrome, vascular and Alzheimer-type dementia, cerebral atrophy, CV disease, ischemic arterial disease after carotid endarterectomy, neurogenic hypertension, fatal familial insomnia, diabetes, catecholamine-producing tumors, exogenous glucocorticoid administration, Cushing's and mineral corticoid excess syndromes, Addison's disease, pseudohypoparathyroidism, sleep apnea, normotensive and hypertensive asthma, chronic renal failure, severe hypertension, Na-sensitive essential hypertension, gestational hypertension, toxemia of pregnancy, essential hypertension with left ventricular hypertrophy, renal, liver, and cardiac transplantation related to immunosuppressive medication, congestive heart failure, and recombinant human erythropoietin therapy. Absence of the normal nocturnal BP decline appears to carry a higher CV and cerebral risk by prolonging the time beyond diurnal waking when the elevated BP load is exerted on target tissues and organs; the average nighttime BP level and magnitude of the nocturnal BP fall are significantly correlated with target organ—cardiac, cerebral, and renal—tissue damage [23].

Evidence of BP Circadian Rhythm Endogenousity: Hypertension Medication Trials

Bedtime vs. Morning-Time Hypertension Therapy: Differential Effects on Asleep and Awake BP and BP Dipping

The peak time of the individual nervous system, endocrine, endothelial, peptide, renal hemodynamic, and other circadian rhythm determinants of the nyctohemeral BP pattern typical of most normotensive and uncomplicated essential hypertensive persons occurs between the last hours of nighttime sleep and initial hours of daytime wakefulness. Clinical trials (Table 6.2) clearly document the BP-lowering effects of conventional long-acting hypertension medications vary, often extensively, according to treatment time [108]. When such medications, especially those that directly or indirectly modulate the SNS and RAAS or their vasomotor effects,

Table 6.2 Ingestion-time awakening vs. bedtime-dependent differences in effect of BP-lowering medications (mmHg from baseline) on awake and asleep SBP/DBP means and sleep-time relative decline of diurnally active hypertension patients[e]

Medication	Dose, mg	No. of patients	Treatment-time reduction in awake SBP/DBP mean		Treatment-time reduction in asleep SBP/DBP mean		Treatment-time effect on sleep-time relative SBP/DBP decline	
			Awakening R_x	Bedtime R_x	Awakening R_x	Bedtime R_x	Awakening R_x	Bedtime R_x
ACEIs								
Ramipril	5	115	-10.1/-6.9	-10.5/-9.0	-4.5/-4.1	-13.5/-11.5*	-3.3/-1.8	3.4/4.9*
Spirapril	6	165	-9.9/-8.0	-8.5/-5.7	-5.7/-4.6	-12.8/-8.6*	-2.5/-2.7	4.1/4.5*
ARBs								
Valsartan	160	90	-17.0/-11.1	-12.0/-9.8	-15.9/-10.8	-17.9/-13.3	0.2/1.3	5.4/6.3*
Valsartan	160	100[a]	-12.8/-6.6	-13.0/-8.5	-10.9/-5.5	-20.5/-11.1*	-1.0/-0.3	6.6/5.4*
Valsartan	160	200[b]	-13.1/-8.3	-12.6/-9.3	-12.9/-8.1	-21.1/-13.9*	0.4/0.9	7.2/7.1*
Olmesartan	20	133	-14.5/-12.1	-13.3/-9.6	-11.2/-8.7	-15.2/-11.5‡	-1.3/-1.4	2.9/4.6*
Olmesartan	40	72	-17.1/-10.1	-16.3/-11.5	-12.6/-8.2	-17.9/-12.5‡	-1.6/-0.2	3.0/3.8*
Telmisartan	80	215	-11.7/-8.8	-11.3/-8.2	-8.3/-6.4	-13.8/-9.7*	-1.6/-1.0	3.1/3.9*
CCBs								
Amlodipine	5	194	-10.2/-7.7	-11.8/-7.2	-9.6/-5.5	-11.2/-6.7	0.1/-1.6	0.2/0.7‡
Nifedipine GITS	30	238	-9.4/-6.3	-12.8/-7.7‡	-7.5/-5.1	-12.8/-7.8*	-0.7/-0.2	1.0/1.5‡
α-Blocker								
Doxazosin GITS	4	39[c]	-2.9/-3.7	-6.0/-5.4	0.7/-1.3	-8.2/-6.5†	-2.3/-2.4	1.9/1.9‡
Doxazosin GITS	4	52[d]	-3.4/-2.9	-5.9/-4.4	0.1/-0.5	-4.9/-5.3‡	-2.3/-2.4	1.7/1.5‡

(continued)

Table 6.2 (continued)

Medication	Dose, mg	No. of patients	Treatment-time reduction in awake SBP/DBP mean		Treatment-time reduction in asleep SBP/DBP mean		Treatment-time effect on sleep-time relative SBP/DBP decline	
			Awakening R_x	Bedtime R_x	Awakening R_x	Bedtime R_x	Awakening R_x	Bedtime R_x
β-Blocker								
Nebivolol	5	173	−14.7/−12.4	−13.4/−10.9	−7.9/−7.4	−10.2/−8.1	−3.6/−3.0	−1.2/−1.4‡
Diuretic								
Torasemide	5	113	−7.3/−3.7	−15.6/−9.9*	−4.3/−2.5	−12.5/−8.0*	−1.6/−0.7	−1.3/−0.2
Combination R_x								
Valsartan/amlodipine	160/5	203	−18.3/−14.5	−22.6/−12.7	−14.4/−10.1	−28.1/−14.7*	−1.3/−2.1	5.5/5.2*
Valsartan/hydrochlorothiazide	160/12.5	204	−17.4/−11.5	−16.7/−11.4	−16.0/−12.0	−20.1/−13.6‡	0.5/2.4	3.9/4.7*

[a]Elderly patients (≥60 years of age)

[b]Non-dipper patients, i.e., sleep-time relative SBP decline <10 %

[c]Doxazosin monotherapy

[d]Doxazosin in combination with other hypertension medications

[e]Table modified from [107]. All studies were conducted by one of the authors (R.C. Hermida) utilizing a prospective, randomized, open label, blinded endpoint (PROBE) design involving grade 1 or 2 essential hypertension (2306 in total) participants. 48 h ABPM and wrist actigraphy were applied at baseline before and again after 12-weeks of timed treatment to accurately derive the awake and asleep SBP/DBP means plus sleep-time relative BP decline ([awake BP mean−asleep BP mean]/awake BP mean x 100), index of extent of BP dipping during nighttime sleep relative to level diurnal waking

*$P<.001$, †$P<.01$, ‡$P<.05$: Statistical significance of comparison of the between treatment-times effects on BP

i.e., angiotensin converting enzyme inhibitors (ACEIs), angiotensin receptor blockers (ARBs), calcium-channel blockers (CCBs), α-blockers, and ß-blockers, are ingested alone or in combination at bedtime rather than morning, reduction of the asleep SBP and DBP means is vastly enhanced as is the sleep-time relative BP decline, thereby greatly improving the BP 24 h profile toward normal. Such findings indicate features of the innate pressor-affecting circadian rhythms are of greater importance than previous appreciated as determinants of the BP 24 h pattern and, therefore, management of hypertension.

Bedtime vs. Morning-Time Hypertension Medication Outcomes Trials: Differential Reduction of Vascular Risk

Several investigations, among them the HOPE [109, 110] and MAPEC [111] trials, have found a bedtime treatment strategy entailing the full daily dose of one or more conventional long-acting hypertension medications affords better 24 h BP control and greater protection against nonfatal and fatal stroke, cardiac, and other CV incidents of hypertensive persons than the traditional morning-time strategy.

The MAPEC study constitutes the first prospective trial expressly designed and conducted to completion to test the hypothesis that so-called bedtime chronotherapy (BTCT: full dose at bedtime of one or more hypertension medications) exerts better 24 h BP control and vascular risk reduction than conventional morning time therapy (CMTT) [111]. A total of 3344 regular clinical patients with baseline SBP and DBP, according to ambulatory BP monitoring (ABPM) threshold criteria, ranging from normotension to sustained hypertension, were randomized to CMTT or BTCT and followed for a median duration of 5.6 years. At baseline and at least annually thereafter, ambulatory BP and physical activity (wrist actigraphy) were assessed simultaneously for 48 h to accurately derive the awake and asleep SBP and DBP means. As expected (Table 6.2) patients randomized to BTCT, in comparison to ones randomized to CMTT, exhibited significantly lower mean asleep BP, greater sleep-time relative BP decline, lesser prevalence of non-dipping (34 % vs. 62 %; $P<.001$), and higher prevalence of controlled ambulatory BP (62 % vs. 53 %, $P<.001$) [112]. Even more important, BTCT, relative to CMTT, better reduced vascular risk—both total CV and major CV events (composite of CV deaths, myocardial infarctions, and ischemic and hemorrhagic strokes), the respective adjusted statistically significant ($P<.001$) hazard ratio (HR) being .39 (.29–.51) and .33 (.19–.55) [112]. The greater incidence of CV events of those randomized to CMTT was independent of the class of BP-lowering single or multiple therapies prescribed. On the other hand, maximum reduction of CV events was attained by the BTCT, relative to CMTT, when it consisted of or included an ARB (HR = .29 [.17–.51]; $P<.001$) or CCB (HR = .46 [.31–.69]; $P<.001$), and lowest HR of CV events was achieved with a BTCT that entailed an ARB, alone or in combination with other classes of hypertension medications [113]. Another notable finding of the MAPEC study [114], and recently verified by a meta-analysis of 9 different cohorts [115], is that the ABPM-derived asleep SBP mean, relative to all the other characteristics and parameters of the BP 24 h profile, most strongly predicts CV risk. Analyses of changes in ambulatory BP that was assessed at least annually during the 5.6-year median follow-up of the MAPEC trial revealed a 17 % reduction in CV risk per each 5-mmHg decrease in the asleep SBP mean ($P<0.001$), by far best achieved with the BTCT approach, independent of change in any other ambulatory BP parameter [114]. The findings were similar also for the higher vascular risk patients, mostly non-dipper, chronic kidney disease [116], type 2 diabetes [117], and resistant hypertensive [118] cohorts. It is hypothesized that the pharmacokinetic and pharmacodynamic behavior of conventionally formulated hypertension medications when ingested at bedtime, as opposed to morning, better aligns with the circadian stage of elevated activity of the ANS, endocrine, endothelial, renal hemodynamic, and other circadian rhythm determinants of the nyctohemeral BP pattern and, assumedly, vascular risk, particularly when BP is abnormal during sleep. The findings of the MAPEC trial showing greatly reduced vascular risk when hypertension medications are optimally timed to the BP circadian determinants have been recently substantiated by a meta-analysis of data of all evening and bedtime treatment outcome trials thus far reported [119, 120].

Mechanisms Underlying the Advantage of Bedtime Chronotherapy

A possible unitary explanation of the ingestion-time differences in effects upon the BP 24 h pattern may entail the classical pressure-natriuresis mechanism [121]. Under usual circumstances, BP is normally lowest at night as is Na excretion. However, in acute and chronic situations when Na intake is excessive or its daytime excretion hampered, BP is adjusted by the pressure-natriuresis mechanism during nighttime sleep to an elevated level as a compensatory response, thereby resulting in abnormal non-dipping 24 h patterning [122]. This is the reason why Na-sensitive hypertensives—patients prone to retain Na to such a degree that BP is significantly increased—tend to be non-dippers. The pressure-natriuresis mechanism and relationship are modulated during the daytime by upright posture and activity, such that it is mainly during the nighttime when Na sensitivity, which is present to varying extent among individuals, most strongly exerts its corrective effects, thus inducing the non-dipping BP patterning. Hence, BP regulation is not constant throughout day and night; on the contrary, it is modulated not only according to the staging of numerous circadian factors and different pathophysiological conditions, but the pharmacological properties of prescribed hypertension medications and circadian time of their ingestion [123]. A modification as simple and inexpensive as switching the ingestion time from morning to evening or bedtime (in diurnally active patients) of one or more hypertension medications may be the only action necessary to achieve proper control of nighttime SBP and DBP, the functional effect being exactly as dietary K supplementation and/or NA restriction, which are known to restore normal dipping [6, 122]. This simple treatment intervention could enhance the effect of therapy not only on sleep-time BP, but also on wake-time BP once an efficient nocturnal excretion of Na is achieved. As a result, the entire circadian BP pattern may be reset to a lower mean level and to a "more normal" day-night variation, simply because natriuresis is enhanced more during the night—the time-of-day for diurnally active persons when it can be most efficient. As discussed in this review, circadian Na excretion patterns also involve multiple, mainly neurohumoral, control mechanisms, such that sleep-time Na retention may entail different underlying pathophysiologic mechanisms. Nonetheless, the pressure-natriuresis mechanism ultimately dominates, due to its infinite gain [121]. Based on the pressure-natriuresis circadian variation, it is possible to explain the remodeling of the BP 24 h pattern of hypertensive patients of differing etiopathophysiologies through the proper administration time of BP-lowering medications.

Discussion and Conclusion

Day/night environmental cycles of temperature and noise; nyctohemeral behavioral patterns of food, liquid, and stimulant consumption, posture, mental stress, and physical activity; and innate circadian rhythms in wakefulness/sleep and autonomic nervous, renin-angiotensin-aldosterone, hypothalamic-pituitary-adrenal, renal hemodynamic, vasoactive peptide, endothelial, and opioid systems are key determinants of the BP 24 h pattern. The current perspective is external environmental and behavioral influences are mostly, if not entirely, responsible for the observed BP 24 h variation of most normotensive and uncomplicated hypertensive persons; nonetheless, as shown here it has a clear genetic basis as substantiated by the large number of determinant endogenous circadian periodicities (Table 6.1) that are orchestrated by the master SCN and peripheral biological time-keeping system. Moreover, that the BP day/night pattern is remodeled with loss of its nocturnal decline in a variety of pathological conditions in which sleep and activity show minor or no alteration constitutes additional evidence of its inherent endogenousity. Finally, studies comparing the BP-lowering and vascular risk sparing effects of BTCT, which entails the ingestion of the full daily dose of one or more conventional long-acting medication(s) approximately 4–8 h prior to the peak time of the SNS, RAAS, and many of the other identified key circadian determinants of the BP 24 h profile, vs. CMTT, which entails the ingestion of medication(s) at or just after the peak time of these determinants, indicate the endogenous circadian components are of much greater importance than previously appreciated. These and other circadian rhythm findings constitute the rationale for the recently proposed guideline recommendations for the management of adult hypertensive patients, including the clinical application of ABPM to diagnose abnormal daytime and sleep-time BP, estimate CV risk, and assess attainment of therapeutic goals [124].

References

1. Hermida RC, Fernández JR, Ayala DE, Artemio A, Smolensky MH. Circadian rhythm of the double (rate-pressure) product in healthy normotensive young adults. Chronobiol Int. 2001;18:477–89.
2. Reinberg A, Ghata J, Halberg F, Gervais P, Abulker C, Dupont J, et al. Rhythmes circadiens du pouls, de la pression areterielle, des excretions urinaires en 17-hydroxycorticosteroides, catecholamines et potassium chez l'hommé adulte sain, actif et au repos. Ann Endocrinol (Paris). 1970;31:277–87.
3. Tuck ML, Stern N, Sowers JR. Enhanced 24-hour norepinephrine and renin secretion in young patients with essential hypertension: relation with the circadian pattern of arterial blood pressure. Am J Cardiol. 1985;55:112–5.
4. Davies AB, Gould BA, Cashman PM, Raftery EB. Circadian rhythm of blood pressure in patients dependent on ventricular demand pacemakers. Br Heart J. 1984;52:93–8.
5. James GD, Pickering TG. The influence of behavioral factors on the daily variation of blood pressure. Am J Hypertens. 1993;6(6 Pt 2):170S–3.
6. Sica DA. What are the influences of salt, potassium, the sympathetic nervous system, and the renin-angiotensin system on the circadian variation in blood pressure? Blood Press Monit. 1999;4 Suppl 2:S9–16.
7. Kario K, Schwartz JE, Pickering TG. Ambulatory physical activity as a determinant of diurnal blood pressure variation. Hypertension. 1999;34(4 Pt 1):685–91.
8. Hermida RC, Calvo C, Ayala DE, Mojón A, López JE. Relationship between physical activity and blood pressure in dipper and nondipper hypertensive patients. J Hypertens. 2002;20: 1097–104.
9. Guessous I, Pruijm M, Ponte B, Ackermann D, Ehret G, Ansermot N, et al. Associations of ambulatory blood pressure with urinary caffeine and caffeine metabolite excretions. Hypertension. 2015;65:691–6.
10. Reppert SM, Weaver DR. Coordination of circadian timing in mammals. Nature. 2002;418: 935e41.
11. Albrecht U. Timing to perfection: the biology of central and peripheral clocks. Neuron. 2012;74:246e60.
12. Arendt J. The pineal gland, circadian rhythms and photoperiodism. In: Redfern P, Lemmer B, editors. Physiology and pharmacology of biological rhythms, Berlin: Springer; Handbook Exp Pharmacol, vol. 125. 1997. p. 375–414.
13. Ekmekcioglu C, Thalhammer T, Humpeler S, Mehrabi MR, Glogar HD, Hölzenbein T, et al. The melatonin receptor subtype MT2 is present in the human cardiovascular system. J Pineal Res. 2003;35:40–4.
14. Peliciari-Garcia RA, Zanquetta MM, Andrade-Silva J, Gomes DA, Barreto-Chaves ML, Cipolla-Neto J. Expression of circadian clock and melatonin receptors within cultured rat cardiomyocytes. Chronobiol Int. 2011;28:21–30.
15. Kitajima T, Kanbayashi T, Saitoh Y, Ogawa Y, Sugiyama T, Kaneko Y, et al. The effects of oral melatonin on the autonomic function in healthy subjects. Psychiatry Clin Neurosci. 2001;55:299–300.
16. Kachi T, Banerji TK, Quay WB. Quantitative cytological analysis of functional changes in adrenomedullary chromaffin cells in normal, sham-operated, and pinealectomized rats in relation to time of day: I. Nucleolar size. J Pineal Res. 1984;1:31–49.
17. Hermida RC, Ayala DE, Fernández JR, Artemio M, Smolensky MH, Fabbian F, et al. Administration-time-differences in effects of hypertension medications on ambulatory blood pressure regulation. Chronobiol Int. 2013;30:280–314.
18. Portaluppi F, Waterhouse J, Minors D. The rhythms of blood pressure in humans. Exogenous and endogenous components and implications for diagnosis and treatment. Ann N Y Acad Sci. 1996;783:1–9.

19. Clark LA, Denby L, Pregibon D, Harshfield GA, Pickering TG, Blank S, et al. A quantitative analysis of the effects of activity and time of day on the diurnal variations of blood pressure. J Chronic Dis. 1987;40:671–81.
20. Sundberg S, Kohvakka A, Gordin A. Rapid reversal of circadian blood pressure rhythm in shift workers. J Hypertens. 1988;6:393–6.
21. McGinty D, Szymusiak R. Neurobiology of sleep. In: Saunders NA, Sullivan CE, editors. Sleep and Breathing. 2nd ed. New York: Marcel Dekker; 1994. p. 1–26.
22. Smolensky MH, Tatar SE, Bergman SA, Losman JG, Barnard CN, Dacso CC, et al. Circadian rhythmic aspects of cardiovascular function. A review by chronobiologic statistical methods. Chronobiologia. 1976;3:337–71.
23. Fabbian F, Smolensky MH, Tiseo R, Pala M, Manfredini R, Portaluppi F. Dipper and non-dipper blood pressure 24-hour patterns: circadian rhythm-dependent physiologic and patho-physiologic mechanisms. Chronobiol Int. 2013;30:17–30.
24. Haus E. Chronobiology in the endocrine system. Adv Drug Deliv Rev. 2007;59:985–1014.
25. Coccagna G, Mantovani M, Brignani F, Manzini A, Lugaresi E. Laboratory note. Arterial pressure changes during spontaneous sleep in man. Electroencephalogr Clin Neurophysiol. 1971;31:277–81.
26. Phillipson EA. Control of breathing during sleep. Am Rev Respir Dis. 1978;118:909–39.
27. Van Someren E. More than a marker: Interaction between the circadian regulation of temperature and sleep, age-related changes, and treatment possibilities. Chronobiol Int. 2000;17:313–54.
28. Krauchi K. The human sleep-wake cycle reconsidered from a thermoregulatory point of view. Physiol Behav. 2007;90:236–45.
29. Talan MI, Engel BT, Kawate R. Overnight increases in haematocrit: additional evidence for a nocturnal fall in plasma volume. Acta Physiol Scand. 1992;144:473–6.
30. Krauchi K, Cajochen C, Wirz-Justice A. Waking up properly: is there a role of thermoregulation in sleep inertia? J Sleep Res. 2004;13:121–7.
31. Suzuki Y, Kuwajima I, Mitani K, Miyao M, Uno A, Matsushita S, et al. The relation between blood pressure variation and daily physical activity in early morning surge in blood pressure. Nippon Ronen Igakkai Zasshi. 1993;30:841–8.
32. Furlan R, Guzzetti S, Crivellaro W, Dassi S, Tinelli M, Baselli G, et al. Continuous 24-hour assessment of the neural regulation of systemic arterial pressure and RR variabilities in ambulant subjects. Circulation. 1990;81:537–47.
33. Somers VK, Dyken ME, Mark AL, Abboud FM. Sympathetic-nerve activity during sleep in normal subjects. N Engl J Med. 1993;328:303–7.
34. van de Borne P, Nguyen H, Biston P, Linkowski P, Degaute JP. Effects of wake and sleep stages on the 24-h autonomic control of blood pressure and heart rate in recumbent men. Am J Physiol. 1994;266(2 Pt 2):H548–54.
35. Lakatua DJ, Haus E, Halberg F, Halberg E, Wendt HW, Sackett-Lundeen LL, et al. Circadian characteristics of urinary epinephrine and norepinephrine from healthy young women in Japan and U.S.A. Chronobiol Int. 1986;3:189–95.
36. Linsell CR, Lightman SL, Mullen PE, Brown MJ, Causon RC. Circadian rhythms of epinephrine and norepinephrine in man. J Clin Endocrinol Metab. 1985;60:1210–5.
37. Sowers JR, Vlachakis N. Circadian variation in plasma dopamine levels in man. J Endocrinol Invest. 1984;7:341–5.
38. Kuchel O, Buu NT. Circadian variations of free and sulfoconjugated catecholamines in normal subjects. Endocr Res. 1985;11:17–25.
39. Yoshida T, Bray GA. Effects of food and light on norepinephrine turnover. Am J Physiol. 1988;254(5 Pt 2):R821–7.
40. Kafka MS, Benedito MA, Roth RH, Steele LK, Wolfe WW, Catravas GN. Circadian rhythms in catecholamine metabolites and cyclic nucleotide production. Chronobiol Int. 1986;3:101–15.
41. Candito M, Pringuey D, Jacomet Y, Souetre E, Salvati E, Ardisson JL, et al. Circadian rhythm in plasma noradrenaline of healthy sleep-deprived subjects. Chronobiol Int. 1992;9:444–7.

42. Veerman DP, Imholz BP, Wieling W, Wesseling KH, van Montfrans GA. Circadian profile of systemic hemodynamics. Hypertension. 1995;26:55–9.
43. Mori H. Circadian variation of haemodynamics in patients with essential hypertension. J Hum Hypertens. 1990;4:384–9.
44. Gordon RD, Wolfe LK, Island DP, Liddle GW. A diurnal rhythm in plasma renin activity in man. J Clin Invest. 1966;45:1587–92.
45. Katz FH, Romfh P, Smith JA. Diurnal variation of plasma aldosterone, cortisol and renin activity in supine man. J Clin Endocrinol Metab. 1975;40:125–34.
46. Liebau H, Manitius J. Diurnal and daily variations of PRA, plasma catecholamines and blood pressure in normotensive and hypertensive man. Contrib Nephrol. 1982;30:57–63.
47. Kool MJ, Wijnen JA, Derkx FH, Struijker Boudier HA, Van Bortel LM. Diurnal variation in prorenin in relation to other humoral factors and hemodynamics. Am J Hypertens. 1994;7:723–30.
48. Veglio F, Pietrandrea R, Ossola M, Vignani A, Angeli A. Circadian rhythm of the angiotensin converting enzyme (ACE) concentration in serum of healthy adult subjects. Chronobiologia. 1987;14:21–5.
49. Cugini P, Letizia C, Scavo D. The circadian rhythmicity of serum angiotensin converting enzyme; phase relation with the circadian cycle of plasma rennin and aldosterone. Chronobiologia. 1988;15:229–32.
50. Gotoh M. Clinical significance of serum angiotensin I-converting enzyme in essential hypertension. Nihon Naibunpi Gakkai Zasshi. 1985;61:1341–57.
51. Li H, Sun NL, Wang J, Liu AJ, Su DF. Circadian expression of clock genes and angiotensin II type 1 receptors in suprachiasmatic nuclei of sinoaortic-denervated rats. Acta Pharmacol Sin. 2007;28:484–92.
52. Stumpe KO, Kolloch R, Vetter H, Gramann W, Kruck F, Ressel C, et al. Acute and long-term studies of the mechanisms of action of beta-blocking drugs in lowering blood pressure. Am J Med. 1976;60:853–65.
53. Lightman SL, James VH, Linsell C, Mullen PE, Peart WS, Sever PS. Studies of diurnal changes in plasma renin activity, and plasma noradrenaline, aldosterone and cortisol concentrations in man. Clin Endocrinol (Oxf). 1981;14:213–23.
54. Brandenberger G, Follenius M, Muzet A, Ehrhart J, Schieber JP. Ultradian oscillations in plasma renin activity: their relationships to meals and sleep stages. J Clin Endocrinol Metab. 1985;61:280–4.
55. Brandenberge G, Follenius M, Simon C, Ehrhart J, Libert JP. Nocturnal oscillations in plasma renin activity and REM-NREM sleep cycles in humans: a common regulatory mechanism? Sleep. 1988;11:242–50.
56. Nicholls MG, Espiner EA, Ikram H, Maslowski AH, Hamilton EJ, Bones PJ. Hormone and blood pressure relationships in primary aldosteronism. Clin Exp Hypertens A. 1984;6:1441–58.
57. Stephenson LA, Kolka MA, Francesconi R, Gonzalez RR. Circadian variations in plasma renin activity, catecholamines and aldosterone during exercise in women. Eur J Appl Physiol. 1989;58:756–64.
58. Richards AM, Nicholls MG, Espiner EA, Ikram H, Cullens M, Hinton D. Diurnal patterns of blood pressure, heart rate and vasoactive hormones in normal man. Clin Exp Hypertens A. 1986;8:153–66.
59. Connell JM, Whitworth JA, Davies DL, Lever AF, Richards AM, Fraser R. Effects of ACTH and cortisol administration on blood pressure, electrolyte metabolism, atrial natriuretic peptide and renal function in normal man. J Hypertens. 1987;5:425–33.
60. Walker BR. Glucocorticoids and cardiovascular disease. Eur J Endocrinol. 2007;157:545–59.
61. Schnackenberg CG, Costell MH, Krosky DJ, Cui J, Wu CW, Hong VS, et al. Chronic inhibition of 11 β-hydroxysteroid dehydrogenase type 1 activity decreases hypertension, insulin resistance, and hypertriglyceridemia in metabolic syndrome. Biomed Res Int. 2013;2013:427640.

62. Girod JP, Brotman DJ. Does altered glucocorticoid homeostasis increase cardiovascular risk? Cardiovasc Res. 2004;64:217–26.
63. Tan KS, McFarlane LC, Lipworth BJ. Effects of oral and inhaled corticosteroid on lymphocyte beta2-adrenoceptor function in asthmatic patients. Br J Clin Pharmacol. 1997;44:565–8.
64. Hamamdzic D, Duzic E, Sherlock JD, Lanier SM. Regulation of alpha 2-adrenergic receptor expression and signaling in pancreatic beta-cells. Am J Physiol. 1995;269(1 Pt 1):E162–71.
65. Langner B, Lemmer B. Circadian changes in the pharmacokinetics and cardiovascular effects of oral propranolol in healthy subjects. Eur J Clin Pharmacol. 1988;33:619–24.
66. Engeland WC, Byrnes GJ, Gann DS. The pituitary-adrenocortical response to hemorrhage depends on the time of day. Endocrinology. 1982;110:1856–60.
67. Whitworth JA, Saines D, Thatcher R, Butkus A, Scoggins BA. Blood pressure and metabolic effects of ACTH in normotensive and hypertensive man. Clin Exp Hypertens A. 1983;5:501–22.
68. Zelinka T, Strauch B, Pecen L, Widimský Jr J. Diurnal blood pressure variation in pheochromocytoma, primary aldosteronism and Cushing's syndrome. J Hum Hypertens. 2004;18:107–11.
69. Biondi B, Klein I. Hypothyroidism as a risk factor for cardiovascular disease. Endocrine. 2004;24:1–13.
70. Dagre AG, Lekakis JP, Papaioannou TG, Papamichael CM, Koutras DA, Stamatelopoulos SF, et al. Arterial stiffness is increased in subjects with hypothyroidism. Int J Cardiol. 2005;103:1–6.
71. Streeten DH, Anderson Jr GH, Howland T, Chiang R, Smulyan H. Effects of thyroid function on blood pressure. Recognition of hypothyroid hypertension. Hypertension. 1988;11:78–83.
72. Kanbay M, Turgut F, Uyar ME, Akcay A, Covic A. Causes and mechanisms of nondipping hypertension. Clin Exp Hypertens. 2008;30:585–97.
73. Dumont M, Ouellette M, Brakier-Gingras L, Lemaire S. Circadian regulation of the biosynthesis of cardiac Met-enkephalin and precursors in normotensive and spontaneously hypertensive rats. Life Sci. 1991;48:1895–902.
74. Shanks MF, Clement-Jones V, Linsell CJ, Mullen PE, Rees LH, Besser GM. A study of 24-hour profiles of plasma met-enkephalin in man. Brain Res. 1981;212:403–9.
75. Wirz-Justice A, Tobler I, Kafka MS, Naber D, Marangos PJ, Borbely AA, et al. Sleep deprivation: effects on circadian rhythms of rat brain neurotransmitter receptors. Psychiatry Res. 1981;5:67–76.
76. Rubin P, Blaschke TF, Guilleminault C. Effect of naloxone, a specific opioid inhibitor, on blood pressure fall during sleep. Circulation. 1981;63:117–21.
77. degli Uberti EC, Salvadori S, Trasforini G, Margutti A, Ambrosio MR, Rossi R, et al. Effect of deltorphin on pituitary-adrenal response to insulin-induced hypoglycemia and ovine corticotropin-releasing hormone in healthy man. J Clin Endocrinol Metab. 1992;75:370–4.
78. degli Uberti EC, Ambrosio MR, Vergnani L, Portaluppi F, Bondanelli M, Trasforini G et al. Stress-induced activation of sympathetic nervous system is attenuated by the selective ∂-opioid receptor agonist deltorphin in healthy man. J Clin Endocrinol Metab. 1993;77:1490–4.
79. Portaluppi F, Montanari L, Bagni B. degli Uberti E, Trasforini G, Margutti A. Circadian rhythms of atrial natriuretic peptide, blood pressure and heart rate in normal subjects. Cardiology. 1989;76:428–32.
80. de los Santos ET, Mazzaferri EL. Calcitonin gene-related peptide: 24-hour profile and responses to volume contraction and expansion in normal men. J Clin Endocrinol Metab. 1991;72:1031–5.
81. Portaluppi F, Vergnani L. degli Uberti EC. Atrial natriuretic peptide and circadian blood pressure regulation: clues from a chronobiological approach. Chronobiol Int. 1993;10:176–89.
82. Portaluppi F, Bagni B. degli Uberti E, Montanari L, Cavallini R, Trasforini G, et al. Circadian rhythms of atrial natriuretic peptide, renin, aldosterone, cortisol, blood pressure and heart rate in normal and hypertensive subjects. J Hypertens. 1990;8:85–95.
83. Portaluppi F, Montanari L, Ferlini M, Vergnani L, D'Ambrosi A, Cavallini AR, et al. Consistent changes in the circadian rhythms of blood pressure and atrial natriuretic peptide in congestive heart failure. Chronobiol Int. 1991;8:432–9.

84. Portaluppi F, Montanari L, Vergnani L, Tarroni G, Cavallini AR, Gilli P, et al. Loss of nocturnal increase in plasma concentration of atrial natriuretic peptide in hypertensive chronic renal failure. Cardiology. 1992;80:312–23.
85. Portaluppi F, Montanari L, Ferlini M, Vergnani L, Bagni B. degli Uberti EC. Differences in blood pressure regulation of congestive heart failure, before and after treatment, correlate with changes in the circulating pattern of atrial natriuretic peptide. Eur Heart J. 1992;13:990–6.
86. Girgis SI, Macdonald DW, Stevenson JC, Bevis PJ, Lynch C, Wimalawansa SJ, et al. Calcitonin gene-related peptide: potent vasodilator and major product of calcitonin gene. Lancet. 1985;2:14–6.
87. Uddman R, Edvinsson L, Ekblad E, Hakanson R, Sundler F. Calcitonin gene-related peptide (CGRP): perivascular distribution and vasodilatory effects. Regul Pept. 1986;15:1–23.
88. Trasforini G, Margutti A, Portaluppi F, Menegatti M, Ambrosio MR, Bagni B, et al. Circadian profile of plasma calcitonin gene-related peptide in healthy man. J Clin Endocrinol Metab. 1991;73:945–51.
89. Portaluppi F, Trasforini G, Margutti A, Vergnani L, Ambrosio MR, Rossi R, et al. Circadian rhythm of calcitonin gene-related peptide in uncomplicated essential hypertension. J Hypertens. 1992;10:1227–34.
90. Itabashi A, Kashiwabara H, Shibuya M, Tanaka, K, Masaoka H, Katayama S, et al. The interaction of calcitonin gene-related peptide with angiotensin II on blood pressure and renin release. J Hypertens. 1988;Suppl 6(4):S418–20.
91. Portaluppi F, Vergnani L, Margutti A, Ambrosio MR, Bondanelli M, Trasforini G, et al. Modulatory effect of the renin-angiotensin system on the plasma levels of calcitonin gene-related peptide in normal man. J Clin Endocrinol Metab. 1993;77:816–20.
92. Trasforin G, Margutti A, Vergnani L, Ambrosio MR, Valentini A, Rossi R, et al. Evidence that enhancement of cholinergic tone increases basal plasma levels of calcitonin gene-related peptide in normal man. J Clin Endocrinol Metab. 1994;78:763–6.
93. Gnaedinger MP, Uehlinger DE, Weidmann P, Sha SG, Muff R, Born W, et al. Distinct hemodynamic and renal effects of calcitonin gene-related peptide and calcitonin in men. Am J Physiol. 1989;257(6 Pt 1):E848–54.
94. Gennari C, Nami R, Agnusdei D, Bianchini C, Pavese G. Acute cardiovascular and renal effects of human calcitonin gene-related peptide. Am J Hypertens. 1989;2(2 Pt 2):45S–9.
95. Otto ME, Svatikova A, Barretto RB, Santos S, Hoffmann M, Khandheria B, et al. Early morning attenuation of endothelial function in healthy humans. Circulation. 2004;109:2507–10.
96. Al Mheid I, Corrigan F, Shirazi F, Veledar E, Li Q, Alexander WR, et al. Circadian variation in vascular function and regenerative capacity in healthy humans. J Am Heart Assoc. 2014;3, e000845.
97. Elherik K, Khan F, McLaren M, Kennedy G, Belch JJ. Circadian variation in vascular tone and endothelial cell function in normal males. Clin Sci (Lond). 2002;102:547–52.
98. Walters JF, Hampton SM, Deanfield JE, Donald AE, Skene DJ, Ferns GA. Circadian variation in endothelial function is attenuated in postmenopausal women. Maturitas. 2006;54:294–303.
99. Kawasaki T, Ueno M, Uezono K, Kawano Y, Abe I, Kawazoe N, et al. The renin-angiotensin-aldosterone system and circadian rhythm of urine variables in normotensive and hypertensive subjects. Jpn Circ J. 1984;48:168–72.
100. Staessen JA, Birkenhager W, Bulpitt CJ, Fagard R, Fletcher AE, Lijnen P, et al. The relationship between blood pressure and sodium and potassium excretion during the day and at night. J Hypertens. 1993;11:443–7.
101. Sirota JH, Baldwin DS, Villareal H. Diurnal variations of renal function in man. J Clin Invest. 1950;29:187–92.
102. Rittig S, Knudsen UB, Nørgaard JP, Pedersen EB, Djurhuus JC. Abnormal diurnal rhythm of plasma vasopressin and urinary output in patients with enuresis. Am J Physiol. 1989;256(4 Pt 2):F664–71.
103. Fukuda M, Urushihara M, Wakamatsu T, Oikawa T, Kobori H. Proximal tubular angiotensinogen in renal biopsy suggests nondipper BP rhythm accompanied by enhanced tubular sodium reabsorption. J Hypertens. 2012;30:1453–9.

104. Kawano Y, Kawasaki T, Kawazoe N, Abe I, Uezono K, Ueno M, et al. Circadian variations of urinary dopamine, norepinephrine, epinephrine and sodium in normotensive and hypertensive subjects. Nephron. 1990;55:277–82.
105. Ueno M, Kawasaki T, Uezono K, Omae T, Matsuoka M. Relationship of urinary kallikrein excretion to renal water and sodium excretion. Metabolism. 1983;32:433–7.
106. Janssen WM, de Zeeuw D, van der Hem GK, de Jong PE. Atrial natriuretic factor influences renal diurnal rhythm in essential hypertension. Hypertension. 1992;20:80–4.
107. Abe K, Sato M, Kasai Y, Haruyama T, Sato K, Miyazaki S, et al. circadian variation in the excretion of urinary kinin, kallikrein and prostaglandin E in normal volunteers. Jpn Circ J. 1981;45:1098–103.
108. Smolensky MH, Hermida RC, Ayala DE, Portaluppi F. Ingestion-time differences in medication effects: Rationale for hypertension chronotherapy to reduce cardiovascular risk and initial proof-of-concept evidence. Curr Pharm Des. 2015;21:773–90.
109. The Heart Outcomes Prevention Evaluation Study Investigators. Effects of angiotensin-converting-enzyme inhibitor, ramipril, on cardiovascular events in high-risk patients. N Engl J Med. 2000;342:145–53.
110. Svensson P, de Faire U, Sleight P, Yusuf S, Ostergren J. Comparative effects of ramipril on ambulatory and office blood pressures: a HOPE Substudy. Hypertension. 2001;38:E28–32.
111. Hermida RC. Ambulatory blood pressure monitoring in the prediction of cardiovascular events and effects of chronotherapy: rationale and design of the MAPEC study. Chronobiol Int. 2007;24:749–75.
112. Hermida RC, Ayala DE, Mojón A, Fernández JR. Influence of circadian time of hypertension treatment on cardiovascular risk: Results of the MAPEC study. Chronobiol Int. 2010;27:1629–51.
113. Hermida RC, Ayala DE, Mojón A, Fernández JR. Cardiovascular risk of essential hypertension: influence of class, number, and treatment-time regimen of hypertension medications. Chronobiol Int. 2013;30:315–27.
114. Hermida RC, Ayala DE, Mojón A, Fernández JR. Decreasing sleep-time blood pressure determined by ambulatory monitoring reduces cardiovascular risk. J Am Coll Cardiol. 2011;58:1165–73.
115. Investigators ABC-H, Roush GC, Fagard RH, Salles GF, Pierdomenico SD. Reboldi G, et al. Prognostic impact from clinic, daytime, and night-time systolic blood pressure in nine cohorts of 13,844 patients with hypertension. J Hypertens. 2014;32:2332–40.
116. Hermida RC, Ayala DE, Mojón A, Fernández JR. Bedtime dosing of antihypertensive medications reduces cardiovascular risk in CKD. J Am Soc Nephrol. 2011;22:2313–21.
117. Hermida RC, Ayala DE, Mojón A, Fernández JR. Influence of time of day of blood pressure-lowering treatment on cardiovascular risk in hypertensive patients with type 2 diabetes. Diabetes Care. 2011;34:1270–6.
118. Ayala DE, Hermida RC, Mojón A, Fernández JR. Cardiovascular risk of resistant hypertension: Dependence on treatment-time regimen of blood pressure-lowering medications. Chronobiol Int. 2013;30:340–52.
119. Zhao P, Xu P, Wan C, Wang Z. Evening versus morning dosing regimen drug therapy for hypertension. Cochrane Database Syst Rev. 2011;10, CD004184.
120. Roush GC, Fapohunda J, Kostis JB. Evening dosing of antihypertensive therapy to reduce cardiovascular events: a third type of evidence based on a systematic review and meta-analysis of randomized trials. J Clin Hypertens (Greenwich). 2014;16:561–8.
121. Guyton AC. Arterial pressure and hypertension. In: Guyton AC, editor. Circulatory physiology. Philadelphia, PA: W.B. Saunders; 1980. p. 44–88.
122. Portaluppi F, Smolensky MH. Perspectives on the chronotherapy of hypertension based on the results of the MAPEC study. Chronobiol Int. 2010;27:1652–67.
123. Fezeu L, Bankir L, Hansel B, Guerrot D. Differential circadian pattern of water and Na excretion rates in the metabolic syndrome. Chronobiol Int. 2014;31:861–7.
124. Hermida R, Smolensky MH, Ayala DE, Fabbian F, Haus E, Fernández JR, et al. Ambulatory blood pressure guidelines for the diagnosis of hypertension and assessment of cardiovascular risk and attainment of treatment goals of adult human beings. Chronobiol Int. 2013;30:1–56.

Chapter 7
Blood Pressure Variability as Elusive Harbinger of Adverse Health Outcomes

Kei Asayama, Fang-Fei Wei, Azusa Hara, Tine W. Hansen, Yan Li, and Jan A. Staessen

Introduction

Blood pressure variability includes short-term, circadian, and long-term components. Assessment of blood pressure variability requires multiple readings obtained within a single or several visits, by conventional office, home or 24-h ambulatory blood pressure monitoring, or by beat-to-beat recordings. Factors that impact visit-to-visit

K. Asayama, M.D., Ph.D.
Studies Coordinating Centre, Research Unit Hypertension and Cardiovascular Epidemiology, KU Leuven Department of Cardiovascular Sciences, University of Leuven, Kapucijnenvoer 35, Box 7001, Leuven 3000, Belgium

Department of Planning for Drug Development and Clinical Evaluation, Tohoku University Graduate School of Pharmaceutical Sciences, Sendai, Japan

Department of Hygiene and Public Health, Teikyo University School of Medicine, Tokyo, Japan

F.-F. Wei, M.D.
Studies Coordinating Centre, Research Unit Hypertension and Cardiovascular Epidemiology, KU Leuven Department of Cardiovascular Sciences, University of Leuven, Kapucijnenvoer 35, Box 7001, Leuven 3000, Belgium

Center for Epidemiological Studies and Clinical Trials and Center for Vascular Evaluations, Shanghai Institute of Hypertension, Shanghai Key Laboratory of Hypertension, Ruijin Hospital, Shanghai Jiaotong University School of Medicine, Shanghai, China

A. Hara, Ph.D.
Studies Coordinating Centre, Research Unit Hypertension and Cardiovascular Epidemiology, KU Leuven Department of Cardiovascular Sciences, University of Leuven, Kapucijnenvoer 35, Box 7001, Leuven 3000, Belgium

T.W. Hansen, M.D., Ph.D.
The Steno Diabetes Center, Gentofte and Research Center for Prevention and Health, Copenhagen, Denmark

© Springer International Publishing Switzerland 2016
W.B. White (ed.), *Blood Pressure Monitoring in Cardiovascular Medicine and Therapeutics*, Clinical Hypertension and Vascular Diseases, DOI 10.1007/978-3-319-22771-9_7

and diurnal blood pressure variability include ethnicity [1], sex [2, 3], age [2, 3], hypertension [3], body mass index [2, 3], use of β-blockers [3, 4], a history of cardiovascular disease [2, 5], renal dysfunction [5], diabetes mellitus [2], a sedentary lifestyle [5], and socioeconomic position [6].

Current indexes of blood pressure variability raise methodological issues related to their poor reproducibility, their interdependence, and their association with the level of blood pressure. Besides methodological problems, the prognostic significance of blood pressure variability remains controversial. Some studies reported associations among end-organ damage [7–9], cardiovascular events [4, 10–15], or mortality [5] with blood pressure variability, whereas others failed to find any association or found variability to be inferior to the level of blood pressure [3, 16, 17]. Several publications proposing that the magnitude of the morning blood pressure surge predicted stroke [18], in particular cerebral hemorrhage [19], or cardiovascular endpoints [20] remained unconfirmed in recently published large-scale observational studies [21–23].

Methodological Issues

Association Between Level and Variability of Blood Pressure

A major problem in many reports is that they assessed target organ damage or the incidence of events as a function of blood pressure variability indexes that are highly dependent on blood pressure level. In the early 1970s, Clement and coworkers assessed blood pressure variability from the standard deviation (SD) and the coefficient of variation (CV) of blood pressure measurements obtained every 5 min for 3 h in 70 untreated hypertensive patients [24]. Sympathetic activity correlated with the level and standard deviation (SD) of blood pressure, but not with the coefficient of variability (CV), a measure of variability that is less dependent on level than the SD [24]. In the 1980s, Mancia and coworker analyzed 24-h continuous intra-arterial recordings and showed that SD correlated positively with blood pressure level and fell with antihypertensive drug treatment, whereas CV was independent of level irrespective of drug intervention [25]. Notwithstanding these initial findings, the

Y. Li, M.D., Ph.D.
Center for Epidemiological Studies and Clinical Trials and Center for Vascular Evaluations, Shanghai Institute of Hypertension, Shanghai Key Laboratory of Hypertension, Ruijin Hospital, Shanghai Jiaotong University School of Medicine, Shanghai, China

J.A. Staessen, M.D., Ph.D. (✉)
VitaK Research and Development, Maastricht University, Maastricht, The Netherlands

Studies Coordinating Centre, Research Unit Hypertension and Cardiovascular Epidemiology, KU Leuven Department of Cardiovascular Sciences, University of Leuven, Kapucijnenvoer 35, Box 7001, Leuven 3000, Belgium
e-mail: jan.staessen@med.kuleuven.be; jan.staessen@maastrichtuniversity.nl

same group used SD rather than CV to estimate the association of blood pressure variability and target organ damage on the incidence of cardiovascular complications [26, 27], and many investigators continue using the SD as the index of blood pressure variability.

Other measures of variability, such as weighted SD [28], the difference between the maximum minus minimum blood pressure level (MMD), and average real variability (ARV) [29], also remain highly dependent on blood pressure level. The weighted SD is the mean of day and night SD values weighted for the number of hours covered by these two periods during ambulatory monitoring. ARV is calculated using the following formula:

$$\text{ARV} = \frac{1}{\sum w_k} \sum_{k=1}^{n-1} w_k \times \left| \text{BP}_{k+1} - \text{BP}_k \right|$$

where n is the number of blood pressure readings, k ranges from 1 to $n-1$, and w_k is the time interval between BP_k and BP_{k+1}. ARV therefore accounts for the order of the measurements and weighs each value according to the measurement interval (Fig. 7.1).

More recently, Rothwell and colleagues proposed blood pressure variability independent of the mean (VIM) as a new index [4, 11]. VIM [4, 11] is the within-subject SD divided by the within-subject mean blood pressure level to the power x and multiplied by the population mean blood pressure level to the power x. The power x is obtained by fitting a curve through a plot of SD against mean blood pressure level, using the model $\text{SD} = a \times \text{mean}^x$, where x is derived by nonlinear regression. The correlation of VIM with the other indexes of blood pressure variability is high [30], but VIM does not correlate with the blood pressure level [4, 11]. VIM therefore allows assessing association of outcome with blood pressure variability with little confounding by blood pressure level [4, 11]. Meanwhile, VIM is tied to the population being examined and cannot be compared across the population because VIM is derived from the distribution of the blood pressure values in each population.

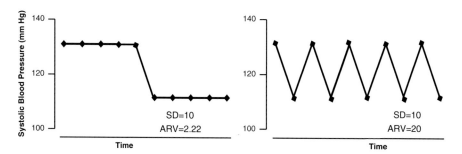

Fig. 7.1 Derivation of the ARV from blood pressure recordings. The ARV averages the absolute differences between consecutive readings and thereby accounts for the order of the blood pressure readings. For distinct blood pressure signals, SD can be the same, whereas ARV is not. ARV denotes average real variability. Reproduced with permission from Hansen TW et al. [17]

Inconsistent Definitions and Poor Reproducibility of Variability Indexes

The morning surge in blood pressure is a good example to highlight how inconsistent definitions and poor reproducibility limit the clinical applicability of indexes of blood pressure variability. In 2003, Kario and colleagues introduced two definitions of the morning surge in blood pressure [18]. The sleep-trough morning surge is the difference between the morning pressure (the average blood pressure during the 2 h after awaking) and the lowest night-time blood pressure (the average of the lowest pressure and the readings immediately preceding and following the lowest value). The pre-awaking morning surge is the difference between the morning blood pressure (the average blood pressure during the 2 h after waking up) and the pre-awakening blood pressure (the average blood pressure during the 2 h before waking up). Other investigators redefined the pre-awakening morning surge as the blood pressure differences over 1-h intervals prior and after awakening or as the blood pressure difference between all readings during sleep and those obtained over 2 h after awakening [31]. Several investigators reported that an exaggerated morning surge predicted outcome [18–20]. However, using a variety of definitions of a single index of blood pressure variability induces confusion and raises the suspicion that definitions were revised to serve the hypothesis to be proven.

In 2008, Wizner and colleagues analyzed the substudy [32] on ambulatory blood pressure monitoring to the Systolic Hypertension in Europe (Syst-Eur) trial [33]. Patients underwent 24-h ambulatory blood pressure monitoring twice before randomization at a 1-month interval and once in 10 months after randomization to double-blind placebo [32]. In 173 patients with repeat recordings within 33 days (median), the short-term repeatability coefficients, expressed as percentages of maximal variation, ranged from 35 to 41 % for the day-time and night-time blood pressure, but from 52 to 75 % for the sleep-trough and the pre-awakening morning surge, higher values represent worse reproducibility. In 219 patients with repeat recordings within 10 months (median), the corresponding long-term estimates ranged from 45 % to 64 % and from 76 % to 83 %, respectively. In categorical analyses of the short-term repeatability of the sleep-trough morning surge and the pre-awakening morning surge, using the 75th percentile as arbitrary cut-off, surging status changed in 28.0 % and 26.8 % of patients (κ-statistic, ≤ 0.33). In the long-term, these proportions were 32.0 % and 32.0 %, respectively (κ-statistic, ≤ 0.20). The κ-statistic indicating moderate reproducibility is 0.4. Stergiou and associates confirmed the poor intra-individual reproducibility of the blood pressure surge in the morning after sleep and in the evening after siesta [31]. Using the four definitions described above [18, 31], the κ-statistics were consistently less than 0.20 [31].

The poor reproducibility of the morning surge and per extension blood pressure variability in general can be ascribed to several factors. Within individuals, blood pressure levels differ between rapid-eye-movement (REM) sleep and non-REM sleep. REM sleep is accompanied by neural sympathetic and electroencephalographic activity similar to that when awake, with distinct cardiovascular effects. In contrast, non-REM sleep is characterized by a suppression in neural sympathetic activity, resulting in a decrease in blood pressure [34]. Ambient temperature and season influence blood pressure levels during sleep and day-time. Cold conditions result in higher surges in the morning blood pressure, later sleep stage transition, and delayed sympathetic activation [35]. The position of the cuff relative to the heart level introduces variability, in particular during sleep, when subjects cannot consciously control body position. Methods of awakening, such as using an alarm clock or natural awakening, affect blood pressure rising at awakening. For patients on antihypertensive drugs, the times of dosing (e.g., morning vs. evening) and the duration of action of the drugs administered influence blood pressure level and the diurnal blood pressure variability, including the magnitude of the morning surge.

Recent Evidence on Blood Pressure Variability

Morning Blood Pressure Surge

Kario and coworkers studied stroke prognosis in 519 patients with hypertension on office measurement (63.6 % women; mean age, 72.5 years) [18]. They assessed silent cerebral infarction by magnetic resonance imaging. For analysis, patients were dichotomized according to the 90th percentile of the sleep-trough distribution (≥55 mmHg). During an average follow-up of 41 months (range, 1–68 months), 44 patients experienced a stroke, of whom two had a silent stroke. The 53 patients in the top tenth of the sleep-trough morning surge distribution, compared with the 466 remaining patients, had a higher baseline prevalence of multiple infarcts (57 % vs. 33 %; $P=0.001$) and a higher stroke incidence (19 % vs. 7.3 %, $P=0.004$) than the 466 remaining patients [18]. The top-ten patients were also older (77 vs. 72 years), had higher office (171 vs. 163 mmHg) and 24-h (143 vs. 138 mmHg) systolic blood pressures, and were followed for a longer period (41 vs. 37 months) [18]. Because of these disparities, 46 patients with exaggerated morning surge were matched with 145 control patients for age and 24-h systolic blood pressure. After matching, the relative risk of stroke in the morning surge compared with the control group was 2.71 (95 % confidence interval [CI], 1.05–7.21; $P=0.047$) [18].

Studies published shortly after this seminal report [18] were not confirmatory [19, 20]. Among 1430 Japanese recruited in the framework of the Ohasama population study, the pre-awakening morning surge in systolic blood pressure marginally predicted cerebral hemorrhage (hazard ratio [HR] per 1–SD increase [+13.8 mmHg], 1.34; CI, 0.95–1.89), whereas the prognostic value for ischemic stroke was far from significant (HR, 0.97; CI, 0.79–1.19). Gosse and colleagues [20] recorded 31 cardiovascular events among 507 White hypertensive patients with a mean follow-up of 92 months [20]. With adjustments applied for age and 24-h systolic blood pressure, the risk of cardiovascular events was not associated with the pre-awakening systolic blood pressure, calculated as the difference of the first systolic blood pressure after standing up minus the last supine systolic blood pressure at awakening. For each 1-mm Hg increase, the estimate of relative risk amounted to 3.3 % (95 % CI, 0.8–5.8 %) [20].

Verdecchia and colleagues [22] investigated the relation between the day–night blood pressure dip and the early morning surge in a cohort of 3012 initially untreated subjects with essential hypertension [22]. The day-to-night reduction in systolic blood pressure showed a direct association ($P<0.0001$) with the sleep-trough ($r=0.56$) and the pre-awakening ($r=0.55$) morning surge in systolic blood pressure [22]. Over a mean follow-up period of 8.4 years, 220 patients died and 268 experienced a cardiovascular event. A blunted sleep-trough (≤ 19.5 mmHg; the lowest quartile) and pre-awakening (≤ 9.5 mmHg) blood pressure surge were both associated with an excess risk of events (HRs, 1.66 [CI, 1.14–2.42] and 1.71 [CI, 1.12–2.71], respectively). However, neither patients with a high sleep-trough (>36.0 mmHg; the highest quartile) nor those with a high pre-awakening (>27.5 mmHg) systolic blood pressure had an increased risk of death or a cardiovascular complication.

Li and colleagues analyzed the International Database on Ambulatory blood pressure monitoring in relation to Cardiovascular Outcomes (IDACO) [21]. This resource included 12 randomly recruited population cohorts with follow-up of both fatal and nonfatal outcomes [21]. During a median follow-up of 11.4 years, 785 deaths and 611 fatal and nonfatal cardiovascular events occurred in 5645 IDACO participants (mean age, 53.0 years; 54.0 % women) [21]. While accounting for covariables and the night-to-day ratio of systolic blood pressure, the HR expressing the risk of all-cause mortality in the top tenth of the sleep-trough morning surge distribution (≥ 37.0 mmHg) compared with the remainder of the study population was 1.32 (CI, 1.09–1.59; Fig. 7.2). For cardiovascular and noncardiovascular mortality, the corresponding HRs were 1.18 (CI, 0.87–1.61) and 1.42 (CI, 1.11–1.80), respectively; for all cardiovascular, cardiac, coronary, and cerebrovascular events, the HRs amounted to 1.30 (CI, 1.06–1.60; Fig. 7.2), 1.52 (CI, 1.15–2.00), 1.45 (CI, 1.04–2.03), and 0.95 (CI, 0.68–1.32), respectively. Analyses of the risk associated with the top tenth of the distribution of the pre-awakening systolic morning surge (≥ 28.0 mmHg) generated similar results (Fig. 7.2). Furthermore, the risk of death or a major cardiovascular event in the 50th percentile group of the sleep-trough morning surge was over 35 % lower ($P<0.01$; Fig. 7.2) than the average risk in the whole study population [21].

In the Pressioni Arteriose Monitorate E Loro Associazioni (PAMELA) study, Bombelli and colleagues [23] analyzed ambulatory blood pressure data of 2011 people. Cardiovascular mortality showed a positive relation with the sleep-trough morning surge in unadjusted analyses (HR, 1.3; CI, 1.1–1.6), which disappeared after adjustment for covariables (HR, 0.9; CI, 0.7–1.1). Cardiovascular mortality, irrespective of adjustment, was unrelated to the pre-awakening morning surge ($P\geq 0.12$). Along similar lines, in this Italian population study [23], there were no differences in the risks of total and cardiovascular mortality when the bottom and top tenths of the distributions of the sleep-trough and pre-awakening morning surge were compared ($P\geq 0.39$).

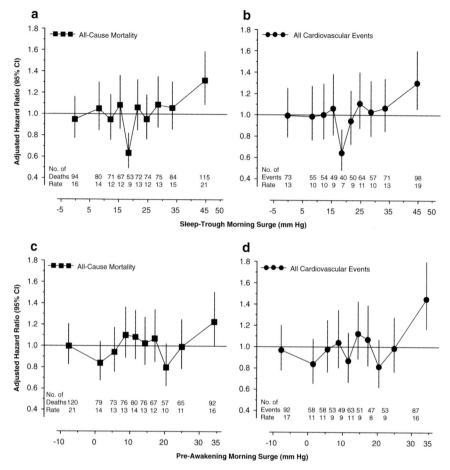

Fig. 7.2 Multivariable-adjusted hazard ratios (95 % CIs) for all-cause mortality (**a, c**) and for all fatal combined with nonfatal cardiovascular events (**b, d**) by ethnic- and sex-specific deciles of the sleep-trough (A and B) and the pre-awakening (**c, d**) morning surge in systolic blood pressure in 5645 participants. The hazard ratios express the risk in deciles compared with the average risk in the whole study population and were adjusted for cohort, sex, age, body mass index, smoking and drinking, serum cholesterol, history of cardiovascular disease, diabetes mellitus, antihypertensive drug treatment, 24-h systolic blood pressure, and the systolic night-to-day blood pressure ratio. The number of events and incidence rates (events per 1000 person–years) are also given for each decile. CI denotes confidence interval. Reproduced with permission from Li Y et al. [21]

Diurnal Blood Pressure Variability

Diurnal blood pressure variability encompasses the day-to-night changes in the blood pressure level and reading-to-reading blood pressure variability in 24-h ambulatory blood pressure recordings. In 1988, O'Brien reported for the first time that an abnormal circadian blood pressure profile with decreased night-time dipping had a more frequent history of stroke [36]. Subsequent studies of populations [37–40] and hypertensive cohorts [41–47] usually corroborated that an elevated nocturnal blood pressure is a harbinger of an unfavorable outcome. In spite of the apparent concordance between these previously published large-scale outcome studies [37–47], several potential limitations required further clarification of the prognostic accuracy of the day-time versus the night-time ambulatory blood pressure. Many studies considered only fatal outcomes [37, 38, 45, 46] or did not have the power to study cause-specific cardiovascular endpoints [37, 38, 40, 44]. Investigators dichotomized the night-to-day blood pressure ratio or applied widely different definitions of dipping status or of the day-time and night-time intervals.

The IDACO consortium therefore assessed the prognostic accuracy of day versus night ambulatory blood pressure in 7458 people enrolled in prospective population studies in Europe, China, and Uruguay [48]. Median follow-up was 9.6 years. Adjusted for day-time blood pressure, confounders, and cardiovascular risk factors, night-time blood pressure predicted ($P<0.01$) total ($n=983$) cardiovascular ($n=387$) and noncardiovascular ($n=560$) mortality [48]. Conversely, adjusted for night-time blood pressure and other covariables, day-time blood pressure predicted only noncardiovascular mortality ($P<0.05$), with lower blood pressure levels being associated with increased risk. Both day-time and night-time blood pressure consistently predicted ($P<0.05$) all cardiovascular events ($n=943$) and stroke ($n=420$) [48]. Adjusted for night-time blood pressure, day-time blood pressure lost prognostic significance for cardiac events ($n=525$; $P≥0.07$). Adjusted for 24-h blood pressure, the night-to-day blood pressure ratio predicted mortality, but not fatal combined with nonfatal events. Participants with a systolic night-to-day blood pressure ratio value of $≥1$ were older, at higher risk of death, and died at an older age than those whose night-to-day ratio was normal ($≥0.80$ to <0.90) [48].

In contrast to commonly held views, the IDACO analysis showed that day-time blood pressure adjusted for night-time blood pressure predicted fatal combined with nonfatal cardiovascular events, except in treated patients, in whom antihypertensive drugs probably reduced blood pressure during the day, but not at night [48]. The increased mortality in patients with higher night-time than day-time blood pressure probably indicated reverse causality. The IDACO findings confirmed that both day-time and night-time blood pressure hold valuable prognostic information [48]. They supported the conclusion that recording blood pressure during the whole day should be the standard in clinical practice. A 2014 IDACO publication [49] highlighted that identification of truly low-risk white coat hypertension requires setting thresholds simultaneously to 24-h, day-time, and night-time blood pressures. In line with the 2007 report [48], Fan and colleagues also demonstrated that isolated nocturnal hypertension predicted cardiovascular outcome even in patients who are normotensive on office or on ambulatory day-time blood pressure measurement [50].

Reading-to-Reading Blood Pressure Variability

Hansen and colleagues also assessed blood pressure variability from the SD and ARV (Fig. 7.3) in 24-h ambulatory recordings in the IDACO population [17]. Higher diastolic ARV in 24-h ambulatory blood pressure recordings predicted

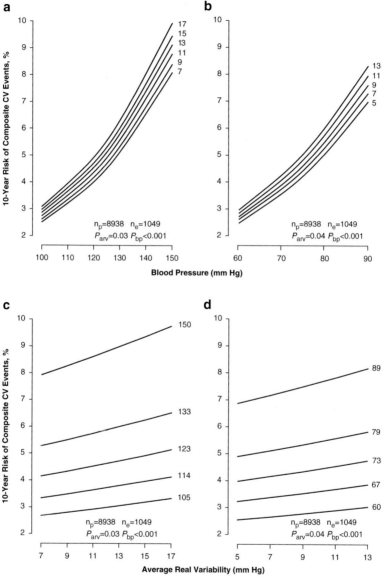

Fig. 7.3 Ten-year absolute risk of combined cardiovascular events in relation to 24-h blood pressure (**a**, **b**) at different levels of systolic and diastolic ARV_{24} (**c**, **d**) at different levels of 24-h systolic and diastolic blood pressure. The analyses were standardized to the distributions (mean or ratio) of cohort, sex, age, 24-h heart rate, body mass index, smoking and drinking, serum cholesterol, history of cardiovascular disease, diabetes mellitus, and treatment with antihypertensive drugs. In panels **a** and **b**, the risk functions span the 5th–95th percentile interval of the 24-h blood pressure and correspond to the 5th, 25th, 50th, 75th, and 95th percentiles of ARV_{24}. In panels **c** and **d**, the risk functions span the 5th–95th percentile interval of ARV_{24} and correspond to the 5th, 25th, 50th, 75th, and 95th percentiles of the 24-h blood pressure. *P*-values are for the independent effect of ARV_{24} (P_{arv}) and 24-h blood pressure (P_{bp}). n_p and n_e indicate the number of participants at risk and the number of events. ARV_{24} denotes average real variability over 24 h. Reproduced with permission from Hansen TW et al. [17]

($P \leq 0.03$) total (HR, 1.13; CI, 1.07–1.19) and cardiovascular (HR, 1.21; CI, 1.12–1.31) mortality and all types of fatal combined with nonfatal endpoints (HR, ≥ 1.07) with the exception of cardiac and coronary events (HR, ≤ 1.02; $P \geq 0.58$). Similarly, higher systolic ARV in 24-h ambulatory recordings predicted ($P < 0.05$) total (HR, 1.11; CI, 1.04–1.18) and cardiovascular (HR, 1.17; CI, 1.07–1.28) mortality and all fatal combined with nonfatal endpoints (HR, ≥ 1.07), with the exception of cardiac and coronary events (HR, ≤ 1.03; $P \geq 0.54$). SD predicted only total and cardiovascular mortality. The incremental cardiovascular risk explained by adding ARV to models already including 24-h ambulatory blood pressure level and other covariables was less than 1 %. This report established that reading-to-reading blood pressure variability is an independent risk factor, significant in a statistical but not in a clinically meaningful manner. It highlighted that the level of the 24-h blood pressure remains the primary blood pressure-related risk factor to account for in clinical practice [17].

Palatini and associates analyzed 7112 untreated hypertensive participants (43.8 % women; mean age, 50.8 years) with day-time and night-time ambulatory blood pressure enrolled in 6 prospective cohorts [51]. During a median of 5.5 years of follow-up, 130 fatal and 455 nonfatal cardiovascular events occurred. In a multivariable-adjusted Cox model, the SD of the night-time systolic blood pressure predicted cardiovascular mortality (HR, 1.48; CI, 1.20–1.84) and morbidity (HR, 1.83; CI, 1.17–2.86), whereas SD of day-time systolic blood pressure did not ($P \geq 0.096$). They proposed as optimal cutoff limits for the night-time SD 12.2 mmHg systolic and 7.9 mmHg diastolic. Participants above these arbitrary thresholds had a 41–132 % higher risk of a composite cardiovascular endpoint than those below these cut-off limits ($P \leq 0.028$). As outlined above, SD as an index of blood pressure variability is closely correlated with blood pressure level. The authors stated that they obtained similar results if they used CV instead of SD, but did not show the data [51].

Within-Visit and Between-Visit Blood Pressure Variability in a Prospective Study

In a randomly recruited Flemish population sample ($n = 2944$; 50.7 % women; mean age, 44.9 years), highly trained observers measured blood pressure five times consecutively at each of two home visits and recorded the incidence of adverse health outcomes in relation to the variability of systolic blood pressure at enrolment [3]. Schutte and colleagues computed VIM, MMD, and ARV for within-visit variability (WVV), between-visit variability, and overall—within-visit combined with between-visit—variability. Over a median follow-up of 12 years, 401 deaths occurred and 311 participants experienced a fatal or nonfatal cardiovascular event. Overall (ten readings over two visits), systolic blood pressure variability averaged (SD) 5.45 (2.82) units for VIM, 15.9 (8.4) mm Hg for MMD, and 4.08 (2.05) mmHg for ARV. In multivariable-adjusted analyses, overall and within- and between-visit blood pressure variability did not predict total or cardiovascular mortality or the composite of any fatal plus nonfatal cardiovascular endpoint. For instance, the HRs for all cardiovascular events combined in relation to overall variability as captured by VIM, MMD, and ARV were 1.05 (CI, 0.96–1.15), 1.06 (CI, 0.96–1.16), and 1.08 (CI, 0.98–1.19), respectively. By contrast, mean systolic blood pressure level was a significant predictor of all endpoints under study, independent of blood pressure variability [3]. These findings suggest that, in the general population, within-subject blood pressure variability does not have any prognostic significance over and beyond systolic blood pressure level [3].

Within-Visit and Between-Visit Blood Pressure Variability in Syst-Eur

Results from randomized clinical trials constitute the strongest evidence for the role and reversibility of any cardiovascular risk factor. In the Syst-Eur trial, Hara and colleagues investigated whether systolic blood pressure variability determines prognosis over and beyond level. Using a double-blind design, 4695 patients ($\geq$60 years) with isolated systolic hypertension (160–219/<95 mmHg) were randomly allocated to active treatment or matching placebo. Active treatment consisted of nitrendipine (10–40 mg/day) with possible addition of enalapril (5–20 mg/day) and/or hydrochlorothiazide (12.5–25.0 mg/day) [52, 53]. They assessed whether on-treatment systolic blood pressure level, visit-to-visit VIM, or WVV predicted total ($n = 286$) or cardiovascular ($n = 150$) mortality or cardiovascular ($n = 347$), cerebrovascular ($n = 133$), or cardiac ($n = 217$) endpoints [54].

Before randomization, patients of the placebo and active-treatment groups had similar characteristics. Of 4695 participants, 3138 (66.8 %) were women. Age averaged 70.2 years and blood pressure 173.8 mmHg systolic and 85.5 mmHg diastolic. Assessed during the run-in period, visit-to-visit blood pressure variability, as captured by SD (mean, 6.4 mmHg), CV (3.65), MMD (12.1 mmHg), and ARV (7.2 mmHg), increased across fourths of the distribution of systolic blood pressure before randomization ($P < 0.0001$). WVV (mean, 3.4 mmHg) during the run-in period also increased with higher systolic blood pressure ($P < 0.0001$), whereas VIM (6.3 units) did not increase with higher run-in systolic blood pressure ($P = 0.084$) [54]. In all 4695 patients, the correlation coefficients of VIM with systolic blood pressure level were 0.01 ($P = 0.59$) during the run-in period and -0.01 ($P = 0.75$) during follow-up after randomization.

At 2 years (median follow-up), active treatment lowered systolic blood pressure by 10.5 mmHg ($P < 0.0001$) more than placebo, whereas the between-group differences in blood pressure variability were not significant, averaging 0.29 units ($P = 0.20$) for VIM and 0.07 mmHg ($P = 0.47$) for WVV (Fig. 7.4) [54]. Active treatment reduced ($P \leq 0.048$) cardiovascular (-28 %), cerebrovascular (-40 %), and cardiac (-24 %) endpoints. In analyses dichotomized by the median, patients with low vs. high VIM had similar event rates ($P \geq 0.14$). Low vs. high WVV was not associated with event rates ($P \geq 0.095$), except for total and cardiovascular mortality on active treatment, which were higher with low WVV ($P \leq 0.0003$). In multivariable-

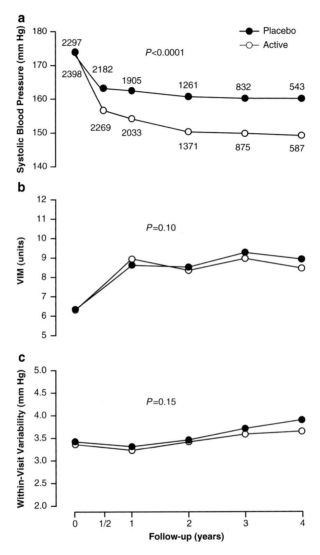

Fig. 7.4 Systolic blood pressure level (**a**), VIM (**b**), and within-visit variability (**c**) at randomization and during follow-up. Values at randomization and at annual intervals during follow-up were derived from at least six blood pressure readings, two at each of three consecutive visits. The blood pressure level at 6 months is the average of four blood pressure readings at two consecutive visits. The computation of variability requires at least three visits. Variability is therefore not plotted at 6 months. *P* values indicate the significance of the average between-group difference throughout follow-up. VIM denotes variability independent of the mean. Reproduced with permission from Hara A et al. [54]

adjusted Cox models, systolic blood pressure level predicted all endpoints ($P \leq 0.0043$), whereas VIM did not predict any adverse outcome ($P \geq 0.058$). Except for an inverse association with total mortality ($P=0.042$), WVV was not predictive ($P \geq 0.15$). Sensitivity analyses, from which the investigators excluded blood pressure readings within 6 months after randomization, 6 months prior to an event, or both, were confirmatory [54]. The double-blind placebo-controlled Syst-Eur trial irrefutably demonstrated that blood-pressure lowering treatment reduces cardiovascular complications by decreasing systolic blood pressure level but not systolic variability and that higher systolic blood pressure level predicted risk without material contribution of variability.

Variability of Self-Measured Home Blood Pressure

Blood pressure variability as captured by self-measurement at home has been assessed for a predictor of target organ damage or cardiovascular complications. Ushigome and colleagues showed significant correlations between macroalbuminuria in type-2 diabetes mellitus and the CV of home blood pressure [55]. On the basis of multivariable-adjusted linear regression analysis including blood pressure level, the same group recently reported that pulse wave velocity was significantly correlated with the SD of three consecutive measurements on one occasion in the morning ($P=0.016$) or evening ($P=0.0099$), but not with the SD of day-to-day home blood pressure ($P \geq 0.78$) [56]. Nishimura and coworkers showed that low-estimated glomerular filtration rate was significantly associated with the SD of home blood pressure [57]. Researchers have been placing expectations on home blood pressure variability as a biomarker for chronic kidney disease [58]. However, as, reported by Okada and colleagues, SD, CV, and ARV of self-measured home blood pressure did not predict the progression of chronic kidney disease [59].

The prognostic significance of self-measured home blood pressure variability was first assessed in the Ohasama population, using the within-participant SD of the morning systolic blood pressure over 26 days (median) [60]. In multivariable-adjusted Cox models also including blood pressure level, the SD was associated with higher risk of total mortality (HR per 1−SD increase of within-participant SD, 1.18; CI, 1.07–1.31), cardiovascular mortality (HR, 1.20; CI, 1.02–1.40), non-cardiovascular mortality (HR, 1.18; CI, 1.04–1.34), stroke mortality (HR, 1.38; CI, 1.12–1.72), but not cardiac mortality (HR, 1.02; CI, 0.89–1.29). The association of blood pressure variability with non-cardiovascular mortality was difficult to interpret, but might reflect reverse causality; subclinical disease leading to greater variability. The Finn-Home investigators assessed the day-to-day variability of the self-measured systolic blood pressure in the morning. The within-participant SD over 7 days predicted total mortality and cardiovascular events [14]. The HRs expressing the incremental risk for a 1−SD increment in variability (3.93 mmHg) were 1.17 (CI, 1.00–1.30; $P=0.03$) and 1.21 (CI, 1.08–1.40; $P=0.006$), respectively [14]. Day-to-day variability in the evening systolic blood pressure was not predictive ($P \geq 0.11$) [14].

Asayama and colleagues explored whether fatal and nonfatal outcomes were associated with the new indexes of blood pressure variability, VIM, ARV, and MMD, derived from the self-measured home blood pressure [61]. They analyzed mortality and stroke risk in 2421 Ohasama residents after excluding high-risk participants with a history of stroke. Participants were asked to record their self-measured home blood pressure for 4 weeks after at least 2 min of rest in the morning within

1 h after awakening and, if applicable, before taking their blood pressure-lowering medications. Participants also obtained the recordings in the evening just before going to bed. Over a median follow-up of 12.0 years, 412 participants died, 139 of cardiovascular causes and 223 had a stroke. In multivariable-adjusted Cox models including morning systolic pressure, VIM and ARV predicted total and cardiovascular mortality in all participants ($P \leq 0.044$), while VIM predicted cardiovascular mortality in treated ($P = 0.014$), but not in untreated ($P = 0.23$) participants. Morning MMD did not predict any endpoint ($P \geq 0.085$). In models already including evening systolic pressure, only VIM predicted cardiovascular mortality in all and in untreated participants ($P \leq 0.046$). When we calculated multivariable-adjusted 10-year risk of cardiovascular mortality and stroke incidence in relation to the mean level and VIM (Fig. 7.5 in all of the participants), both morning and evening systolic blood pressure were consistent predictors ($P \leq 0.032$) with the exception of cardiovascular mortality in treated participants for morning systolic pressure ($P = 0.082$). Being on antihypertensive drug treatment seemed to be the main driver of the significant

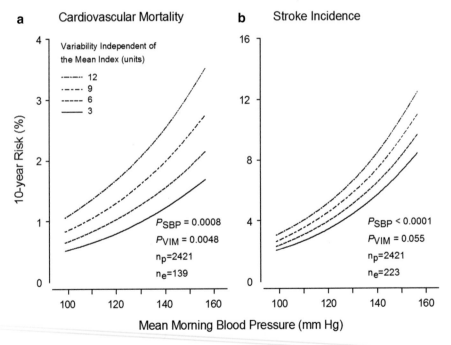

Fig. 7.5 Absolute 10-year risk of cardiovascular mortality (**a**) and stroke incidence (**b**) in relation to the mean level of systolic blood pressure measured at home in the morning in 2421 participants. The analyses were standardized to the distributions (mean or ratio) of sex, age, body mass index, heart rate, smoking and drinking, total cholesterol, diabetes mellitus, history of cardiovascular diseases, and treatment with antihypertensive drugs. Four continuous lines represent the risk independently associated with VIM equal to 3, 6, 9, and 12 units. P values are for the independent effect of SBP (P_{SBP}) and VIM (P_{VIM}). n_p and n_e indicate the number of participants at risk and the number of events. Reproduced with permission from Asayama K et al. [61]

associations between cardiovascular mortality and blood pressure variability [61], whereas the new indexes of blood pressure variability, VIM, derived from self-measured home blood pressure did not incrementally predict outcome over and beyond mean systolic pressure.

Beat-to-Beat Blood Pressure Variability

Beat-to-beat recordings allow capturing blood pressure variability, even over short time intervals [62]. In 256 untreated Chinese patients referred to a hypertension clinic, Wei and colleagues assessed the association of target organ with VIM, MMD, and ARV, determined from 10-min beat-to-beat, 24-h ambulatory, and 7-day home blood pressure recordings [62]. Effect sizes (standardized β) were computed using multivariable regression models. In beat-to-beat recordings, left ventricular mass index ($n=128$) was not ($P \geq 0.18$) associated with systolic blood pressure level, but increased with all three systolic variability indices (+2.97–3.53 g/m [2]; $P < 0.04$). The urinary albumin-to-creatinine ratio increased ($P \leq 0.03$) with systolic blood pressure level (+1.14–1.17 mg/mmol, according to the model) and MMD (+1.18 mg/mmol); and aortic pulse wave velocity increased with systolic blood pressure level (+0.69 m/s; $P < 0.001$). In 24-h recordings, all three indexes of organ damage increased ($P < 0.03$) with systolic blood pressure level, whereas the associations with systolic blood pressure variability were nonsignificant ($P \geq 0.15$) except for an increase in aortic pulse wave velocity ($P < 0.05$) with VIM (+0.16 m/s) and MMD (+0.17 m/s). In home blood pressure recordings, the urinary albumin-to-creatinine ratio (+1.27–1.30 mg/mmol) and aortic pulse wave velocity (+0.36–0.40 m/s) increased ($P < 0.05$) with systolic blood pressure level, whereas all associations of target organ damage with the variability indexes were nonsignificant ($P \geq 0.07$). In summary, while accounting for systolic blood pressure level, associations of target organ damage with systolic blood pressure variability were readily detectable in beat-to-beat recordings, least noticeable in home recordings, with 24-h ambulatory monitoring being informative only for aortic pulse wave velocity [62].

Conclusions

Recent publications [4, 11–13] reviewed elsewhere [63, 64] suggested that clinicians might reduce stroke incidence more by targeting systolic blood pressure variability along with level, preferentially using calcium-channel blockers [4, 11–13, 65], which might result in less blood pressure variability than other antihypertensive drugs classes. These recommendations, not endorsed by current guidelines [66], largely originated from observational population studies [5, 51, 67], or cohort analyses that enrolled high-risk patients with hypertension [4, 11], diabetes mellitus [55–57, 68, 69], a history of stroke or transient ischemic attack [11], or renal failure

[59, 70–73]. Other methodological issues that might have confounded the issue are categorization of continuous variability measures for risk prediction [5, 11], the application of variability indexes that are dependent on blood pressure level [5, 11], and the limitation of endpoints to mortality. While addressing these issues in the aforementioned population studies [3, 17], one was never able to identify blood pressure variability as a clinically meaningful cardiovascular risk factor. In particular, the recent evidence demonstrates that the morning surge is only a weak predictor of cardiovascular risk, attaining significance only in the top tenth of the distribution in studies with large sample size [19–23]. As Bombelli and coworkers concluded, the morning surge *"appears to be an epiphenomenon of 24-hour blood pressure variability,"* and that the morning surge represents only a tiny part of the whole-day blood pressure variability [23].

Although this does not preclude that blood pressure variability remains a target in clinical research, in particular if captured by beat-to-beat recordings [62], the current large international population studies do not support blood pressure variability as a prime target in the management of hypertension. The analysis of the Syst-Eur randomized clinical trial [54], in line with current recommendations, is strong evidence supporting the idea that blood pressure level, not variability, remains center-fold in the primary and secondary prevention of blood pressure-related cardiovascular complications. Blood pressure variability currently remains a research tool that needs further prospective studies with hard endpoints to define potential application, where it might be of use in daily clinical practice.

References

1. White WB. Diagnostic evaluation: ambulatory blood pressure monitoring in clinical hypertension management. J Am Soc Hypertens. 2014;8:939–41.
2. de la Sierra A, Redon J, Banegas JR, Segura J, Parati G, Gorostidi M, de la Cruz JJ, Sobrino J, Llisterri JL, Alonso J, Vinyoles E, Pallarés V, Sarria A, Aranda P, Ruilope LM, Spanish Society of Hypertension Ambulatory Blood Pressure Monitoring Registry Investigators. Prevalence and factors associated with circadian blood pressure patterns in hypertensive patients. Hypertension. 2009;53:466–72.
3. Schutte R, Thijs L, Liu Y, Asayama K, Jin Y, Odili AN, Gu YM, Kuznetsova T, Jacobs L, Staessen JA. Within-subject blood pressure level—not variability - predicts fatal and nonfatal outcomes in a general population. Hypertension. 2012;60:1138–47.
4. Rothwell PM, Howard SC, Dolan E, Dobson JE, Dahlöf B, Poulter NR, Sever PS, on behalf of the ASCOT-BPLA and MRC Trial Investigators. Effects of β blockers and calcium-channel blockers on within-individual variability in blood pressure and risk of stroke. Lancet Neurol. 2010;9:469–80.
5. Muntner P, Shimbo D, Tonelli M, Reynolds K, Arnett DK, Oparil S. The relationship between visit-to-visit variability in systolic blood pressure and all-cause mortality in general population. Findings from NHANES III, 1988 to 1994. Hypertension. 2011;57:160–6.
6. Hickson DA, Diez Roux AV, Wyatt SB, Gebreab SY, Ogedegbe G, Sarpong DF, Taylor HA, Wofford MR. Socioeconomic position is positively associated with blood pressure dipping among African-American adults : the Jackson Heart Study. Am J Hypertens. 2011;24:1015–21.
7. Parati G, Pomidossi G, Albini F, Malaspina D, Mancia G. Relationship of 24-hour blood pressure mean and variability to severity of target-organ damage in hypertension. J Hypertens. 1987;5:93–8.

8. Tatasciore A, Renda G, Zimarino M, Soccio M, Bilo G, Parati G, Schillaci G, De Caterina R. Awake systolic blood pressure variability correlates with target-organ damage in hypertensive subjects. Hypertension. 2007;50:325–32.
9. Matsui Y, Ishikawa J, Eguchi K, Shibasaki S, Shimada S, Kario K. Maximum value of home blood pressure: a novel indocator of target organ damage in hypertension. Hypertension. 2011;57:1087–93.
10. Kikuya M, Hozawa A, Ohokubo T, Tsuji I, Michimata M, Matsubara M, Ota M, Nagai K, Araki T, Satoh H, Ito S, Hisamichi S, Imai Y. Prognostic significance of blood pressure and heart rate variabilities. The Ohasama Study. Hypertension. 2000;36:901–6.
11. Rothwell PM, Howard SC, Dolan E, O'Brien E, Dobson JE, Dahlöf B, Sever PS, Poulter NR. Prognostic significance of visit-to-visit variability, maximum systolic blood pressure, and episodic hypertension. Lancet. 2010;375:895–905.
12. Rothwell PM. Limitations of the usual blood-pressure hypothesis and importance of variability, instability, and episodic hypertension. Lancet. 2010;375:938–48.
13. Webb AJS, Fischer U, Mehta Z, Rothwell PM. Effects of antihypertensive-drug class on interindividual variation in blood pressure and risk of stroke : a systematic review and meta-analysis. Lancet. 2010;375:906–15.
14. Johansson JK, Niiranen TJ, Puukka PJ, Jula AM. Prognostic value of the variability in home-measured blood pressure and heart rate. The Finn-Home study. Hypertension. 2012;59:212–8.
15. Shimbo D, Newman JD, Aragaki AK, LaMonte MJ, Bavry AA, Allison M, Manson JE, Wassertheil-Smoller S. Association between annual visit-to-visit blood pressure variability and stroke in postmenopausal women. Data from the Women's Health Initiative. Hypertension. 2012;60:625–30.
16. Pierdomenico SD, Lapenna D, Di Tommaso R, Di Carlo S, Esposito AL, Di Mascio R, Ballone E, Cuccurullo F, Mezzetti A. Blood pressure variability and cardiovascular risk in treated hypertensive patients. Am J Hypertens. 2006;19:991–7.
17. Hansen TW, Thijs L, Li Y, Boggia J, Kikuya M, Björklund-Bodegård K, Richart T, Ohkubo T, Jeppesen J, Pedersen CT, Dolan E, Kuznetsova T, Stolarz-Skrzypek K, Tikhonoff V, Malyutina S, Casiglia E, Nikitin Y, Lind L, Sandoya E, Kawecka-Jaszcz K, Imai Y, Wang J, Ibsen H, O'Brien E, Staessen JA, for the International Database on Ambulatory Blood Pressure in Relation to Cardiovascular Outcome Investigators. Prognostic value of reading-to-reading blood pressure variability over 24 hours in 8938 subjects from 11 populations. Hypertension. 2010;55:1049–57.
18. Kario K, Pickering TG, Umeda Y, Hoshide S, Hoshide Y, Morinari M, Murata M, Kuroda T, Schwartz JE, Shimada K. Morning surge in blood pressure as predictor of silent and clinical cerebrovascular disease in elderly hypertensives: a prospective study. Circulation. 2003;107:1401–6.
19. Metoki H, Ohkubo T, Asayama K, Obara T, Hashimoto J, Totsune K, Hoshi H, Satoh H, Imai K. Prognostic significance for stroke of a morning pressor surge and a nocturnal blood pressure decline: The Ohasama Study. Hypertension. 2006;47:149–54.
20. Gosse P, Lasserre R, Minifie C, Lemetayer P, Clementy J. Blood pressure surge on rising. J Hypertens. 2004;22:1113–8.
21. Li Y, Thijs L, Hansen TW, Kikuya M, Boggia J, Richart T, Metoki H, Ohkubo T, Pedersen CT, Kuznetsova T, Stolarz-Skrzypek K, Tikhonoff V, Malyutina S, Casiglia E, Nikitin Y, Sandoya E, Kawecka-Jaszcz K, Ibsen H, Imai Y, Wang J, Staessen JA, for International Database on Ambulatory Blood Pressure in Relation to Cardiovascular Outcome Investigators. Prognostic value of the morning blood pressure surge in 5645 subjects from 8 populations. Hypertension. 2010;55:1040–8.
22. Verdecchia P, Angeli F, Mazzotta G, Garofoli M, Ramundo E, Gentile G, Ambrosio G, Reboldi G. Day-night dip and early-morning surge in blood pressure in hypertension: prognostic implications. Hypertension. 2014;60:34–42.
23. Bombelli M, Fodri D, Toso E, Macchiarulo M, Cairo M, Facchetti R, Dell'Oro R, Grassi G, Mancia G. Relationship among morning blood pressure surge, 24-hour blood pressure variability, and cardiovascular outcomes in a white population. Hypertension. 2014;64:943–50.

24. Clement DL, Mussche MM, Vanhoutte G, Pannier R. Is blood pressure variability related to activity of the sympathetic system? Clin Sci. 1979;57:217s–9.
25. Mancia G, Ferrari A, Gregorini L, Parati G, Pomidossi G, Bertinieri G, Grassi G, Zanchetti A. Blood pressure variability in man : its relation to high blood pressure, age and baroreflex sensitivity. Clin Sci (Lond). 1980;59 Suppl 6:401s–4.
26. Parati G, Pomidossi G, Casadei R, Groppelli A, Trazzi S, Di Rienzo M, Mancia G. Role of heart rate variability in the production of blood pressure variability in man. J Hypertens. 1987;5:557–60.
27. Frattola A, Parati G, Cuspidi C, Albini F, Mancia G. Prognostic value of 24-hour blood pressure variability. J Hypertens. 1993;11:1133–7.
28. Bilo G, Giglio A, Styczkiewicz K, Caldara G, Maronati A, Kawecka-Jaszcz K, Mancia G, Parati G. A new method for assessing 24-h blood pressure variability after excluding the contribution of nocturnal blood pressure fall. J Hypertens. 2007;25:2058–66.
29. Mena L, Pintos S, Queipo NV, Aizpúrua JA, Maestre G, Sulbarán T. A reliable index for the prognostic significance of blood pressure variability. J Hypertens. 2005;23:505–11.
30. Levitan EB, Kaciroti N, Oparil S, Julius S, Muntner P. Relationships between metrics of visit-to-visit variability of blood pressure. J Hum Hypertens. 2013;27(10):589–93.
31. Stergiou GS, Mastorantonakis SE, Roussias LG. Intraindividual reproducibility of blood pressure surge upon rising after nighttime sleep and siesta. Hypertens Res. 2014;31:1859–64.
32. Wizner B, Dechering DG, Thijs L, Atkins N, Fagard R, O'Brien E, de Leeuw PW, Parati G, Palatini P, Clement D, Grodzicki T, Kario K, Staessen JA. Short-term and long-term reproducibility of the morning blood pressure in older patients with isolated systolic hypertension. J Hypertens. 2008;26:1328–35.
33. Staessen JA, Fagard R, Thijs L, Celis H, Arabidze GG, Birkenhager WH, Bulpitt CJ, de Leeuw PW, Dollery CT, Fletcher AE, Forette F, Leonetti G, Nachev C, O'Brien ET, Rosenfeld J, Rodicio JL, Tuomilehto J, Zanchetti A, for the Systolic Hypertension in Europe (Syst-Eur) Trial Investigators. Randomised double-blind comparison of placebo and active treatment for older patients with isolated systolic hypertension [correction published in Lancet 1997, volume 350, November 29, p 1636]. Lancet. 1997;350:757–64.
34. Wolk R, Gami AS, Garcia-Touchard A, Somers VK. Sleep and cardiovascular disease. Curr Probl Cardiol. 2005;30:625–62.
35. Kuo TB, Hong CH, Hsieh IT, Lee GS, Yang CC. Effects of cold exposure on autonomic changes during the last rapid eye movement sleep transition and morning blood pressure surge in humans. Sleep Med. 2014;15:986–97.
36. O'Brien E, Sheridan J, O'Malley K. Dippers and non-dippers. Lancet. 1988;2:397.
37. Ohkubo T, Hozawa A, Yamaguchi J, Kikuya M, Ohmori K, Michimata M, Matsubara M, Hashimoto J, Hoshi H, Araki T, Tsuji I, Satoh H, Hisamichi S, Imai Y. Prognostic significance of the nocturnal decline in blood pressure in individuals with and without high 24-h blood pressure : the Ohasama study. J Hypertens. 2002;20:2183–9.
38. Hansen TW, Jeppesen J, Rasmussen F, Ibsen H, Torp-Pedersen C. Ambulatory blood pressure monitoring and mortality : a population-based study. Hypertension. 2005;45:499–504.
39. Ingelsson E, Björklund K, Lind L, Ärnlöv J, Sundström J. Diurnal blood pressure pattern and risk of congestive heart failure. JAMA. 2006;295:2859–66.
40. Mancia G, Facchetti R, Bombelli M, Grassi G, Sega R. Long-term risk of mortality associated with selective and combined elevation in office, home, and ambulatory blood pressure. Hypertension. 2006;47:846–53.
41. Verdecchia P, Porcellati C, Schillaci G, Borgioni C, Ciucci A, Battistelli M, Guerrieri M, Gatteschi C, Zampi I, Santucci A, Santucci C, Reboldi G. Ambulatory blood pressure. An independent predictor of prognosis in essential hypertension. Hypertension. 1994;24:793–801.
42. Staessen JA. Thijs L, Fagard R, O'Brien ET, Clement D, de Leeuw PW, Mancia G, Nachev C, Palatini P, Parati G, Tuomilehto J, Webster J, for the Systolic Hypertension in Europe Trial Investigators. Predicting cardiovascular risk using conventional vs ambulatory blood pressure in older patients with systolic hypertension. JAMA. 1999;282:539–46.

43. Kario K, Pickering TG, Matsuo T, Hoshide S, Schwartz JE, Shimada K. Stroke prognosis and abnormal nocturnal blood pressure falls in older hypertensives. Hypertension. 2001;38:852–7.
44. Clement DL, De Buyzere ML, De Bacquer DA, de Leeuw PW, Duprez DA, Fagard RH, Gheeraert PJ, Missault LH, Braun JJ, Six RO, Van der Niepen P, O'Brien E, for the Office versus Ambulatory Pressure Study investigators. Prognostic value of ambulatory blood-pressure recordings in patients with treated hypertension. N Engl J Med. 2003;348:2407–15.
45. Dolan E, Stanton A, Thijs L, Hinedi K, Atkins N, McClory S, Den Hond E, McCormack P, Staessen JA, O'Brien E. Superiority of ambulatory over clinic blood pressure measurement in predicting mortality. The Dublin Outcome Study. Hypertension. 2005;46:156–61.
46. Ben-Dov IZ, Kark JD, Ben-Ishay D, Mekler J, Ben-Arie L, Bursztyn M. Predictors of all-cause mortality in clinical ambulatory monitoring. Unique aspects of blood pressue during sleep. Hypertension. 2007;167(19):2116–21.
47. Schwartz GL, Bailey KR, Mosley T, Knopman DS, Jack Jr CR, Canzanello VJ, Turner ST. Association of ambulatory blood pressure with ischemic brain injury. Hypertension. 2007;49:1228–34.
48. Boggia J, Li Y, Thijs L, Hansen TW, Kikuya M, Björklund-Bodegård K, Richart T, Ohkubo T, Kuznetsova T, Torp-Pedersen C, Lind L, Ibsen H, Imai Y, Wang JG, Sandoya E, O'Brien E, Staessen JA, on behalf of the International Database on Ambulatory blood pressure monitoring in relation to Cardiovascular Outcomes (IDACO) investigators. Prognostic accuracy of day versus night ambulatory blood pressure : a cohort study. Lancet. 2007;370:1219–29.
49. Asayama K, Thijs L, Li Y, Gu YM, Hara A, Liu YP, Zhang Z, Wei FF, Lujambio I, Mena LJ, Boggia J, Hansen TW, Björklund-Bodegård K, Nomura K, Ohkubo T, Jeppesen J, Torp-Pedersen C, Dolan E, Stolarz-Skrzypek K, Malyutina S, Casiglia E, Nikitin Y, Lind L, Luzardo L, Kawecka-Jaszcz K, Sandoya E, Filipovský J, Maestre GE, Wang J, Imai Y, Franklin SS, O'Brien E, Staessen JA, on behalf of the Ambulatory blood pressure monitoring in relation to Cardiovascular Outcomes (IDACO) Investigators. Setting thresholds to varying blood pressure monitoring intervals differentially affects risk estimates associated with white-coat and masked hypertension in the population. Hypertension. 2014;64:935–42.
50. Fan HQ, Li Y, Thijs L, Hansen TW, Boggia J, Kikuya M, Björklund-Bodegård K, Richart T, Ohkubo T, Jeppesen J, Torp-Pedersen C, Dolan E, Kuznetsova T, Stolarz-Skrzypek K, Tikhonoff V, Malyutina S, Casiglia E, Nikitin Y, Lind L, Sandoya E, Kawecka-Jaszcz K, Imai Y, Ibsen H, O'Brien E, Wang J, Staessen JA. Prognostic value of isolated nocturnal hypertension on ambulatory measurement in 8711 subjects from 10 populations. J Hypertens. 2010;28:2036–45.
51. Palatini P, Reboldi G, Beilin LJ, Casiglia E, Eguchi K, Imai Y, Kario K, Ohkubo T, Pierdomenico SD, Schwartz JE, Wing L, Verdecchia P. Added predictive value of night-time blood pressure variability for cardiovascular events and mortality: the Ambulatory Blood Pressure–International study. Hypertension. 2014;64:487–93.
52. Staessen JA, Byttebier G, Buntinx F, Celis H, O'Brien ET, Fagard R. for the Ambulatory Blood Pressure Monitoring and Treatment of Hypertension Investigators. Antihypertensive treatment based on conventional or ambulatory blood pressure measurement. A randomized controlled trial. JAMA. 1997;278:1065–72.
53. Staessen JA, Thijs L, Birkenhäger WH, Bulpitt CJ, Fagard R, on behalf of the Syst-Eur Investigators. Update on the Systolic Hypertension in Europe (Syst-Eur) Trial. Hypertension. 1999;33:1476–9.
54. Hara A, Thijs L, Asayama K, Jacobs L, Wang JG, Staessen JA. Randomised double-blind comparison of placebo and active drugs for effects on risks associated with blood pressure variability in the Systolic Hypertension in Europe trial. PLoS One. 2014;9, e103169.
55. Ushigome E, Fukui M, Hamaguchi M, Senmaru T, Sakabe K, Tanaka M, Yamazaki M, Hasegawa G, Nakamura N. The coefficient variation of home blood pressure is a novel factor associated with macroalbuminuria in type 2 diabetes mellitus. Hypertens Res. 2011;34:1271–5.
56. Fukui M, Ushigome E, Tanaka M, Hamaguchi M, Tanaka T, Atsuta H, Ohnishi M, Oda Y, Hasegawa G, Nakamura N. Home blood pressure variability on one occasion is a novel factor associated with arterial stiffness in patients with type 2 diabetes. Hypertens Res. 2013;36:219–25.

57. Nishimura M, Kato Y, Tanaka T, Todo R, Tone A, Yamada K, Ootani S, Kawabe Y, Yoshizumi H, Hoshiyama Y. Significance of estimating the glomerular filtration rate for the management of hypertension in type 2 diabetes with microalbuminuria. Hypertens Res. 2013;36:705–10.

58. Romero MJ. Home blood pressure variability: a new target to monitor in chronic kidney disease patients with low eGFR? Hypertens Res. 2013;36:673–5.

59. Okada T, Matsumoto H, Nagaoka Y, Nakao T. Association of home blood pressure variability with progression of chronic kidney disease. Blood Press Monit. 2012;17:1–7.

60. Kikuya M, Ohkubo T, Metoki H, Asayama K, Hara H, Obara T, Inoue R, Hoshi H, Hashimoto J, Totsune K, Satoh H, Imai K. Day-by-day variability of blood pressure and heart rate at home as a novel predictor of prognosis. The Ohasama study. Hypertension. 2008;52:1045–50.

61. Asayama K, Kikuya M, Schutte R, Thijs L, Hosaka M, Satoh M, Obara T, Inoue R, Metoki H, Hoshi H, Ohkubo T, Staessen JA, Imai Y. Home blood pressure variability as cardiovascular risk factor in the population of Ohasama. Hypertension. 2013;61:61–9.

62. Wei FF, Li Y, Xi TY, Ding FH, Wang JG, Staessen JA. Beat-to-beat, reading-to-reading, and day-to-day blood pressure variability in relation to organ damage in untreated Chinese. Hypertension. 2014;63:790–6.

63. Parati G, Ochoa JE, Lombardi C, Bilo G. Assessment and management of blood-pressure variability. Nat Rev Cardiol. 2013;10:143–55.

64. Muntner P, Levitan EB. Visit-to-visit variability of blood pressure: current knowledge and future research directions. Blood Press Monit. 2013;18:232–8.

65. Webb AJS, Wilson M, Lovett N, Paul N, Fischer U, Rothwell PM. Response of day-to-day home blood pressure variability by antihypertensive drug class after transient ischemic attack or nondisabling stroke. Stroke. 2014;45:2967–73.

66. Mancia G, Fagard R, Narkiewicz K, Redón J, Zanchetti A, Böhm M, Christiaens T, Cifkova R, De Backer G, Dominiczak A, Galderisi M, Grobbee DE, Jaarsma T, Kirchhof P, Kjeldsen SE, Laurent S, Manolis AJ, Nilsson PM, Ruilope LM, Schmieder RE, Sirnes PA, Sleight P, Viigimaa M, Waeber B, Zannad F. 2013 ESH/ESC Guidelines for the management of arterial hypertension: The Task Force for the management of arterial hypertension of the European Society of Hypertension (ESH) and of the European Society of Cardiology (ESC). Eur Heart J. 2013;34:2159–219.

67. Grove JS, Reed DM, Yano K, Hwang LJ. Variability in systolic blood pressure — a risk factor for coronary heart disease ? Am J Epidemiol. 1997;145:771–6.

68. Hsieh YT, Tu ST, Cho TJ, Chang SJ, Chen JF, Hsieh MC. Visit-to-visit variability in blood pressure strongly predicts all-cause mortality in patients with type 2 diabetes : a 5.5-year prospective analysis. Eur J Clin Invest. 2012;42:245–53.

69. Kilpatrick ES, Rigby AS, Atkin SL. The role of blood pressure variability in the development of nephropathy in type 1 diabetes. Diabetes Care. 2010;33:2442–7.

70. Tozawa M, Iseki K, Yoshi S, Fujiyama K. Blood pressure variability as an adverse prognostic risk factor in end-stage renal disease. Nephrol Dial Transplant. 1999;14:1976–81.

71. Brunelli SM, Thadhani RI, Lynch KE, Ankers ED, Joffe MM, Boston R, Chang Y, Feldman HI. Association between long-term blood pressure variability and mortality among incident hemodialysis patients. Am J Kidney Dis. 2008;52:716–26.

72. Rossignol P, Cridlig J, Lehert P, Kessler M, Zannad F. Visit-to-visit variability is a strong variability is a strong predictor of cardiovascular events in hemodialysis : insights from FOSIDIAL. Hypertension. 2012;60:339–46.

73. McMullan CJ, Lambers Heerspink HJ, Parving HH, Dwyer JP, Forman JP, de Zeeuw D. Visit-to-visit variability in blood pressure and kidney and cardiovascular outcomes in patients with type 2 diabetes and nephropathy: a post hoc analysis from the RENAAL study and the Irbesartan Diabetic Nephropathy Trial. Am J Kidney Dis. 2014;64:714–22.

Chapter 8
Physiologic Control of the Circadian Variability in Blood Pressure

Michel Burnier, Olivier Bonny, and Gregoire Wuerzner

Introduction

Many biological or physiological processes follow a rhythm with a period length which may vary from a fraction of seconds to hours, days, or even seasons [1]. Such rhythmic variations have been described in a vast range of organisms from bacteria to humans [1]. Blood pressure (BP) is a physiological parameter with a high short term variability, but also a well-recognized circadian rhythm with a period length of about 24 h [2, 3]. Indeed continuous measurements of BP have shown that BP rises in the early morning upon awakening, fluctuates during the day depending on mental and physical activities [4], and decreases by 10–15 % during the night while sleeping [3]. A second peak in BP is often seen early in the evening. For many decades, the circadian rhythm of BP has largely been ignored by physicians mainly because BP was measured almost uniquely during medical terms and not outside the physician's office. With the development of ambulatory blood pressure monitoring (ABPM) in the 1980s, more information were gathered on the circadian variations of BP and it became apparent that patients exhibited a variety of patterns in night-time BP leading to the concept of dippers with a normal fall in night-time BP (10–15 %), non-dippers with no decrease in BP at night (<10 %), extreme dippers with a fall in BP greater than 20 % at night, and reverse dippers with an increase in BP at night [5, 6]. In recent years, the clinical interest for the circadian rhythm of BP has grown rapidly with the recognition that the onset of adverse cardiovascular events

M. Burnier, M.D. (✉) • G. Wuerzner, M.D.
Department of Medicine, Service of Nephrology and Hypertension, Centre Hospitalier Universitaire Vaudois, Rue du Bugnon 17, Lausanne 1011, Switzerland
e-mail: michel.burnier@chuv.ch

O. Bonny, M.D., Ph.D.
Department of Pharmacology and Toxicology, Universite de Lausanne, Lausanne, Switzerland

© Springer International Publishing Switzerland 2016
W.B. White (ed.), *Blood Pressure Monitoring in Cardiovascular Medicine and Therapeutics*, Clinical Hypertension and Vascular Diseases,
DOI 10.1007/978-3-319-22771-9_8

demonstrates a circadian pattern which follows quite closely that of BP [7]. Moreover, patients with a blunted or absent circadian rhythm, and in particular those with no dipping at night, are at higher risk of developing cardiovascular, cerebral, or renal complications probably because of a pressure overload during sleep leading to long-term organ dysfunction [8–13]. At last, recent data has suggested that an antihypertensive therapy restoring or maintaining a normal circadian rhythm of BP might be associated with a better control of BP and lesser complications of hypertension. This latter observation is the basis of the concept of chronotherapy in hypertension which has gain a great clinical interest recently [14–16].

The circadian variations of blood pressure are under the influence of numerous physiological and biological factors originating from various organs including the brain, the heart, the kidney, and the neuro-endocrine system. Moreover, environmental factors such as light, temperature, and even air pollution affect the day–night cycle of BP. The purpose of the present article is to review the physiological determinants of the circadian rhythm of BP and how these factors may be modulated clinically in order to maintain a normal circadian rhythm.

Central and Peripheral Clocks and the Circadian Rhythm of Blood Pressure

Classically, circadian variations of BP were explained primarily by the existence of a unique circadian pacemaker located in the suprachiasmatic nucleus of the hypothalamus and coordinating all overt rhythms in the body including blood pressure and heart rate. This view has changed considerably with the discovery that circadian clocks are operative not only centrally (master clock), but also in peripheral tissues and cells where they create a network of peripheral clocks controlling physiological processes [17, 18].

The daily light/dark cycle is the major factor affecting the master clock which then transmit synchronizing signals to clocks located in peripheral tissues [19]. As far as BP rhythm is concerned, evidence has accumulated to suggest that cardiac, vascular, and renal tissues possess local clocks which have similarities to the central clock and may contribute to the circadian variations in BP [20–23]. Metabolic cycles may also contribute to the BP rhythm [24].

At the molecular levels, the central and peripheral clock systems are composed of interconnected feedback loops of gene transcription and translation factors in which the heterodimeric CLOCK/BMAL1 transcription factor complex activates the transcription of repressor clock genes such as the *Period* genes (*Per1* and *Per2*) and *Cryptochrome* genes (*Cry1* and *Cry2*). The products of these genes in turn inhibit CLOCK/BMAL1 transcriptional activity, thereby reducing their own transcription [19] (Fig. 8.1). These core clock components regulate a large number of output genes, either directly or by driving the rhythmic expression of downstream transcription factors, such as albumin D-site-binding protein (DBP), hepatic leukemia factor (HLF), and thyrotroph embryonic factor (TEF), three members of

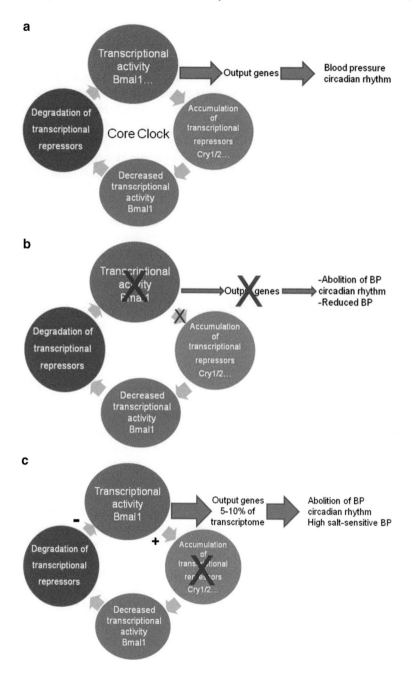

Fig. 8.1 Schematic representation of the impact of Bmal1 and Cry1/Cry2 on the circadian variations in blood pressure in mice. (**a**) Normal situation, (**b**) Bmal1 knockout mice, (**c**) Cry1/Cry2 knockout mice. (**a**) Normal situation. For explanations see text. (**b**) Impact of Bmal1 knockout. Note that the circadian rhythm disappears and BP decreases. (**c**) Impact of dual Cry1/Cry2 knockout. Note that the circadian rhythm disappears and BP increases

the proline- and acidic amino acid-rich basic leucine zipper (PAR bZip) protein family [25]. The majority of studies having assessed the impact of central and peripheral clock systems on the circadian variability of BP have been conducted in genetically engineered mice. Interestingly, in many knock-out mice the single or multiple deletions of clock genes or of their downstream transcription factors have been associated with either a decrease or an increase in BP, but a rather preserved circadian rhythm. However, recent studies have reported a complete disruption of the BP circadian rhythm in *Bmal1* knockout and *Cry1/Cry2* double knockout mice animals, indicating that genetic components of the circadian system are crucial in the maintenance of a diurnal BP rhythm [26, 27]. More recently, evidence has published suggesting that clock gene expression in smooth muscle and not in the brain is involved in maintaining a norma BP circadian rhythm [28]. Moreover, several factors such as salt [29], angiotensin II [30], and catecholamines [26], which also contribute to the circadian rhythm of BP as will be discussed below, have been reported to modulate the expression of clock genes. These results therefore suggest that the central and peripheral clock systems are determinant to maintain circadian variations of BP, but there are definitively other external factors that affect the BP rhythm beyond the central and tissue clocks.

Sleep/Activity Cycle and Circadian Variations of Blood Pressure

As mentioned earlier, the sleep/activity cycle is one of the main determinants of the circadian variations of BP in humans. In fact, many factors explain the reduction of BP associated with sleep. This includes not only the reduction in physical activity, but also the change in body position (supine vs. standing), the reduction in mental stress and activity, and a lower activity of neuro-endocrine systems such as the autonomic nervous system. The reduction in physical activity is a well-recognized factor contributing to the decrease in night-time BP [4]. Indeed, physical activity is not only a determinant of BP variability during daytime accounting for 20–60 % of daytime variability, it is also a major factor affecting the reduction of BP during night-time as demonstrated recently using new techniques to evaluate physical activity such as actimeters [31, 32]. Thus, blunted or absent reductions of night-time BP have been reported in subjects physically active at night such as subjects working during the night or doing night shifts [33, 34]. Interestingly, an increased physical activity during daytime has been associated with a greater dipping of BP at night, an effect which has been attributed to a greater reduction in sympathetic tone during the night [31, 35]. Of note, physical activity appears to affect essentially the changes in night-time systolic BP and to a much lesser degree diastolic BP.

Beyond the lack of nocturnal physical activity, the quality of sleep per se has an important impact on the changes in BP measured during the night. In fact, the definition of the dipping of BP at night is highly dependent on the quality of sleep.

The apparently poor reproducibility of the dipping pattern has been attributed in part to the impact of BP measuring devices on sleep quality [36]. Thus, when the dipping of BP at night was assessed on several occasions using short-term or long-term repeated ambulatory BP monitoring, about 20–40 % of patients classified as non-dippers actually changed category and became dippers on the second assessment [37–39]. The interference of monitoring devices with sleep is certainly contributing to this poor reproducibility, but many other factors may play a role as will be discussed below.

A lack of physiological decrease in night-time BP is a hallmark of patients with sleep disturbances such as sleep apnea. Normally during sleep, there is an inhibition of cardiovascular sympathetic tone resulting in a reduction in heart rate and BP [40]. In patients with obstructive sleep apnea, oxygen desaturation and carbon dioxide retention cause a peripheral vasoconstriction and a rise in systolic BP at the end of the apnea. When a new respiratory cycle starts with the resolution of the airway obstruction, there is an increase in venous return and cardiac output on a background of peripheral vascular vasoconstriction leading to marked increases in BP [41]. The elevated BP and sympathetic activity with each apneic event contribute to the lack of fall in night-time BP in patients with sleep apnea. Among the other factors that contribute to the development of a high BP at night and consequently hypertension in patients with sleep apnea, one must also cite an elevated muscle tone and micro-arousals [41].

Interestingly, the increased sympathetic nerve activity occurring during the night in patients with obstructive sleep apnea persists during daytime because of the activation of chemoreceptors, a decrease in baroreceptor reflex sensitivity, and endothelial dysfunction [42–46]. In addition to these cardiovascular factors, the stimulation of hormonal systems such as the rennin–angiotensin system, aldosterone, or endothelin appears to participate in the increase in night-time BP observed in patients with sleep apnea syndrome [47]. A summary of the pathophysiological link between obstructive sleep apnea and night-time BP and hypertension is presented in Fig. 8.2.

Neuro-hormonal Factors and the Circadian Rhythm of Blood Pressure

Most if not all hormonal systems are characterized by a certain rhythmicity of their secretion during the 24 h of a day. Neuro-hormonal systems have a well-known influence on blood pressure control mediated by direct vascular effects, but also by metabolic and renal effects such as the regulation of renal sodium and water balance. Hence, the day/night profile of neuro-hormonal systems may have an impact on the circadian variations of BP. The diurnal variations in plasma renin activity, aldosterone, angiotensin II, cortisol, ACTH, and melatonin have been well-studied in healthy subjects investigated in standard conditions, but also after sleep deprivation or shifts in sleeping hours. The goal of these studies was not only to

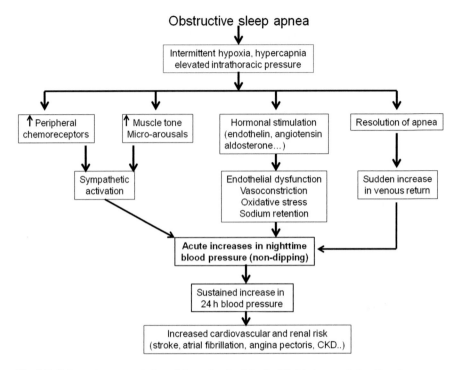

Fig. 8.2 Schematic representation of the pathophysiological link between obstructive sleep apnea and an altered circadian rhythm of blood pressure leading to a high cardiovascular risk

characterize the 24 h profile of each of these hormones, but also to assess the precise role of sleep on the 24 h profile variations [48, 49]. Today, it is well established that plasma renin activity and plasma aldosterone and cortisol levels peak in the early morning upon awakening and decrease progressively during the day. Yet the factors contributing to the diurnal variations of these hormones appear to differ between the rennin–angiotensin–aldosterone system and the adrenocorticotrophic system. Indeed, whereas the former is essentially linked to the changes in sleep processes [48], the variations in plasma cortisol and ACTH are independent of sleep and appear to be modulated primarily by a circadian rhythmicity [49]. Other hormonal systems such as endothelin, atrial natriuretic peptide, or brain natriuretic peptide have been investigated as well and were found to follow a certain rhythm with differences between day and night concentrations. However, it seems that the circadian variations of these hormones are more prominent in disease states such as hypertension, chronic kidney disease, or obstructive sleep apnea than in normal healthy subjects [47, 50, 51]. Whether these systems participate in the generation of a circadian rhythm of BP is not clear and it may well be that most of these hormonal systems, with the exception of cortisol, rather follow the sleep/activity cycle of BP than determine a circadian rhythm of BP.

Among all neuro-endocrine systems, the sympathetic nervous system appears to be one of the main determinants of the circadian rhythm of BP. Both plasma epinephrine and norepinephrine follow a diurnal rhythm in humans, but once again it appears that the circadian variations in epinephrine and norepinephrine cannot be explained by a single controlling influence, the variations in norepinephrine being tightly linked to changes in posture and sleep [52], whereas the variations in plasma epinephrine appear to be under the control of a central oscillator [53]. The activity of the sympathetic nervous system increases markedly in the early morning and then fluctuates depending on posture, physical activity, and mental stress. The activity of sympathetic nervous system has been associated with the circadian variations in vascular tone [54] and the early morning rise in sympathetic tone has been related to the early morning BP surge, which is one of the factors implicated in the increased incidence of cardiovascular events (myocardial infarction, sudden death, stroke) observed in the early morning hours of the day [55–57].

Thus, taken together, the data available so far suggest that some of the neuro-hormonal systems such as the sympathetic nervous system or cortisol have a clear circadian rhythm, which appears to be independent of the sleep/activity cycle and may therefore influence directly the circadian rhythm of BP. As far as other hormonal systems are concerned, the variability of their day/night plasma concentrations appears to be a consequence of the circadian variations in sleeping and active periods rather than a cause of the circadian rhythm of blood pressure.

Sodium Balance and the Circadian Rhythm of Blood Pressure

The renal excretion of water, sodium, and other solutes has also been shown to follow a circadian pattern with higher excretion rates during daytime than during night-time [58]. Recently, Firsov et al. have also demonstrated in mice that renal sodium excretion follows a circadian rhythm and that this rhythm is under the influence of circadian clocks [59]. Their data suggest that the circadian clock affects BP, at least in part, by exerting dynamic control over renal sodium handling. The same authors found that many major parameters of kidney function, including tubular reabsorption and secretion, exhibit strong circadian oscillations that might contribute to the circadian variations in BP [60].

One of the first observations relating sodium excretion and the dipping pattern of BP was made by Uzu et al. in a small group of 42 patients with essential hypertension characterized for their salt sensitivity [61]. In this study, the authors first show that the fall in BP during the night is blunted in salt-sensitive patients and that sodium restriction using a low sodium diet can shift the circadian rhythm of blood pressure from a non-dipper to a dipper pattern [61]. In a subgroup of the same patients, the administration of a thiazide diuretic, which induced a negative sodium balance, also reversed the non-dipping pattern of night-time BP [62]. We assessed whether the night-time BP and the dipping are associated with the circadian pattern of sodium excretion in 325 individuals of African descent from 73 families.

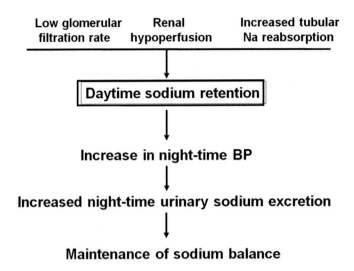

Fig. 8.3 Schematic representation of the effect of a reduced renal capacity to excrete sodium on night-time blood pressure according to the pressure–natriuresis relationship

In each subject, ambulatory BP and daytime and night-time urinary electrolyte excretion were measured simultaneously. In this study, we found indeed that the capacity to excrete sodium during daytime was a significant determinant of nocturnal BP and dipping [63]. Moreover, these data provide some insights on the lack of reproducibility of the dipping pattern in individuals. Indeed, if the night-time dip is influenced by urinary sodium excretion during the day, the decrease in night-time blood pressure will depend on the daytime sodium intake which may vary considerably from day to day. Hence, dietary factors will directly influence the reproducibility of the dipping profile of an individual. Taken together these findings indicated that the ability to excrete sodium during the day is an important determinant of night-time blood pressure as well as of the dipping pattern at least in the normotensive and hypertensive population and particularly among salt-sensitive hypertensive patients.

Later on, the impact of renal function on the night/day ratio of blood pressure and urinary water and electrolyte excretion was investigated. Interestingly, Fukuda et al. found that in patients with renal diseases and a reduced renal function, the lower the glomerular filtration the higher the day/night ratio of blood pressure, urinary sodium excretion, and urinary protein excretion [64]. In this population, the night/day ratio increases mainly in order to eliminate sodium and osmoles rather than water [65]. These data emphasize the importance of glomerular filtration, which affects the capacity to excrete sodium as a determinant of night-time BP. These observations have been summarized in a hypothesis paper of the renal mechanisms of the dipping pattern of BP [66]. According to this hypothesis, the increase in night-time blood pressure represents the classical pressure–natriuresis

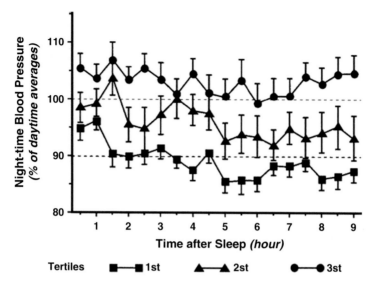

Fig. 8.4 Duration until nocturnal mean arterial pressure begins to fall to <90 % of daytime in patients with chronic kidney disease divided into three tertiles according to creatinine clearance (tertile 1 had the highest clearance and tertile 3 the lowest)—From reference [67])

phenomenon whereby sodium balance is maintained in patients with a limited capacity to excrete salt (Fig. 8.3). In line with this hypothesis, additional observations were made indicating that patients with renal dysfunction require a longer duration until BP falls during the night and that a delayed decrease in night-time BP can be considered as a marker of excessive sodium retention [67, 68] (Fig. 8.4).

Yet, whether these renal mechanisms account for the non-dipping pattern frequently observed in an unselected population has not been conclusively demonstrated so far. Nevertheless, renal sodium retention is a clinical characteristic of several disease conditions associated with a blunted or absence of fall in BP during the night. As shown in Table 8.1, a non-dipping profile of 24-h BP has been reported in several clinical conditions. These include secondary forms of hypertension such as malignant hypertension, primary hyperaldosteronism, Cushing syndrome, or pheochromocytoma [69, 70]. A blunted decrease in night-time blood pressure has also been described in patients with a reduced renal function such as patients with diabetic and nondiabetic nephropathies, congestive heart failure, organ transplantation, or elderly patients [69]. At last, drugs like cyclosporin and non-steroidal anti-inflammatory agents have been shown to increase night-time blood pressure and to blunt the nocturnal dip [69]. These various clinical conditions share a common feature: they are all associated with a reduced capacity of excreting sodium either because of a reduction in glomerular filtration rate (primary or secondary) or because of an increased tubular sodium reabsorption as observed in primary hyperaldosteronism or following the administration of drugs such as NSAIDs, COX-2 inhibitors.

Table 8.1 Diseases
associated with an increased
renal reabsorption of sodium
and impaired decrease in
blood pressure during the
night (non-dipping)

Malignant hypertension
Obstructive sleep apnea syndrome
Pheochromocytoma
Toxemia of pregnancy
Cushing's syndrome
Diabetes (type 1 and 2)
Chronic kidney disease
Renal and cardiac transplantation
Congestive heart failure
Elderly patients with a reduced glomerular filtration
Drugs such as non-steroidal anti-inflammatory agents or calcineurin inhibitors

Overall, these data tend to confirm that sodium intake, and in particular the capacity to excrete salt, is an important determinant of the physiological control of the circadian variations in BP in humans.

Metabolic and Environmental Factors Contributing to the Circadian Variations in Blood Pressure

The impact of sodium intake and excretion on the diurnal variations of BP actually points out the potential roles of the feeding/fast cycle and of the metabolic processes on BP variability [71]. Indeed, depending on the time of food intake, the time-pattern of sodium excretion may vary from day to day or between populations. Moreover, the involvement of gastrointestinal hormones and metabolic factors may vary. The role of the feeding/fasting cycle on BP variability has retained relatively little attention so far. In rats, studies have shown that restricted feeding resulted in an essentially complete loss of coupling of cardiovascular variability to the light cycle. Instead, rats showed increased BP and heart rate and behavioral activity associated with the availability of food [72]. This is not entirely surprising as changes in feeding regimens can profoundly alter the circadian rhythms of body temperature, hormone release, behavioral activity, and peptide levels in the brain [72]. Yet similar observations have not been done in all species and whether the feeding schedule indeed plays a role in variations of BP during day- and night-time remains unclear. Nonetheless, it is clear that several hormonal factors regulating the metabolism such as leptin, adiponectin, insulin, and glucagon follow a circadian rhythm that appears to be independent of plasma glucose concentrations and hence centrally mediated [73, 74]. Whether the circadian production of these metabolic hormones affects BP directly is uncertain. However, disruption of the normal rhythm of some of these hormones has been associated with the development of obesity and metabolic syndrome, which in turn may lead to hypertension and an abnormal dipping of BP during the night.

Interestingly, some specific components of the nutrition may have an impact on BP and its diurnal rhythm. Thus, in a recent cross-sectional study, a high reported caffeine intake was associated with a lower prevalence of hypertension only in non-smokers [75]. In a subsequent analysis of the same subjects, it appeared that caffeine induced a more pronounced reduction in night-time BP than daytime, thus reinforcing the dipping pattern [76]. It is also worth noting that the benefits of caffeine consumption on BP are probably mediated by the renal properties of caffeine metabolites on adenosine receptors, which induce a diuresis and natriuresis. This observation reemphasizes the role of the kidney in the regulation of the circadian pattern of BP.

The circadian variations of BP blood pressure are also influenced by the environment, which induces short-term as well as long-term fluctuations of BP. Thus beyond the light cycle, BP variability is modulated by the external temperature, the altitude and latitude, and the air quality. Studies focusing on external temperature and weather conditions have clearly shown a seasonality of diurnal BP changes and the complexity of the interactions between weather and BP [77, 78]. A more recent study conducted in 1897 patients referred to a hypertension unit using simultaneously a device that enables to monitor personal-level environmental temperature and a 24-h ambulatory BP monitor has actually reported that temperature not only modulates the seasonal variations of BP, but also the everyday BP rhythm, Thus, the authors found that air temperature measured at personal level negatively affects daytime systolic BP, whereas seasonality mainly affects night-time SBP and morning BP surge [79]. These data indicate that external temperature can modify the variability of BP during the day and the night and thereby modulate the circadian rhythm of BP.

Air pollution has been associated with BP in several studies and positive associations between particulate matter and BP have been reported [80, 81]. Recently, we have analyzed the association of exposure to particulate matter with aerodynamic diameters <10 μm (PM10) on the day of examination and ≤7 days before with ambulatory blood pressure and with sodium excretion in 359 adults from the general population using multiple linear regression [82]. We found that short-term exposure to PM10 was significantly associated with higher night-time SBP, DBP, and a blunted nocturnal SBP dipping in adults from the general population. The mechanism whereby air pollution increases BP appears to be linked to an increase in renal sodium reabsorption by the proximal, and interestingly, the sodium reabsorption precedes the increase in night-time BP. Unfortunately, this study investigated only the short-term effects of air pollution on BP and the real impact on a long-term exposure to air pollution remains to be investigated. In any case, air pollution has been clearly associated with an increased risk of cardiovascular events and reduction in air pollution may be associated with a reduced incidence of complications associated with hypertension.

Conclusions

The physiological control of the circadian variations of BP is very complex and involved many apparently redundant systems. Yet experimental studies on the clock control systems have revealed that the day/night variations in BP are very well preserved and maintained throughout species. The recognition of the various factors that can modulate or blunt the circadian rhythm of BP, and in particular abolish the night-time fall in BP leading to a non-dipping pattern, is of high clinical relevance. Indeed, some of these factors can be corrected, for example, by treating sleep apnea or by reducing salt intake leading to a recovery of the normal circadian rhythm of BP. Moreover, a great interest for chronotherapy has emerged in recent years. This therapeutic approach emphasizes the need to maintain or restore a normal day/night rhythm of BP by prescribing drugs not only in the morning, but also in the evening. At last, the first evidence suggesting that patients with normal circadian variations in BP may develop less cardiovascular and renal complications may be strong incentive to pay more attention to the physiological factors involved in the circadian variability of BP.

References

1. Gachon F, Nagoshi E, Brown SA, Ripperger J, Schibler U. The mammalian circadian timing system: from gene expression to physiology. Chromosoma. 2004;113(3):103–12.
2. Agarwal R. Regulation of circadian blood pressure: from mice to astronauts. Curr Opin Nephrol Hypertens. 2010;19(1):51–8.
3. Millar-Craig MW, Bishop CN, Raftery EB. Circadian variation of blood-pressure. Lancet. 1978;1(8068):795–7.
4. Clark LA, Denby L, Pregibon D, et al. A quantitative analysis of the effects of activity and time of day on the diurnal variations of blood pressure. J Chronic Dis. 1987;40(7):671–81.
5. Burnier M, Wuerzner G. What is the hypertension "phenotype"? Curr Cardiovasc Risk Rep 2015;9(9).
6. Routledge F, McFetridge-Durdle J. Nondipping blood pressure patterns among individuals with essential hypertension: a review of the literature. Eur J Cardiovasc Nurs. 2007;6(1):9–26.
7. Weber MA. The 24-hour blood pressure pattern: does it have implications for morbidity and mortality? Am J Cardiol. 2002;89(2A):27A–33.
8. Cuspidi C, Macca G, Sampieri L, et al. Target organ damage and non-dipping pattern defined by two sessions of ambulatory blood pressure monitoring in recently diagnosed essential hypertensive patients. J Hypertens. 2001;19(9):1539–45.
9. Kario K, Matsuo T, Kobayashi H, Imiya M, Matsuo M, Shimada K. Nocturnal fall of blood pressure and silent cerebrovascular damage in elderly hypertensive patients. Advanced silent cerebrovascular damage in extreme dippers. Hypertension. 1996;27(1):130–5.
10. Lurbe E, Redon J, Kesani A, et al. Increase in nocturnal blood pressure and progression to microalbuminuria in type 1 diabetes. N Engl J Med. 2002;347(11):797–805.
11. Davidson MB, Hix JK, Vidt DG, Brotman DJ. Association of impaired diurnal blood pressure variation with a subsequent decline in glomerular filtration rate. Arch Intern Med. 2006;166(8):846–52.
12. Cuspidi C, Sala C, Valerio C, Negri F, Mancia G. Nocturnal hypertension and organ damage in dippers and nondippers. Am J Hypertens. 2012;25(8):869–75.

13. Routledge FS, McFetridge-Durdle JA, Dean CR. Night-time blood pressure patterns and target organ damage: a review. Can J Cardiol. 2007;23(2):132–8.
14. Stranges PM, Drew AM, Rafferty P, Shuster JE, Brooks AD. Treatment of hypertension with chronotherapy: is it time of drug administration? Ann Pharmacother. 2015;49(3):323–34.
15. Carter BL, Chrischilles EA, Rosenthal G, Gryzlak BM, Eisenstein EL, Vander Weg MW. Efficacy and safety of nighttime dosing of antihypertensives: review of the literature and design of a pragmatic clinical trial. J Clin Hypertens (Greenwich). 2014;16(2):115–21.
16. Hermida RC, Ayala DE, Smolensky MH, et al. Chronotherapy improves blood pressure control and reduces vascular risk in CKD. Nat Rev Nephrol. 2013;9(6):358–68.
17. Reppert SM, Weaver DR. Coordination of circadian timing in mammals. Nature. 2002;418(6901):935–41.
18. Schibler U, Sassone-Corsi P. A web of circadian pacemakers. Cell. 2002;111(7):919–22.
19. Lowrey PL, Takahashi JS. Mammalian circadian biology: elucidating genome-wide levels of temporal organization. Annu Rev Genomics Hum Genet. 2004;5:407–41.
20. Tokonami N, Mordasini D, Pradervand S, et al. Local renal circadian clocks control fluid-electrolyte homeostasis and BP. J Am Soc Nephrol. 2014;25(7):1430–9.
21. Young ME. The circadian clock within the heart: potential influence on myocardial gene expression, metabolism, and function. Am J Physiol Heart Circ Physiol. 2006;290(1):H1–16.
22. McNamara P, Seo SB, Rudic RD, Sehgal A, Chakravarti D, FitzGerald GA. Regulation of CLOCK and MOP4 by nuclear hormone receptors in the vasculature: a humoral mechanism to reset a peripheral clock. Cell. 2001;105(7):877–89.
23. Takeda N, Maemura K. Circadian clock and cardiovascular disease. J Cardiol. 2011;57(3):249–56.
24. Cui H, Kohsaka A, Waki H, Bhuiyan ME, Gouraud SS, Maeda M. Metabolic cycles are linked to the cardiovascular diurnal rhythm in rats with essential hypertension. PLoS One. 2011;6(2), e17339.
25. Gachon F. Physiological function of PARbZip circadian clock-controlled transcription factors. Ann Med. 2007;39(8):562–71.
26. Curtis AM, Cheng Y, Kapoor S, Reilly D, Price TS, Fitzgerald GA. Circadian variation of blood pressure and the vascular response to asynchronous stress. Proc Natl Acad Sci U S A. 2007;104(9):3450–5.
27. Masuki S, Todo T, Nakano Y, Okamura H, Nose H. Reduced alpha-adrenoceptor responsiveness and enhanced baroreflex sensitivity in Cry-deficient mice lacking a biological clock. J Physiol. 2005;566(Pt 1):213–24.
28. Xie Z, Su W, Liu S, et al. Smooth-muscle BMAL1 participates in blood pressure circadian rhythm regulation. J Clin Invest. 2015;125(1):324–36.
29. Mohri T, Emoto N, Nonaka H, et al. Alterations of circadian expressions of clock genes in Dahl salt-sensitive rats fed a high-salt diet. Hypertension. 2003;42(2):189–94.
30. Herichova I, Soltesova D, Szantoova K, et al. Effect of angiotensin II on rhythmic per2 expression in the suprachiasmatic nucleus and heart and daily rhythm of activity in Wistar rats. Regul Pept. 2013;187:49–56.
31. Wuerzner G, Bochud M, Zweiacker C, Tremblay S, Pruijm M, Burnier M. Step count is associated with lower nighttime systolic blood pressure and increased dipping. Am J Hypertens. 2013;26(4):527–34.
32. Agarwal R, Light RP. Physical activity is a determinant of circadian blood pressure variation in chronic kidney disease. Am J Nephrol. 2010;31(1):15–23.
33. Yamasaki F, Schwartz JE, Gerber LM, Warren K, Pickering TG. Impact of shift work and race/ethnicity on the diurnal rhythm of blood pressure and catecholamines. Hypertension. 1998;32(3):417–23.
34. Su TC, Lin LY, Baker D, et al. Elevated blood pressure, decreased heart rate variability and incomplete blood pressure recovery after a 12-hour night shift work. J Occup Health. 2008;50(5):380–6.
35. Ling C, Diaz KM, Kretzschmar J, et al. Chronic aerobic exercise improves blood pressure dipping status in African American nondippers. Blood Press Monit. 2014;19(6):353–8.

36. Hinderliter AL, Routledge FS, Blumenthal JA, et al. Reproducibility of blood pressure dipping: relation to day-to-day variability in sleep quality. J Am Soc Hypertens. 2013;7(6):432–9.
37. Cuspidi C, Meani S, Valerio C, et al. Reproducibility of dipping/nondipping pattern in untreated essential hypertensive patients: impact of sex and age. Blood Press Monit. 2007;12(2):101–6.
38. Omboni S, Parati G, Palatini P, et al. Reproducibility and clinical value of nocturnal hypotension: prospective evidence from the SAMPLE study. Study on Ambulatory Monitoring of Pressure and Lisinopril Evaluation. J Hypertens. 1998;16(6):733–8.
39. Hernandez-del Rey R, Martin-Baranera M, Sobrino J, et al. Reproducibility of the circadian blood pressure pattern in 24-h versus 48-h recordings: the Spanish Ambulatory Blood Pressure Monitoring Registry. J Hypertens. 2007;25(12):2406–12.
40. Somers VK, Dyken ME, Mark AL, Abboud FM. Sympathetic-nerve activity during sleep in normal subjects. N Engl J Med. 1993;328(5):303–7.
41. Baguet JP, Narkiewicz K, Mallion JM. Update on Hypertension Management: obstructive sleep apnea and hypertension. J Hypertens. 2006;24(1):205–8.
42. Hedner JA, Wilcox I, Laks L, Grunstein RR, Sullivan CE. A specific and potent pressor effect of hypoxia in patients with sleep apnea. Am Rev Respir Dis. 1992;146(5 Pt 1):1240–5.
43. Narkiewicz K, Montano N, Cogliati C, van de Borne PJ, Dyken ME, Somers VK. Altered cardiovascular variability in obstructive sleep apnea. Circulation. 1998;98(11):1071–7.
44. Narkiewicz K, van de Borne PJ, Pesek CA, Dyken ME, Montano N, Somers VK. Selective potentiation of peripheral chemoreflex sensitivity in obstructive sleep apnea. Circulation. 1999;99(9):1183–9.
45. Carlson JT, Hedner JA, Sellgren J, Elam M, Wallin BG. Depressed baroreflex sensitivity in patients with obstructive sleep apnea. Am J Respir Crit Care Med. 1996;154(5):1490–6.
46. Phillips BG, Narkiewicz K, Pesek CA, Haynes WG, Dyken ME, Somers VK. Effects of obstructive sleep apnea on endothelin-1 and blood pressure. J Hypertens. 1999;17(1):61–6.
47. Moller DS, Lind P, Strunge B, Pedersen EB. Abnormal vasoactive hormones and 24-hour blood pressure in obstructive sleep apnea. Am J Hypertens. 2003;16(4):274–80.
48. Brandenberger G, Follenius M, Goichot B, et al. Twenty-four-hour profiles of plasma renin activity in relation to the sleep-wake cycle. J Hypertens. 1994;12(3):277–83.
49. Charloux A, Gronfier C, Lonsdorfer-Wolf E, Piquard F, Brandenberger G. Aldosterone release during the sleep-wake cycle in humans. Am J Physiol. 1999;276(1 Pt 1):E43–9.
50. Dhaun N, Moorhouse R, MacIntyre IM, et al. Diurnal variation in blood pressure and arterial stiffness in chronic kidney disease: the role of endothelin-1. Hypertension. 2014;64(2):296–304.
51. Jensen LW, Pedersen EB. Nocturnal blood pressure and relation to vasoactive hormones and renal function in hypertension and chronic renal failure. Blood Press. 1997;6(6):332–42.
52. Dodt C, Breckling U, Derad I, Fehm HL, Born J. Plasma epinephrine and norepinephrine concentrations of healthy humans associated with nighttime sleep and morning arousal. Hypertension. 1997;30(1):71–6.
53. Linsell CR, Lightman SL, Mullen PE, Brown MJ, Causon RC. Circadian rhythms of epinephrine and norepinephrine in man. J Clin Endocrinol Metab. 1985;60(6):1210–5.
54. Panza JA, Epstein SE, Quyyumi AA. Circadian variation in vascular tone and its relation to alpha-sympathetic vasoconstrictor activity. N Engl J Med. 1991;325(14):986–90.
55. Muller JE, Stone PH, Turi ZG, et al. Circadian variation in the frequency of onset of acute myocardial infarction. N Engl J Med. 1985;313(21):1315–22.
56. Muller JE, Ludmer PL, Willich SN, et al. Circadian variation in the frequency of sudden cardiac death. Circulation. 1987;75(1):131–8.
57. Marler JR, Price TR, Clark GL, et al. Morning increase in onset of ischemic stroke. Stroke. 1989;20(4):473–6.
58. Staessen JA, Birkenhager W, Bulpitt CJ, et al. The relationship between blood pressure and sodium and potassium excretion during the day and at night. J Hypertens. 1993;11(4):443–7.
59. Nikolaeva S, Pradervand S, Centeno G, et al. The circadian clock modulates renal sodium handling. J Am Soc Nephrol. 2012;23(6):1019–26.

60. Firsov D, Tokonami N, Bonny O. Role of the renal circadian timing system in maintaining water and electrolytes homeostasis. Mol Cell Endocrinol. 2012;349(1):51–5.
61. Uzu T, Ishikawa K, Fujii T, Nakamura S, Inenaga T, Kimura G. Sodium restriction shifts circadian rhythm of blood pressure from nondipper to dipper in essential hypertension. Circulation. 1997;96(6):1859–62.
62. Uzu T, Kimura G. Diuretics shift circadian rhythm of blood pressure from nondipper to dipper in essential hypertension. Circulation. 1999;100(15):1635–8.
63. Bankir L, Bochud M, Maillard M, Bovet P, Gabriel A, Burnier M. Nighttime blood pressure and nocturnal dipping are associated with daytime urinary sodium excretion in African subjects. Hypertension. 2008;51(4):891–8.
64. Fukuda M, Munemura M, Usami T, et al. Nocturnal blood pressure is elevated with natriuresis and proteinuria as renal function deteriorates in nephropathy. Kidney Int. 2004;65(2):621–5.
65. Fukuda M, Motokawa M, Miyagi S, et al. Polynocturia in chronic kidney disease is related to natriuresis rather than to water diuresis. Nephrol Dial Transplant. 2006;21(8):2172–7.
66. Fukuda M, Goto N, Kimura G. Hypothesis on renal mechanism of non-dipper pattern of circadian blood pressure rhythm. Med Hypotheses. 2006;67(4):802–6.
67. Fukuda M, Mizuno M, Yamanaka T, et al. Patients with renal dysfunction require a longer duration until blood pressure dips during the night. Hypertension. 2008;52(6):1155–60.
68. Fukuda M, Uzu T, Kimura G. Duration until nighttime blood pressure fall indicates excess sodium retention. Chronobiol Int. 2012;29(10):1412–7.
69. Burnier M, Coltamai L, Maillard M, Bochud M. Renal sodium handling and nighttime blood pressure. Semin Nephrol. 2007;27(5):565–71.
70. Uzu T, Nishimura M, Fujii T, et al. Changes in the circadian rhythm of blood pressure in primary aldosteronism in response to dietary sodium restriction and adrenalectomy. J Hypertens. 1998;16(12 Pt 1):1745–8.
71. Beard TC, Blizzard L, O'Brien DJ, Dwyer T. Association between blood pressure and dietary factors in the dietary and nutritional survey of British adults. Arch Intern Med. 1997;157(2):234–8.
72. van den Buuse M. Circadian rhythms of blood pressure and heart rate in conscious rats: effects of light cycle shift and timed feeding. Physiol Behav. 1999;68(1-2):9–15.
73. Jauch-Chara K, Hallschmid M, Schmid SM, et al. Plasma glucagon decreases during night-time sleep in Type 1 diabetic patients and healthy control subjects. Diabet Med. 2007;24(6):684–7.
74. Merl V, Peters A, Oltmanns KM, et al. Preserved circadian rhythm of serum insulin concentration at low plasma glucose during fasting in lean and overweight humans. Metabolism. 2004;53(11):1449–53.
75. Guessous I, Dobrinas M, Kutalik Z, et al. Caffeine intake and CYP1A2 variants associated with high caffeine intake protect non-smokers from hypertension. Hum Mol Genet. 2012;21(14):3283–92.
76. Guessous I, Pruijm M, Ponte B, et al. Associations of ambulatory blood pressure with urinary caffeine and caffeine metabolite excretions. Hypertension. 2015;65(3):691–6.
77. Modesti PA. Season, temperature and blood pressure: a complex interaction. Eur J Intern Med. 2013;24(7):604–7.
78. Morabito M, Crisci A, Orlandini S, Maracchi G, Gensini GF, Modesti PA. A synoptic approach to weather conditions discloses a relationship with ambulatory blood pressure in hypertensives. Am J Hypertens. 2008;21(7):748–52.
79. Modesti PA, Morabito M, Massetti L, et al. Seasonal blood pressure changes: an independent relationship with temperature and daylight hours. Hypertension. 2013;61(4):908–14.
80. Brook RD. Why physicians who treat hypertension should know more about air pollution. J Clin Hypertens (Greenwich). 2007;9(8):629–35.
81. Brook RD, Urch B, Dvonch JT, et al. Insights into the mechanisms and mediators of the effects of air pollution exposure on blood pressure and vascular function in healthy humans. Hypertension. 2009;54(3):659–67.
82. Tsai DH, Riediker M, Wuerzner G, et al. Short-term increase in particulate matter blunts nocturnal blood pressure dipping and daytime urinary sodium excretion. Hypertension. 2012;60(4):1061–9.

Chapter 9
Prognostic Value of Ambulatory Blood Pressure Monitoring

Fabio Angeli and Paolo Verdecchia

Introduction

Ambulatory monitoring provides a direct record of blood pressure (BP) throughout the whole day in patients engaged in their usual activities [1]. Frequent readings during wakefulness and sleep enable clinicians to obtain a more precise estimation of a patient's BP, to assess BP levels in the outpatient setting, and to study BP variability and circadian BP profile [1].

Ambulatory BP measurements have high reproducibility, avoid the transient rise in BP in response to a medical environment, and show a remarkable clinical value in assessing the extent of cardiovascular damage and prognosis [1–3]. Furthermore, the evidence that ambulatory BP monitoring gives information over and above conventional BP measurement has been growing steadily over the past 25 years and the rationale for its use in clinical practice is soundly based.

We aimed to specifically address the evidence provided in this regard by cross-sectional and longitudinal studies. We also critically discussed the available data supporting the concept that not only 24-h average BP values, but also specific BP patterns occurring within the 24 h may have clinical relevance.

To this purpose, we searched for clinical studies using research Methodology Filters [4]. The following research terms were used: "BP determination," "hypertension," "masked hypertension," "white coat hypertension," "BP monitoring,

F. Angeli, M.D.
Division of Cardiology and Cardiovascular Pathophysiology,
Hospital "S.M. della Misericordia", Perugia, Italy
e-mail: angeli.internet@gmail.com

P. Verdecchia, M.D. (✉)
Department of Internal Medicine, Hospital of Assisi,
Via Valentin Muller 1, Assisi 06081, Italy
e-mail: verdec@tin.it

© Springer International Publishing Switzerland 2016
W.B. White (ed.), *Blood Pressure Monitoring in Cardiovascular Medicine and Therapeutics*, Clinical Hypertension and Vascular Diseases,
DOI 10.1007/978-3-319-22771-9_9

ambulatory," and "prognosis." We also checked the reference list of identified articles and previous systematic reviews to find other relevant studies.

Office and Ambulatory Blood Pressure

Office-based BP readings are limited in the amount of information they provide, as they represent a single snapshot in time. Conversely, BP readings recorded at pre-defined intervals throughout the 24 h portray a better picture of BP fluctuations [5]. Thus, ambulatory BP is superior to clinic BP to reflect the true pattern of BP during usual daily life. Average ambulatory BP levels generally show a weak association with office BP values taken by a doctor or a nurse. For example, by plotting office BP versus the average daytime ambulatory BP in a large population of patients with office hypertension, for any given value of office BP, the observed ambulatory BP may vary considerably from the predicted value by linear regression equation (Fig. 9.1).

From a practical standpoint, the combined use of office and ambulatory BP identifies four different clinical categories of untreated subjects [6, 7]:

1. Subjects who are normotensive by clinic BP and hypertensive by ambulatory BP (masked hypertension; Fig. 9.2, upper left panel).

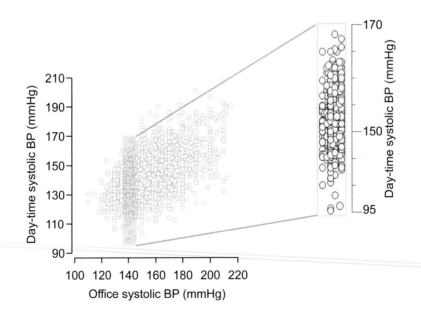

Fig. 9.1 Relation between office and ambulatory systolic blood pressure in untreated hypertensive subjects enrolled in the "Progetto Ipertensione Umbria monitoraggio Ambulatoriale" (PIUMA) study. For any given value of office BP, the observed ambulatory BP varies considerably from the predicted value by linear regression equation. *BP* blood pressure

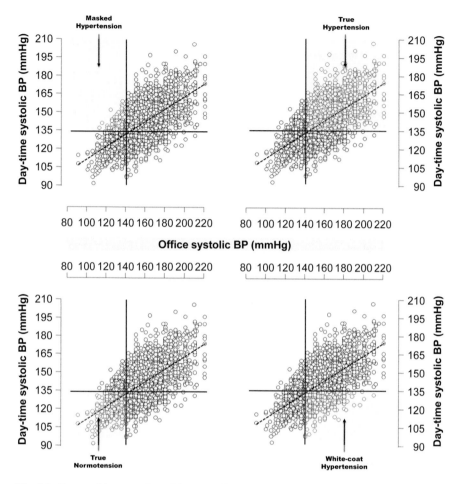

Fig. 9.2 Untreated hypertensive subjects enrolled in the "Progetto Ipertensione Umbria monitoraggio Ambulatoriale" (PIUMA) classified into 4 groups according to office (<140 or ≥140 mmHg) and day-time ambulatory (<135 or ≥135 mmHg) systolic blood pressure levels. *BP* blood pressure

2. Subjects hypertensive by both methods (true hypertension; Fig. 9.2, upper right panel).
3. Subjects normotensive by both methods (true normotension; Fig. 9.2, lower left panel).
4. Subjects who are hypertensive based on office BP and normotensive by ambulatory BP (white coat hypertension, or isolated office hypertension; Fig. 9.2, lower right panel).

Notably, for both masked hypertension and white coat hypertension, the definition should be preferentially restricted to untreated patients. In treated patients, the office-ambulatory BP discrepancy might be conditioned by a different drop in one vs. the other pressure (because of the time of drug administration, the duration of the effect, and other reasons) and patients may have had originally a sustained rather than a white coat or masked hypertension condition.

Masked Hypertension

The phenomenon of masked hypertension (also referred to as "reverse white coat hypertension" or "white coat normotension") is defined as a clinical condition in which a patient's office BP level is normal (<140/90 mmHg), but ambulatory BP readings are in the hypertensive range (for instance; ambulatory daytime BP ≥135/85 mmHg).

This condition underlines the concept that hypertension may not be detected in these subjects on the grounds of traditional BP measurement. Reactivity to daily life stressors and some behavioral factors can selectively influence the phenomenon of masked hypertension. As depicted in a recent algorithm [6] proposed for the identification and management of subjects with masked hypertension (Fig. 9.3), several factors may be involved as potential determinants of masked hypertension [6]. They include pre-hypertension or high-normal BP, smoking status, regular alcohol consumption, male sex, diabetes, obesity, contraceptive use in women, sedentary habits, and exposure to high environmental stress [6].

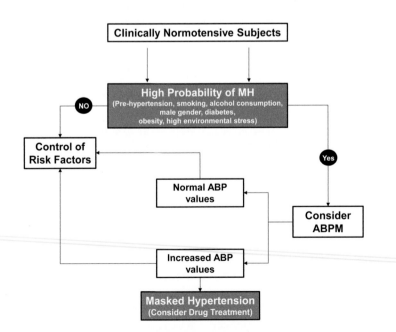

Fig. 9.3 Suggested algorithm for evaluating and treating masked hypertension. *MH* masked hypertension, *ABP* ambulatory blood pressure, *ABPM* ambulatory blood pressure monitoring

According to recent observations from cross-sectional studies, prevalence of masked hypertension ranges between 8 and 38 % [8]. Such variability has been attributed to different patient characteristics, populations studied, and different definitions of masked hypertension. Indeed, some studies were conducted in the general population, other in referred subjects with normotension, other in untreated or treated hypertensive patients, and other in elderly people, or specifically in men [6].

Individuals with masked hypertension present a higher prevalence of organ damage, particularly metabolic risk factors, left ventricular (LV) hypertrophy, increased carotid intima-media thickness, and impaired large artery distensibility when compared with subjects with a normal BP level both inside and outside the clinic or office [9].

Moreover, outcome studies have documented that masked hypertension increases cardiovascular risk, which appears to be comparable to that found in patients with concomitant in-office and out-of-office hypertension [6]. Available evidences show that subjects with masked hypertension have a 1.5–3-fold higher risk of major cardiovascular disease than those with normotension, and their risk is not different from that of patients with sustained hypertension [6, 8].

Some systematic overviews [6, 10, 11] evaluated the prognostic impact of masked hypertension. In this regard, the most recent meta-analysis [6] including 8 cohort studies (Table 9.1) reported quantitative data for cardiovascular prognosis. It showed that the risk of major cardiovascular disease was higher in subjects with masked hypertension than in the normotensive subjects regardless of the definition of masked hypertension based on self-measured BP (hazard ratio [HR]: 2.13; 95 % confidence interval [CI]: 1.35–3.35; $p=0.001$) or 24-h ambulatory BP (HR: 2.00; 95 % CI: 1.54–2.60; $p<0.001$) [6].

The high prevalence of masked hypertension remarks the priority of measuring out-of-office BP in a consistent proportion of people with apparently normal or well-controlled office BP. Nevertheless, the optimal strategy for detecting this condition is not yet clear and it is virtually impossible to screen for masked hypertension the totality of the general population [12]. Thus, it appears reasonable to restrict screening to those individuals at increased risk for cardiovascular complications

Table 9.1 Clinical studies that addressed the adverse prognostic impact of masked hypertension

Study	Selection criteria	MH detected by
Bjorklund et al. [114]	70-year-old men	ABPM
Bobrie et al. [115]	Age ≥60 years	Home BP
Fagard et al. [116]	Age ≥60 years	ABPM
Hansen et al. [39]	Population sample aged 41–72 years	ABPM
Ohkubo et al. [117]	Population sample aged ≥40 years	ABPM
Mancia et al. [118]	Population sample aged 25–74 years	ABPM
Mancia et al. [118]	Population sample aged 25–74 years	Home BP
Pierdomenico et al. [17]	Age: 60 years (mean)	ABPM

ABPM ambulatory blood pressure monitoring, *BP* blood pressure (including patients with kidney disease or diabetes) and with potentially high pre-screen probability of masked hypertension (Fig. 9.3) [6].

Finally, since the cardiovascular risk in masked hypertension seems to be equivalent to that in sustained hypertension, it is reasonable that people with masked hypertension should undergo lifestyle changes and antihypertensive drug therapy targeted on out-of office BP [5, 6, 13] (Fig. 9.3).

White Coat Hypertension

White coat hypertension, also referred to as isolated office hypertension, is generally defined as a persistently elevated office BP ($\geq$140/90 mmHg) with concomitant normal BP outside the office (<130–135/85 mmHg for daytime BP) [1].

Despite a large number of studies, it's not easy to give an unequivocal definition of white coat hypertension based on results of 24-h ambulatory BP monitoring. While the usual definition of elevated office BP is out of discussion ($\geq$140 mmHg for systolic and/or 90 mmHg for diastolic BP) [1–3], the upper reference limits of ambulatory BP used to define white coat hypertension differed across the available studies. The definition was based on both systolic and diastolic values in some studies and solely on diastolic values in others; some studies used the average ambulatory BP during the day and other used the average 24-h ambulatory BP [7, 8].

Such differences might seem clinically unimportant, but the prevalence of white coat hypertension and of the associated cardiac target-organ damage increased markedly when moving from more restrictive (lower) to more liberal (higher) limits of ambulatory BP normalcy over a relatively narrow range [14]. For example, the prevalence of LV hypertrophy, virtually absent below 120 mmHg and very low below 130 mmHg (6 %) for systolic BP, increases to 10.5 % when the limit was set to a more liberal value (140 mmHg) [14].

In addition, modest swings over a narrow range of presumably normal or nearly normal ambulatory BP may result in remarkable differences in the predicted cardiovascular risk [8, 15–18].

In some reports from our group [8, 15, 16], the subset with white coat hypertension was subdivided into two groups with low ambulatory BP values (average daytime ambulatory BP <130/80 mmHg) or values intermediate (between 130/80 and 131/86 mmHg in women or 136/87 mmHg in men). The differences in event-free survival between the normotensive group and the group with white coat hypertension defined restrictively were not significant, whereas the differences between the normotensive group and the white coat hypertension group defined more liberally were significant [8, 15, 16].

These data suggest that a daytime ambulatory BP <130 mmHg systolic and <80 mmHg diastolic may be defined "optimal" to identify individuals with white coat hypertension and low cardiovascular risk (i.e., risk not dissimilar from that of clinically normotensive subjects). To add further insight into the long-term clinical relevance of white coat hypertension, an International Collaborative Study examined individual data from 4 prospective cohort studies from the United States, Italy, and Japan [19]. In this study, 4,406 initially untreated subjects with essential hypertension and 1,549 healthy normotensive controls were followed for a median of 5.4 years [19]. Using the same restrictive ambulatory limits for the definition of white coat hypertension (average awake ambulatory BP <130/80 mmHg), the adjusted HR for stroke was 1.15 (95 % CI: 0.61–2.16) in the white coat hypertension group (p=0.66) and 2.01 (95 % CI: 1.31–3.08) in the ambulatory hypertension group (p=0.001) compared with the normotensive group. However, the incidence of stroke tended to increase in the white coat hypertension group in the long run, and the corresponding hazard curve crossed that of the ambulatory hypertension group by the ninth year of follow-up [19]. These data raised the hypothesis, to be tested in future studies, that white coat hypertension might not be a fully benign condition on the long-term, being a sort of intermediate condition between normotension and established hypertension [20–25].

Although controversy still exists regarding the prognostic impact of this condition, current evidence suggests a treatment based on lifestyle measures in the low-risk stratum of subjects with white coat hypertension under the conditions of restricted definition (daytime ambulatory BP <130/80 mmHg), absence of important comorbid conditions and target organ damage, and adequate follow-up [20–25].

Surrogate Outcome Markers

Surrogate outcome markers may provide a significant contribution to early diagnosis and outcome prediction in hypertension. They are useful noninvasive tools for designing and evaluating therapeutic programs and are increasingly employed as predictive endpoints for treatment [26].

In this context, the association between office BP and hypertensive target organ damage (TOD) usually is relatively poor. Conversely, the closer correlation between TOD and ambulatory BP is well-established regardless of whether the damage is quantified in the heart (LV hypertrophy or dysfunction), in the kidney (microalbuminuria or overt proteinuria), in the brain (cerebral lacunae or white matter lesions as identified by nuclear magnetic resonance), or in the small and large arteries [27].

Left Ventricular Hypertrophy

In the earlier studies by Drayer et al. [28] and Devereux et al. [29], ambulatory BP correlated more closely with LV mass than did office BP. Subsequently, several studies confirmed these results and actually there is a general consensus regarding the closer correlation between LV mass and ambulatory over clinic BP (Fig. 9.4) [30–32].

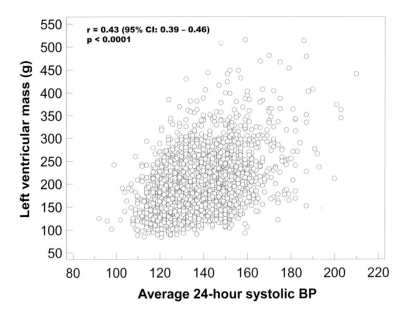

Fig. 9.4 Association between average 24-h systolic blood pressure and left ventricular mass in untreated hypertensive subjects enrolled in the "Progetto Ipertensione Umbria Monitoraggio Ambulatoriale" (PIUMA) study. *BP* blood pressure

More recent data have also provided evidence that serial changes in LV mass show a closer association with the changes in ambulatory BP than with those in clinic BP [33].

In this context, the Study on Ambulatory Monitoring of Pressure and Lisinopril Administration (SAMPLE) evaluated whether in hypertensive patients with a marked echocardiographic LV hypertrophy regression of hypertrophy by a 12-month treatment was more closely related to reduction in 24-h average than in office BP [34]. Treatment consistently reduced office BP, 24-h average BP, and LV mass index. The reductions in office and 24-h BP showed a limited relationship to each other, while only the latter, but not the former, showed a significant relationship with the degree of the LV hypertrophy regression [34].

More recently, a report from the Progetto Ipertensione Umbria Monitoraggio Ambulatoriale (PIUMA) study [33] demonstrated that the changes in LV mass during BP-lowering treatment was significantly associated with the changes in 24-h systolic BP ($r=0.40$), diastolic BP ($r=0.33$), and pulse pressure ($r=0.35$). Weaker associations were found with the changes in clinic BP ($r=0.32$, 0.31 and 0.16, respectively). When 24-h systolic BP and 24-h diastolic BP were forced into the same model, only 24-h systolic BP achieved significance. Similarly, when 24-h systolic BP and 24-h pulse pressure were included into the same model as covariates, only 24-h systolic BP was associated to statistical significance [33].

Other Organ Damages

A large number of studies have investigated whether, on a cross-sectional basis, other organ damages accompanying hypertension are more closely related to ambulatory than to office BP. Microalbuminuria and albumin excretion rate are better predicted by ambulatory BP than by office BP [35].

The European Lacidipine Study on Atherosclerosis (ELSA) [34] demonstrated that either the number of plaques or the size of the thickening was more closely related to 24-h average systolic BP and ambulatory pulse pressure than to the corresponding office values. Indeed, 24-h average systolic BP or pulse pressure values were only second to age in their correlation with carotid artery wall status, their importance being also greater than that seen for serum cholesterol and other components of the lipid profile [34].

Similarly, Asmar et al. found a closer association of arterial distensibility by carotid-femoral pulse velocity with ambulatory BP than with office BP [36].

Taken together, these data provide substantial evidence that the adverse effects of hypertension are related to the average ambulatory BP level to which target organs have been exposed over time and that the more accurate prognostic value of ambulatory over clinic BP is partially due to a more strict association with hypertension-related organ damage.

Ambulatory Blood Pressure Components

Historically, average 24-h, daytime (awake), and night-time (asleep) BP values have been the principal components of the ambulatory BP profile to be investigated as prognostic markers [5, 37]. However, new statistical techniques and the ability to handle large volumes of data with computer-assisted analysis have led to studies that described different aspects of ambulatory readings and several information provided by ambulatory BP monitoring [2, 3].

A new language emerged, with such terms as "nocturnal BP dipping," "morning surge in BP," "ambulatory pulse pressure," "ambulatory arterial stiffness index (AASI)," "average heart rate and heart rate period," "BP variability and variability-ratios," and "BP load" [1, 5, 37]. Health professionals have thus to adjust and incorporate this new knowledge into their clinical practice.

Average Blood Pressure

One of the first studies that addressed the prognostic value of ambulatory BP in a general population sample was the Ohasama study [38]. In this Japanese population (1542 subjects, 565 men and 977 women, aged ≥40 years), the association between BP levels and mortality was more distinctive for the 24-h ambulatory BP than it was for the office BP. Specifically, when both 24-h and office BP values were included in a multivariable Cox model, only the systolic ambulatory BP was related significantly to the increased risk of cardiovascular mortality [38].

Similar results were also observed in a Danish general population cohort [39]. A recent meta-analysis of 7,030 subjects [40] showed that average day-time ambulatory BP was superior to office BP in predicting cardiovascular events. In multivariate-adjusted continuous analyses, both office and ambulatory BP predicted cardiovascular outcome. However, in fully adjusted models, including both office and ambulatory BP, office BP lost its predictive value, whereas systolic day-time ambulatory BP retained their prognostic significance.

More recently, measurement of night-time BP proved to yield additional prognostic data in terms of all-cause mortality and cardiovascular events. In the Dublin Outcome Study [41], a large observational registry of subjects who underwent ambulatory BP before treatment, after correction for several confounders, ambulatory BP was superior to office BP for prediction of cardiovascular mortality and night-time ambulatory BP was the most potent ambulatory BP component for prediction of outcome [41].

A cohort study of 7458 patients in six countries from Europe, Asia, and South America [42] found that both day-time and night-time BP predicted all cardiovascular events. Nevertheless, night-time BP, adjusted for day-time BP, independently predicted total, cardiovascular, and non-cardiovascular mortality [42].

In elderly subjects with isolated systolic hypertension [43], ambulatory systolic BP was a significantly better predictor of cardiovascular and cerebrovascular events than conventional BP measurement. During follow-up, 98 patients developed a major cardiovascular event and after adjustment for age, sex, office BP, active treatment, previous events, cigarette smoking, and residence in the western Europe, the average night-time systolic BP was a significant predictor of total, cardiac, and cerebrovascular future events, whereas the average daytime BP did not yield statistical significance [43]. In this study, for every 10 mmHg increase in night-time systolic BP, the hazard rate for cardiovascular events was 1.20 (95 % CI: 1.08–1.35), while those for cardiac and cerebrovascular events were 1.16 (95 % CI: 1.02–1.33) and 1.31 (95 % CI: 1.06–1.62), respectively [43].

Notably, the interpretation of these averages in clinical practice is obviously dependent on the definition of normalcy. Although reference values for average ambulatory BP are still uncertain for the paucity of data allowing a shared definition dividing up normotension from hypertension, currently accepted limits of normalcy for average ambulatory BP based on several population-based data banks and longitudinal studies in hypertension are reported in Table 9.2 [1].

Table 9.2 Recommended limits of normalcy for ambulatory blood pressure

Limits of normalcy	Value
Average 24-h	<130/80 mmHg
Average day-time	<135/85 mmHg (optimal: <130/80 mmHg)
Average night-time	<120/70 mmHg

Day–Night Blood Pressure Changes

Intra-arterial studies with beat-to-beat recording in ambulant subjects showed that, in normotensive individuals, BP is characterized by a circadian pattern, with values tending to peak during the day-time hours and then falling to a nadir at night [44, 45]. In this context, 24-h ambulatory BP monitoring appears to be a valid tool to investigate the diurnal BP changes associated with the sleep–wake cycle, because it has been demonstrated that intra-arterial 24-h BP profile is similar in the absence and in the presence of concomitant noninvasive BP monitoring [46].

Several studies addressed the issue of the prognostic value of night-time BP and day–night BP changes, particularly in individuals whose nocturnal BP remains elevated [47]. Typically, "non-dippers" are defined by a reduction in BP by less than a given percentage from day to night, and the subjects out of this definition are classified as "dippers." The threshold values for classification ranged from 10 % to 10/5 mmHg, up to 0 % (i.e., no reduction in BP from day to night or a higher BP during night than during day) [48].

Several reports from independent centers showed that prevalence of LV hypertrophy [49], cerebrovascular disease [50, 51], and microalbuminuria [52] was higher among subjects with blunted or abolished fall in BP from day to night than individuals with normal day–night BP difference.

Furthermore, day–night BP changes significantly refined cardiovascular risk stratification above office BP and other traditional risk markers [53, 54].

Yamamoto et al. [55] demonstrated that the degree of ambulatory BP reduction from day to night at the baseline assessment was significantly ($p < 0.01$) smaller in the group with subsequent cerebrovascular events than in the group with no future events. In older patients with isolated systolic hypertension, the Syst-Eur study found that cardiovascular risk increased with a higher night:day ratio of systolic BP (i.e., in patients more likely to be non-dippers) independent of the average 24-h BP [43]. Similarly, Ohkubo et al [56] showed an increased cardiovascular mortality in "non-dippers" (relative risk [RR]: 2.56, $p = 0.02$) and "reverse-dippers" (RR: 3.69, $p = 0.004$) in comparison with "dippers."

Nevertheless, it is important to mention that night-time BP may lose its prognostic significance in hypertensive subjects with significant sleep disturbances during overnight monitoring, which may occur for the compressive, tactile, and sonorous stimuli produced by repeated cuff inflations [57].

Recent findings from our group supported this hypothesis, suggesting that the prognostic impact of day–night BP changes should be investigated including the perceived quantity of sleep as effect modifier in outcome analyses [57]. Specifically, we followed 2934 initially untreated hypertensive subjects and we assessed the perceived quantity of sleep during overnight BP monitoring [57]. Overall, 58.7, 27.7, 9.7, and 4.0 % of subjects reported a sleep duration perceived as usual (group A), <2 h less than usual (group B), 2–4 h less than usual (group C), and >4 h less than usual (group D). Daytime BP did not differ across the groups (all p not significant). Night-time BP increased from group A to D (124/75, 126/76, 128/77, and 129/79 mmHg, respectively; all p for trend <0.01). Over a median follow-up period of 7 years, there were 356 major cardiovascular events and 176 all-cause deaths. Incidence of total cardiovascular events and deaths was higher in the subjects with a night/day ratio in systolic BP >10 % compared with those with a greater day–night BP drop in the group with perceived sleep duration as usual or <2 h less than usual (both p <0.01), not in the group with duration of sleep ≥2 h less than usual (all p not significant). Notably, in a Cox model, the independent prognostic value of night-time BP for total cardiovascular end points and all-cause mortality disappeared in the subjects with perceived sleep deprivation ≥2 h.

Blood Pressure Variability

BP is characterized by marked fluctuations occurring within a 24-h period. Rather than representing "background noise," or a phenomenon occurring at random, these variations are thought to be the result of complex interactions between extrinsic environmental and behavioral factors and intrinsic cardiovascular regulatory mechanisms [58].

Although the adverse cardiovascular consequences of hypertension are thought to depend largely on mean BP values, the hypothesis that increased short-term BP variability may contribute to a worse prognosis in hypertensive patients received a great deal of attention.

Ambulatory BP variability is generally estimated by computing the standard deviation (SD) of the mean systolic and diastolic BP values over a 24-h period or, more appropriately, day-time and night-time periods separately in order to exclude the day–night BP dip from the estimate of this kind of variability. However, other estimates, including weighted standard deviation and coefficient of variation, have been proposed in the last years [59–61].

Importantly, prospective studies have provided evidence that an increase in BP variability within 24-h independently predicts progression of subclinical organ damage, cardiovascular events, and cardiovascular mortality [62–64]. Overall, these evidences support the concept that the adverse cardiovascular consequences of high BP depend on BP variability as well as on mean BP [62–64].

Of particular interest are the findings of a 2007 analysis of the PIUMA study [64]. In this study, BP variability was estimated by the SD of daytime or night-time systolic and diastolic BP. A BP variability ≤ or > the group median (12.7/10.4 mmHg for day-time systolic and diastolic BP and 10.8/8.9 mmHg for night-time systolic and diastolic BP) identified subjects at low or high BP variability. During follow-up, there were 167 new cardiac and 122 new cerebrovascular events. The rate of cardiac events (×100 person–years) was higher (all p <0.05) in the subjects with high than in those with low BP variability (day-time systolic BP: 1.45 vs. 0.72, day-time diastolic BP: 1.29 vs. 0.91; night-time systolic BP: 1.58 vs. 0.62; night-time diastolic BP: 1.32 vs. 0.85). The rate of cerebrovascular events was also higher (all p <0.05) in the subjects with high than in those with low BP variability [64].

In a multivariate analysis, after adjustment for several confounders, a high night-time systolic BP variability was associated with a 51 % ($p=0.024$) excess risk of cardiac events. The relation of day-time BP variability to cardiac events and that of day-time and night-time BP variability to cerebrovascular events lost significance in the multivariate analysis [64].

More recently, these findings have been examined in a large multinational cooperative database including 7,112 untreated hypertensive patients enrolled in 6 prospective studies [65]. In a multivariable Cox model, night-time BP variability (as estimated by SD) was an independent predictor of all-cause mortality, cardiovascular mortality, and cardiovascular events. In contrast, day-time BP variability was not an independent predictor of outcomes in any model. In fully adjusted models, a night-time systolic BP SD ≥ 12.2 mmHg was associated with a 41 % greater risk of cardiovascular events, a 55 % greater risk of cardiovascular death, and a 59 % increased risk of all-cause mortality compared with an SD < 12.2 mmHg. The corresponding values for a diastolic BP SD of ≥ 7.9 mmHg were 48 %, 132 %, and 77 %, respectively. The addition of night-time BP variability to fully adjusted models had a significant impact on risk reclassification and integrated discrimination for all outcomes (relative integrated discrimination improvement for systolic BP variability: 9 % cardiovascular events, 14.5 % all-cause death, 8.5 % cardiovascular death; for diastolic BP variability: 10 % cardiovascular events, 19.1 % all-cause death, 23 % cardiovascular death, all $P<0.01$).

Pulse Pressure

Age-related increases in BP are mainly attributable to an increase in systolic BP with a parallel steadiness, or slight decrease in diastolic BP [66]. This leads to a widening in pulse pressure. Stiffening of large arteries and decreased arterial compliance are recognized key features of aging, which largely account for the changes in pulse pressure occurring from 50 years of age onwards [66].

Because pulse pressure is strongly affected by the alerting reaction evoked by the clinical visit [67], it has been suggested that 24-h ambulatory pulse pressure may better reflect "true" pulse pressure during normal daily life.

A significant association has been noted in several studies between pulse pressure and subsequent rate of cardiovascular morbid events, and such association was in part independent from the effects of systolic and diastolic BP [68–75]. In this context, some analyses of the PIUMA study elucidated the independent prognostic value of ambulatory pulse pressure [73, 74]. The first report included 2,010 initially untreated and uncomplicated subjects with essential hypertension (mean age, 51.7 years; 52 % men) [74]. All subjects underwent baseline procedures including 24-h noninvasive ambulatory BP monitoring and the mean duration of follow-up was 3.8 years (range, 0–11 years). In the three tertiles of the distribution of average 24-h pulse pressure (Fig. 9.5, right panel), the rate of total cardiovascular events was 1.19, 1.81, and 4.92, respectively (log-rank test, $p<0.01$). Similar results were

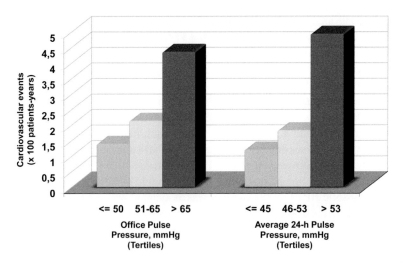

Fig. 9.5 Progressive increase in total cardiovascular events from the first to the third tertile of the distribution of office (*left*) and ambulatory (*right*) pulse pressure

obtained for office pulse pressure (Fig. 9.5, left panel). However, after controlling for several independent risk markers including white coat hypertension and non-dipper status, we found that ambulatory pulse pressure was associated with the biggest reduction in the −2 log likelihood statistics for cardiovascular morbidity ($p < 0.05$ versus office pulse pressure). For any given level of office pulse pressure, cardiovascular morbidity and mortality markedly increased with average 24-h ambulatory pulse pressure.

In a subsequent study, we demonstrated that in subjects with hypertension, ambulatory mean BP and pulse pressure exert a different predictive effect on cardiac and cerebrovascular outcome [73]. While pulse pressure was the dominant predictor of cardiac events, mean BP was the major independent predictor of cerebrovascular events [73]. Specifically, after adjustment for age, sex, diabetes, serum cholesterol, and cigarette smoking (all $p < 0.01$), for each 10 mmHg increase in 24-h pulse pressure, there was an independent 35 % increase in the risk of cardiac events (95 % CI: 17–55 %). Twenty-four-hour mean BP was not a significant predictor of cardiac events after controlling for pulse pressure. Conversely, for every 10 mmHg increase in 24-h mean BP, the risk of cerebrovascular events increased by 42 % (95 % CI: 19–69 %), and 24-h pulse pressure did not yield significance after controlling for 24-h mean BP.

Early Morning Blood Pressure Surge

It is well-known that a marked diurnal variation exists in the time of onset of cardiovascular events, with a peak in early morning [76, 77]. BP also exhibits a similar diurnal variation, with a decrease during sleep and a surge in the morning [76, 77].

Dynamic diurnal variations in pressor stress from a nadir in the night to a peak in the morning (the morning surge in BP) have attracted attention as trigger for cardiovascular events.

In the last few years, the following two different estimates of the morning surge in BP proved prognostic significance [78, 79]: (1) the sleep-trough morning BP surge computed as the difference between the average BP during the 2 h following awakening and the lowest night-time BP (i.e., the average of the lowest BP and the two readings immediately preceding and after the lowest value); and (2) the pre-awakening morning BP surge as the difference between the average BP during the 2 h after awakening and the average BP during the 2 h before awakening (Fig. 9.6).

In a population of 519 older hypertensive subjects from Japan who contributed 44 stroke events, during an average follow-up of 41 months, a higher morning BP rise (sleep-through morning surge ≥55 mmHg) was associated with stroke risk independently of ambulatory BP, nocturnal BP falls, and silent cerebral infarct ($p=0.008$) [78].

More recently, an analysis by the International Database of Ambulatory Blood Pressure in Relation to Cardiovascular Outcome (IDACO) demonstrated that the morning surge above the 90th percentile (sleep-through morning surge ≥37 mmHg) significantly and independently predicted cardiovascular outcome and might contribute to risk stratification by ambulatory BP monitoring [79].

In contrast, a recent analysis of the PIUMA study [53] showed that a greater morning BP surge, either expressed as sleep-trough or pre-awakening surge, did not predict a greater cardiovascular risk in a large sample of 3012 subjects with hypertension. Unexpectedly, in a multivariable Cox model (after adjustment for several predictive covariates, including age, sex, diabetes mellitus, cigarette smoking, total cholesterol, LV hypertrophy, estimated glomerular filtration rate, and average 24-h systolic BP), a blunted sleep trough (≤19.5 mmHg) and pre-awakening (≤9.5 mmHg) BP surge were associated with an excess risk of events (HR: 1.66, 95 % CI: 1.14–2.42, and HR: 1.71, 95 % CI: 1.12–2.71, respectively). These findings were explained by the evidence that the day–night reduction in systolic BP showed a direct association with the sleep trough ($r=0.564; p<0.0001$) and the pre-awakening ($r=0.554; p<0.0001$) systolic BP surge: the greater the day–night dip, the greater the morning BP surge and vice versa [53] (Fig. 9.6).

Heart Rate

Epidemiological evidences demonstrate that heart rate correlates with cardiovascular morbidity [80]. However, much less is known about the independent prognostic value of ambulatory heart rate in hypertensive patients. Only data from three main longitudinal studies underlined the prognostic importance of elevated ambulatory heart rate for cardiovascular events.

The first report was an analysis of the PIUMA study published in 1998 [81]. In a subset of 1,942 initially untreated and uncomplicated subjects with essential

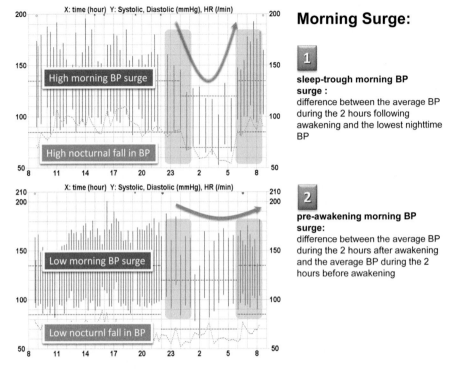

Morning Surge:

1

sleep-trough morning BP surge :
difference between the average BP during the 2 hours following awakening and the lowest nighttime BP

2

pre-awakening morning BP surge:
difference between the average BP during the 2 hours after awakening and the average BP during the 2 hours before awakening

Fig. 9.6 Different estimates of the morning blood pressure surge. The figure also suggests that day–night reduction in systolic blood pressure may be directly associated with the sleep trough or the pre-awakening systolic blood pressure surge (see text for details). *BP* blood pressure

hypertension, a blunted reduction of heart rate from day to night during the baseline examination was associated to an increased risk of death [81]. In a multivariable model, after adjustment for age, diabetes, and average 24-h systolic BP (all $p < 0.01$), for each 10 % less reduction in the heart rate from day to night the RR of mortality was 1.30 (95 % CI: 1.02–1.65, $p = 0.04$) [81].

Similar results have been obtained by Ben-Dov and coworkers [82] in a large sample of 3,957 patients and by the IDACO investigators [83]. Hansen and coworkers demonstrated that the night:day heart rate ratio predicted total and non-cardiovascular mortality, while day-time heart rate did not predict mortality or any fatal combined with nonfatal event [83].

Newer Measures

In the last few years, other summary measures have been proposed for describing different aspects of ambulatory readings. They include novel advanced techniques for the estimation of BP variability, ambulatory arterial stiffness index (AASI), and BP load.

Nevertheless, controversy exists as to which components have independent prognostic significance over and beyond average ambulatory BP [5].

Novel Indices of Blood Pressure Variability

Ambulatory BP variability is traditionally assessed from the SD of BP measurements. However, other advanced indices have been proposed. Calculation of the "weighted" SD of the 24-h mean value (computed as the average of the day-time and night-time BP SD, each weighted for the duration of the respective day or night period) has been analyzed as a method of excluding day-to-night BP changes from the quantification of overall 24-h SD, without discarding either daytime or nighttime values [84].

Average real variability (ARV) is computed as the average of the absolute differences between consecutive BP measurements [85, 86].

Some investigators also proposed maximum minus minimum blood pressure (MMD) as alternative index of BP variability [87].

Variability of BP independent of the mean (VIM) [88] is calculated as the SD divided by the mean to the power x and multiplied by the population mean to the power x. The power x is obtained by fitting a curve through a plot of SD against mean, using the model $SD = a \times mean^x$, where x was derived by nonlinear regression analysis.

Finally, Gavish et al. [89] suggested a variability ratio as an alternative index of BP variability for risk stratification in elderly patients with slower heart rate.

Some of these parameters have been shown to be better predictors of organ damage and cardiovascular risk than the conventional 24-h SD of BP [58, 90]. Nevertheless, computation of these indices appears somewhat complicated for routine clinical practice, requires ad-hoc software, and can be affected by artifacts during ambulatory BP monitoring recording.

Furthermore, it is not clear whether the addition of these novel indices improves risk stratification after adjustment for traditional risk factors and 24-h average BP levels [5].

Ambulatory Arterial Stiffness Index

This parameter has been conceived as novel index of vascular stiffness. Computing the slope of diastolic on systolic pressure from 24-h ambulatory recordings, the AASI is defined as 1 minus this regression slope [91].

Dolan and coworkers demonstrated that AASI predicts cardiovascular mortality in hypertensive patients and provides prognostic information complementary to pulse pressure, independent of mean arterial pressure [92].

However, AASI seems to be not independently related to other widely accepted measures of arterial compliance (such as pulse wave velocity [93]) and it is significantly influenced by nocturnal BP reduction [94]. Moreover, it has been shown to predict stroke and cardiovascular death, but not cardiac death, in a number of independent populations [92, 95, 96].

Blood Pressure Load

As originally defined [97, 98], BP load is the percentage of BP>140/90 mmHg by day and >120/80 mmHg at night. More recently, BP load has been computed as the percentage of ambulatory BP readings above threshold values of 135/85 mmHg for day-time and 120/70 mmHg for night-time BP or as the percentage area under the BP curve above these set limits [1]. Some studies have reported significant associations between BP load, end-organ damage, and cardiovascular events [98, 99], whereas others failed to demonstrate the ability of BP load to refine the risk of developing target organ damage and cardiovascular disease [100, 101].

Interpretation of Ambulatory Blood Pressure Monitoring: A Pragmatic Approach

The clinical use of ambulatory BP monitoring in individual subjects to optimize their management is not so simple and immediate and measurements should be interpreted carefully. Moreover, there is no consensus on the summary measures that should be used in clinical decision making.

Interpretation of ambulatory BP monitoring in individual patients to optimize their management must be kept simple and clinicians should concentrate on ambulatory components which proved to substantially refine risk profiling over and beyond the BP level.

In such a context, the addition of ambulatory pulse pressure, dipping status, and SD of night-time BP variability to models of long-term outcomes improves risk stratification after accounting for the impact of average ambulatory BP levels.

To this purpose, we developed some algorithms for the clinical use of ambulatory BP monitoring [5, 20–25, 37] and suggested the acronym "Ambulatory Does Prediction Valid" (ADPV) [102]:

- **A**verage ambulatory BP
- **D**ipping pattern
- **P**ulse pressure
- **V**ariability of night-time systolic BP

Figure 9.7 shows an algorithm that may be used to refine cardiovascular risk stratification and guide treatment strategies [102]. As recommended by current Guidelines [1–3, 103], office BP (or home BP if available) is the first line procedure to identify subjects who could be candidate for commencing drug treatment.

In the subjects with increased office BP, 24-h ambulatory BP identifies low-risk individuals with normal or optimal values of daytime ambulatory BP (i.e., white coat hypertension). These subjects are generally suitable for lifestyle measures without antihypertensive drug treatment. However, indications from current guidelines should remain mandatory in subjects with associated risk factors or target organ damage [1–3, 104].

In the context of a high clinical suspicion of masked hypertension, ambulatory BP monitoring may be useful to identify subjects with hypertension undetected on the grounds of usual methods. Since the cardiovascular outcome in masked hypertension is equivalent to that in sustained hypertension, subjects with masked hypertension should undergo lifestyle changes and antihypertensive drug therapy targeted on ambulatory BP levels [6].

In subjects with elevated daytime BP (i.e., ambulatory hypertension), one (or more) of the following conditions identifies high-risk individuals, regardless of

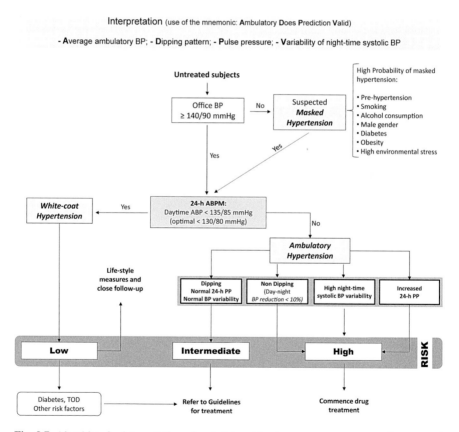

Fig. 9.7 Algorithm for interpretation of ambulatory blood pressure measurements in untreated hypertensive subjects. *BP* blood pressure, *ABPM* ambulatory blood pressure monitoring, *PP* pulse pressure, *TOD* target organ damage

office BP values (office hypertension or masked hypertension): a non-dipping status, an increased 24-h pulse pressure, or a high night-time systolic BP variability. In these subjects, drug treatment is highly recommended [102].

Conclusion and Perspectives

The main advantage of 24-h ambulatory BP monitoring relies in the high number of readings obtained in an outpatient setting, which results in a closer estimate of the "true" BP [105, 106]. Ambulatory BP monitoring appears to be most useful when the diagnosis of hypertension is uncertain, to detect masked hypertension or white coat hypertension, to evaluate patients who are apparently resistant to treatment, and to assess symptomatic episodes of hypotension or hypertension (Table 9.3). However, a policy of offering 24-h ambulatory BP monitoring to all patients with hypertension, particularly if untreated, is generating growing attention. The National Institute for Health and Care Excellence (NICE) was the first to state unequivocally that 24-h ambulatory BP monitoring should be offered to all people with elevated office BP [107]. The U.S. Preventive Services Task Force (USPSTF), an independent panel of experts in prevention and evidence-based medicine recently suggested to offer 24-h ambulatory BP monitoring to all subjects with elevated office BP at screening and to offer antihypertensive treatment solely to subjects with elevated ambulatory BP, not to those with white coat hypertension [108].

The position of USPSTF and NICE is shared, in principle, by a recent Position Paper of the European Society of Hypertension. The paper states that an accurate diagnosis of white coat hypertension "can best be achieved by performing 24-hour ambulatory BP monitoring and/or home BP monitoring in all patients with uncom-

Table 9.3 Generally accepted indications for ambulatory blood pressure monitoring	Clinical indications
	Suspected white coat hypertension
	Suspected masked hypertension
	High risk of future cardiovascular events
	Identifying abnormal blood pressure patterns
	Daytime hypertension
	Suspected nocturnal hypertension or no night-time reduction in BP
	Increased blood pressure variability
	Increased pulse pressure
	Assessment of treatment (and titration of antihypertensive treatment)
	Assessing hypertension in the elderly
	Identifying ambulatory hypotension
	Suspected orthostatic hypotension
	Endocrine hypertension

plicated, stage 1 and 2 essential hypertension before prescribing antihypertensive drug therapy" [1].

However, at least three areas in the field of ambulatory BP monitoring require specific studies in the field. First, it remains to be proved that tailoring treatment on the basis of ambulatory BP provides a better cardiovascular protection than traditional treatment based on office BP. This would require a large, multinational, randomized, outcome-based study that, unfortunately, is unlikely to be ever planned and conducted because of its magnitude and expense [109]. Only a few studies have addressed the prognostic value of in-treatment ambulatory BP [22, 105, 106, 110–112]. For instance, in the PIUMA study [110] only 27 % of subjects achieved office BP control, defined as BP <140/90 mmHg, and 37 % of subjects achieved ambulatory BP control, defined as daytime BP <135/85 mmHg. Ambulatory BP control significantly predicted a lesser risk for subsequent cardiovascular disease, whereas office BP control did not. Similarly, in the Office Versus Ambulatory blood pressure (OvA) study [111], higher mean values for 24-h BP were independent risk factors for new cardiovascular events.

Secondly, the "dipper"/"non-dipper" classification has been criticized because it implies an arbitrary dichotomization of a continuous variable. It is also unclear whether systolic and diastolic BP should be considered separately, or together, in the definition of day–night BP changes [113]. Outcome studies are thus needed to derive universally accepted outcome-driven thresholds of normalcy for day–night BP changes.

Finally, randomized intervention studies are also needed in persons with white coat hypertension in order to compare a regimen based on lifestyle measures versus a standard based on office BP. Again, such a trial is unlikely to be ever performed because of its complexity and cost.

Conflict of Interest None of the authors of this study has financial or other reasons that could lead to a conflict of interest.

References

1. O'Brien E, Parati G, Stergiou G, et al. European society of hypertension position paper on ambulatory blood pressure monitoring. J Hypertens. 2013;31:1731–68.
2. Mancia G, Fagard R, Narkiewicz K, et al. 2013 ESH/ESC guidelines for the management of arterial hypertension: the Task Force for the Management of Arterial Hypertension of the European Society of Hypertension (ESH) and of the European Society of Cardiology (ESC). Eur Heart J. 2013;34:2159–219.
3. James PA, Oparil S, Carter BL, et al. 2014 Evidence-Based Guideline for the Management of High Blood Pressure in Adults: Report From the Panel Members Appointed to the Eighth Joint National Committee (JNC 8). JAMA. 2014;311(5):507–20.
4. Haynes RB, Wilczynski N, McKibbon KA, Walker CJ, Sinclair JC. Developing optimal search strategies for detecting clinically sound studies in MEDLINE. J Am Med Inform Assoc. 1994;1(6):447–58.
5. Angeli F, Reboldi G, Verdecchia P. Interpretation of ambulatory blood pressure profile: a prognostic approach for clinical practice. J Hypertens. 2015;33:454–7.

6. Angeli F, Reboldi G, Verdecchia P. Masked hypertension: evaluation, prognosis, and treatment. Am J Hypertens. 2010;23:941–8.
7. Angeli F, Verdecchia P, Gattobigio R, Sardone M, Reboldi G. White-coat hypertension in adults. Blood Press Monit. 2005;10:301–5.
8. Verdecchia P, Angeli F, Gattobigio R, et al. The clinical significance of white-coat and masked hypertension. Blood Press Monit. 2007;12:387–9.
9. Kawano Y, Horio T, Matayoshi T, Kamide K. Masked hypertension: subtypes and target organ damage. Clin Exp Hypertens. 2008;30:289–96.
10. Bobrie G, Clerson P, Menard J, Postel-Vinay N, Chatellier G, Plouin PF. Masked hypertension: a systematic review. J Hypertens. 2008;26:1715–25.
11. Fagard RH, Cornelissen VA. Incidence of cardiovascular events in white-coat, masked and sustained hypertension versus true normotension: a meta-analysis. J Hypertens. 2007;25:2193–8.
12. Papadopoulos DP, Makris TK. Masked hypertension definition, impact, outcomes: a critical review. J Clin Hypertens (Greenwich). 2007;9:956–63.
13. Angeli F, Verdecchia P, Poltronieri C, et al. Ambulatory blood pressure monitoring in the elderly: features and perspectives. Nutr Metab Cardiovasc Dis. 2014;24:1052–6.
14. Verdecchia P, Schillaci G, Boldrini F, Zampi I, Porcellati C. Variability between current definitions of 'normal' ambulatory blood pressure. Implications in the assessment of white coat hypertension. Hypertension. 1992;20:555–62.
15. Verdecchia P, Porcellati C, Schillaci G, et al. Ambulatory blood pressure. An independent predictor of prognosis in essential hypertension. Hypertension. 1994;24:793–801.
16. Verdecchia P, Schillaci G, Borgioni C, Ciucci A, Porcellati C. White-coat hypertension. Lancet. 1996;348:1444–5. author reply 1445-6.
17. Pierdomenico SD, Lapenna D, Bucci A, et al. Cardiovascular outcome in treated hypertensive patients with responder, masked, false resistant, and true resistant hypertension. Am J Hypertens. 2005;18:1422–8.
18. Kario K, Shimada K, Schwartz JE, Matsuo T, Hoshide S, Pickering TG. Silent and clinically overt stroke in older Japanese subjects with white-coat and sustained hypertension. J Am Coll Cardiol. 2001;38:238–45.
19. Verdecchia P, Reboldi GP, Angeli F, et al. Short- and long-term incidence of stroke in white-coat hypertension. Hypertension. 2005;45:203–8.
20. Angeli F, Reboldi G, Repaci S, Garofoli M, Casavecchia M, Ambrosio G, Verdecchia P. Ambulatory blood pressure monitoring in clinical practice. G Ital Cardiol (Rome). 2008;9:402–7.
21. Verdecchia P, Angeli F. How can we use the results of ambulatory blood pressure monitoring in clinical practice? Hypertension. 2005;46:25–6.
22. Verdecchia P, Angeli F, Cavallini C. Ambulatory blood pressure for cardiovascular risk stratification. Circulation. 2007;115:2091–3.
23. Verdecchia P, Angeli F, Gattobigio R. Clinical usefulness of ambulatory blood pressure monitoring. J Am Soc Nephrol. 2004;15 Suppl 1:S30–3.
24. Verdecchia P, Angeli F, Gattobigio R, Porcellati C. Ambulatory blood pressure monitoring and prognosis in the management of essential hypertension. Expert Rev Cardiovasc Ther. 2003;1:79–89.
25. Verdecchia P, Angeli F, Staessen JA. Compared with whom? Addressing the prognostic value of ambulatory blood pressure categories. Hypertension. 2006;47:820–1.
26. Verdecchia P, Angeli F, Achilli P, et al. Echocardiographic left ventricular hypertrophy in hypertension: marker for future events or mediator of events? Curr Opin Cardiol. 2007;22:329–34.
27. Mancia G, Parati G. Ambulatory blood pressure monitoring and organ damage. Hypertension. 2000;36:894–900.
28. Drayer JI, Weber MA, DeYoung JL. BP as a determinant of cardiac left ventricular muscle mass. Arch Intern Med. 1983;143:90–2.

29. Devereux RB, Pickering TG, Harshfield GA, et al. Left ventricular hypertrophy in patients with hypertension: importance of blood pressure response to regularly recurring stress. Circulation. 1983;68:470–6.
30. Verdecchia P, Schillaci G, Boldrini F, et al. Risk stratification of left ventricular hypertrophy in systemic hypertension using noninvasive ambulatory blood pressure monitoring. Am J Cardiol. 1990;66:583–90.
31. Moulopoulos SD, Stamatelopoulos SF, Zakopoulos NA, et al. Effect of 24-hour blood pressure and heart rate variations on left ventricular hypertrophy and dilatation in essential hypertension. Am Heart J. 1990;119:1147–52.
32. Fagard R, Staessen J, Thijs L, Amery A. Multiple standardized clinic blood pressures may predict left ventricular mass as well as ambulatory monitoring. A metaanalysis of comparative studies. Am J Hypertens. 1995;8:533–40.
33. Verdecchia P, Angeli F, Gattobigio R, Guerrieri M, Benemio G, Porcellati C. Does the reduction in systolic blood pressure alone explain the regression of left ventricular hypertrophy? J Hum Hypertens. 2004;18 Suppl 2:S23–8.
34. Mancia G, Zanchetti A, Agabiti-Rosei E, et al. Ambulatory blood pressure is superior to clinic blood pressure in predicting treatment-induced regression of left ventricular hypertrophy. SAMPLE Study Group. Study on Ambulatory Monitoring of Blood Pressure and Lisinopril Evaluation. Circulation. 1997;95:1464–70.
35. Reboldi G, Gentile G, Angeli F, Verdecchia P. Microalbuminuria and hypertension. Minerva Med. 2005;96:261–75.
36. Asmar RG, Brunel PC, Pannier BM, Lacolley PJ, Safar ME. Arterial distensibility and ambulatory blood pressure monitoring in essential hypertension. Am J Cardiol. 1988;61:1066–70.
37. Reboldi G, Angeli F, Verdecchia P. Interpretation of ambulatory blood pressure profile for risk stratification: keep it simple. Hypertension. 2014;63:913–4.
38. Ohkubo T, Imai Y, Tsuji I, et al. Prediction of mortality by ambulatory blood pressure monitoring versus screening blood pressure measurements: a pilot study in Ohasama. J Hypertens. 1997;15:357–64.
39. Hansen TW, Jeppesen J, Rasmussen S, Ibsen H, Torp-Pedersen C. Ambulatory blood pressure monitoring and risk of cardiovascular disease: a population based study. Am J Hypertens. 2006;19:243–50.
40. Hansen TW, Kikuya M, Thijs L, et al. Prognostic superiority of daytime ambulatory over conventional blood pressure in four populations: a meta-analysis of 7,030 individuals. J Hypertens. 2007;25:1554–64.
41. Dolan E, Stanton A, Thijs L, et al. Superiority of ambulatory over clinic blood pressure measurement in predicting mortality: the Dublin outcome study. Hypertension. 2005;46:156–61.
42. Boggia J, Li Y, Thijs L, et al. Prognostic accuracy of day versus night ambulatory blood pressure: a cohort study. Lancet. 2007;370:1219–29.
43. Staessen JA, Thijs L, Fagard R, et al. Predicting cardiovascular risk using conventional vs ambulatory blood pressure in older patients with systolic hypertension. Systolic Hypertension in Europe Trial Investigators. JAMA. 1999;282:539–46.
44. Littler WA, West MJ, Honour AJ, Sleight P. The variability of arterial pressure. Am Heart J. 1978;95:180–6.
45. Mancia G, Ferrari A, Gregorini L, Parati G, Pomidossi G, Bertinieri G, et al. Blood pressure and heart rate variabilities in normotensive and hypertensive human beings. Circ Res. 1983;53:96–104.
46. Parati G, Pomidossi G, Casadei R, et al. Ambulatory blood pressure monitoring does not interfere with the haemodynamic effects of sleep. J Hypertens Suppl. 1985;3:S107–9.
47. Fagard RH, Staessen JA, Thijs L. Prediction of cardiac structure and function by repeated clinic and ambulatory blood pressure. Hypertension. 1997;29:22–9.

48. Pickering TG. How should the diurnal changes of blood pressure be expressed? Am J Hypertens. 1995;8:681–2.
49. Verdecchia P, Schillaci G, Guerrieri M, et al. Circadian blood pressure changes and left ventricular hypertrophy in essential hypertension. Circulation. 1990;81:528–36.
50. Kario K, Matsuo T, Kobayashi H, Imiya M, Matsuo M, Shimada K. Nocturnal fall of blood pressure and silent cerebrovascular damage in elderly hypertensive patients. Advanced silent cerebrovascular damage in extreme dippers. Hypertension. 1996;27:130–5.
51. O'Brien E, Sheridan J, O'Malley K. Dippers and non-dippers. Lancet. 1988;2:397.
52. Bianchi S, Bigazzi R, Baldari G, Sgherri G, Campese VM. Diurnal variations of blood pressure and microalbuminuria in essential hypertension. Am J Hypertens. 1994;7:23–9.
53. Verdecchia P, Angeli F, Mazzotta G, et al. Day-night dip and early-morning surge in blood pressure in hypertension: prognostic implications. Hypertension. 2012;60:34–42.
54. Verdecchia P, Angeli F, Borgioni C, et al. Prognostic value of circadian blood pressure changes in relation to differing measures of day and night. J Am Soc Hypertens. 2008;2:88–96.
55. Yamamoto Y, Akiguchi I, Oiwa K, Hayashi M, Kimura J. Adverse effect of nighttime blood pressure on the outcome of lacunar infarct patients. Stroke. 1998;29:570–6.
56. Ohkubo T, Imai Y, Tsuji I, et al. Relation between nocturnal decline in blood pressure and mortality. The Ohasama Study. Am J Hypertens. 1997;10:1201–7.
57. Verdecchia P, Angeli F, Borgioni C, Gattobigio R, Reboldi G. Ambulatory blood pressure and cardiovascular outcome in relation to perceived sleep deprivation. Hypertension. 2007;49:777–83.
58. Parati G, Ochoa JE, Lombardi C, Bilo G. Assessment and management of blood-pressure variability. Nat Rev Cardiol. 2013;10:143–55.
59. Mancia G. Short- and long-term blood pressure variability: present and future. Hypertension. 2012;60:512–7.
60. Zakopoulos NA, Tsivgoulis G, Barlas G, et al. Impact of the time rate of blood pressure variation on left ventricular mass. J Hypertens. 2006;24:2071–7.
61. Zakopoulos NA, Toumanidis ST, Barlas GJ, et al. A pressure-time index' for assessing the severity of essential hypertension. J Hypertens. 1999;17:1387–93.
62. Mancia G, Bombelli M, Facchetti R, et al. Long-term prognostic value of blood pressure variability in the general population: results of the Pressioni Arteriose Monitorate e Loro Associazioni Study. Hypertension. 2007;49:1265–70.
63. Hansen TW, Thijs L, Li Y, et al. Prognostic value of reading-to-reading blood pressure variability over 24 hours in 8938 subjects from 11 populations. Hypertension. 2010;55:1049–57.
64. Verdecchia P, Angeli F, Gattobigio R, Rapicetta C, Reboldi G. Impact of blood pressure variability on cardiac and cerebrovascular complications in hypertension. Am J Hypertens. 2007;20:154–61.
65. Palatini P, Reboldi G, Beilin LJ, et al. Added predictive value of night-time blood pressure variability for cardiovascular events and mortality: the Ambulatory Blood Pressure-International Study. Hypertension. 2014;64:487–93.
66. Verdecchia P, Angeli F. Does brachial pulse pressure predict coronary events? Adv Cardiol. 2007;44:150–9.
67. Mancia G, Bertinieri G, Grassi G, et al. Effects of blood-pressure measurement by the doctor on patient's blood pressure and heart rate. Lancet. 1983;2:695–8.
68. Dyer AR, Stamler J, Shekelle RB, et al. Pulse pressure-III. Prognostic significance in four Chicago epidemiologic studies. J Chronic Dis. 1982;35:283–94.
69. Madhavan S, Ooi WL, Cohen H, Alderman MH. Relation of pulse pressure and blood pressure reduction to the incidence of myocardial infarction. Hypertension. 1994;23:395–401.
70. Benetos A, Safar M, Rudnichi A, et al. Pulse pressure: a predictor of long-term cardiovascular mortality in a French male population. Hypertension. 1997;30:1410–5.
71. Franklin SS, Khan SA, Wong ND, Larson MG, Levy D. Is pulse pressure useful in predicting risk for coronary heart Disease? The Framingham heart study. Circulation. 1999;100:354–60.

72. Angeli F, Angeli E, Ambrosio G, et al. Neutrophil count and ambulatory pulse pressure as predictors of cardiovascular adverse events in postmenopausal women with hypertension. Am J Hypertens. 2011;24:591–8.
73. Verdecchia P, Schillaci G, Reboldi G, Franklin SS, Porcellati C. Different prognostic impact of 24-hour mean blood pressure and pulse pressure on stroke and coronary artery disease in essential hypertension. Circulation. 2001;103:2579–84.
74. Verdecchia P, Schillaci G, Borgioni C, Ciucci A, Pede S, Porcellati C. Ambulatory pulse pressure: a potent predictor of total cardiovascular risk in hypertension. Hypertension. 1998;32:983–8.
75. Verdecchia P, Angeli F, Taddei S. At the beginning of stiffening: endothelial dysfunction meets "pulsology". Hypertension. 2006;48:541–2.
76. Willich SN, Levy D, Rocco MB, Tofler GH, Stone PH, Muller JE. Circadian variation in the incidence of sudden cardiac death in the Framingham Heart Study population. Am J Cardiol. 1987;60:801–6.
77. Muller JE, Stone PH, Turi ZG, et al. Circadian variation in the frequency of onset of acute myocardial infarction. N Engl J Med. 1985;313:1315–22.
78. Kario K, Pickering TG, Umeda Y, et al. Morning surge in blood pressure as a predictor of silent and clinical cerebrovascular disease in elderly hypertensives: a prospective study. Circulation. 2003;107:1401–6.
79. Li Y, Thijs L, Hansen TW, et al. Prognostic value of the morning blood pressure surge in 5645 subjects from 8 populations. Hypertension. 2010;55:1040–8.
80. Goldberg RJ, Larson M, Levy D. Factors associated with survival to 75 years of age in middle-aged men and women. The Framingham Study. Arch Intern Med. 1996;156:505–9.
81. Verdecchia P, Schillaci G, Borgioni C, et al. Adverse prognostic value of a blunted circadian rhythm of heart rate in essential hypertension. J Hypertens. 1998;16:1335–43.
82. Ben-Dov IZ, Kark JD, Ben-Ishay D, Mekler J, Ben-Arie L, Bursztyn M. Blunted heart rate dip during sleep and all-cause mortality. Arch Intern Med. 2007;167:2116–21.
83. Hansen TW, Thijs L, Boggia J, et al. Prognostic value of ambulatory heart rate revisited in 6928 subjects from 6 populations. Hypertension. 2008;52:229–35.
84. Bilo G, Giglio A, Styczkiewicz K, et al. A new method for assessing 24-h blood pressure variability after excluding the contribution of nocturnal blood pressure fall. J Hypertens. 2007;25:2058–66.
85. Mena L, Pintos S, Queipo NV, Aizpurua JA, Maestre G, Sulbaran T. A reliable index for the prognostic significance of blood pressure variability. J Hypertens. 2005;23:505–11.
86. Parati G, Rizzoni D. Assessing the prognostic relevance of blood pressure variability: discrepant information from different indices. J Hypertens. 2005;23:483–6.
87. Masugata H, Senda S, Murao K, et al. Visit-to-visit variability in blood pressure over a 1-year period is a marker of left ventricular diastolic dysfunction in treated hypertensive patients. Hypertens Res. 2011;34:846–50.
88. Rothwell PM, Howard SC, Dolan E, et al. Prognostic significance of visit-to-visit variability, maximum systolic blood pressure, and episodic hypertension. Lancet. 2010;375:895–905.
89. Gavish B, Bursztyn M. Blood pressure and heart period variability ratios derived from 24-h ambulatory measurements are predictors of all-cause mortality. J Hypertens. 2015;33:491–8.
90. Asayama K, Schutte R, Li Y, Hansen TW, Staessen JA. Blood pressure variability in risk stratification: What does it add? Clin Exp Pharmacol Physiol. 2014;41:1–8.
91. Dolan E, Li Y, Thijs L, et al. Ambulatory arterial stiffness index: rationale and methodology. Blood Press Monit. 2006;11:103–5.
92. Dolan E, Thijs L, Li Y, et al. Ambulatory arterial stiffness index as a predictor of cardiovascular mortality in the Dublin Outcome Study. Hypertension. 2006;47:365–70.
93. Angeli F, Reboldi G, Verdecchia P. More than a REASON to use arterial stiffness as risk marker and therapeutic target in hypertension. Hypertens Res. 2011;34:445–7.
94. Baumann M, Dan L, Nurnberger J, Heemann U, Witzke O. Association of ambulatory arterial stiffness index and brachial pulse pressure is restricted to dippers. J Hypertens. 2008;26:210–4.

95. Hansen TW, Staessen JA, Torp-Pedersen C, et al. Ambulatory arterial stiffness index predicts stroke in a general population. J Hypertens. 2006;24:2247–53.
96. Kikuya M, Staessen JA, Ohkubo T, et al. Ambulatory arterial stiffness index and 24-hour ambulatory pulse pressure as predictors of mortality in Ohasama, Japan. Stroke. 2007;38:1161–6.
97. Zachariah PK, Sheps SG, Ilstrup DM, et al. Blood pressure load—a better determinant of hypertension. Mayo Clinic Proc. 1988;63:1085–91.
98. White WB, Dey HM, Schulman P. Assessment of the daily blood pressure load as a determinant of cardiac function in patients with mild-to-moderate hypertension. Am Heart J. 1989;118:782–95.
99. Andrade SS, Serro-Azul JB, Nussbacher A, et al. Daytime systolic blood pressure load and previous stroke predict cardiovascular events in treated octogenarians with hypertension. J Am Geriatr Soc. 2010;58:2232–4.
100. Liu M, Li Y, Wei FF, Zhang L, Han JL, Wang JG. Is blood pressure load associated, independently of blood pressure level, with target organ damage? J Hypertens. 2013;31:1812–8.
101. Parati G, Liu X, Ochoa JE. What matters is not only how often but also how much blood pressure rises. Limitations of blood pressure load. J Hypertens. 2013;31:1776–9.
102. Angeli F, Reboldi G, Poltronieri C, et al. Clinical utility of ambulatory blood pressure monitoring in the management of hypertension. Expert Rev Cardiovasc Ther. 2014;12:623–34.
103. Parati G, Stergiou G, O'Brien E, et al. European Society of Hypertension practice guidelines for ambulatory blood pressure monitoring. J Hypertens. 2014;32:1359–66.
104. Verdecchia P, Angeli F. [The Seventh Report of the Joint National Committee on the Prevention, Detection, Evaluation and Treatment of High Blood Pressure: the weapons are ready]. Rev Esp Cardiol (Engl Ed). 2003;56:843–7.
105. Verdecchia P, Angeli F, Mazzotta G, Gentile G, Reboldi G. Home Blood Pressure Measurements Will Not Replace 24-Hour Ambulatory Blood Pressure Monitoring. Hypertension. 2009.
106. Verdecchia P, Angeli F, Mazzotta G, Gentile G, Reboldi G. Home blood pressure measurements will or will not replace 24-hour ambulatory blood pressure measurement. Hypertension. 2009.
107. National Clinical Guideline Centre. Hypertension: The Clinical Management of Primary Hypertension in Adults: Update of Clinical Guidelines 18 and 34 London; London: Royal College of Physicians; 2011.
108. Piper MA, Evans CV, Burda BU, Margolis KL, O'Connor E, Whitlock EP. Diagnostic and predictive accuracy of blood pressure screening methods with consideration of rescreening intervals: a systematic review for the U.S. Preventive services task force. Ann Intern Med. 2015;162:192–204.
109. Mancia G, Verdecchia P. Clinical value of ambulatory blood pressure – evidence and limits. Circ Res. 2015;116(6):1034–45.
110. Verdecchia P, Reboldi G, Porcellati C, et al. Risk of cardiovascular disease in relation to achieved office and ambulatory blood pressure control in treated hypertensive subjects. J Am Coll Cardiol. 2002;39:878–85.
111. Clement DL, De Buyzere ML, De Bacquer DA, et al. Prognostic value of ambulatory blood-pressure recordings in patients with treated hypertension. N Engl J Med. 2003;348:2407–15.
112. Redon J, Campos C, Narciso ML, Rodicio JL, Pascual JM, Ruilope LM. Prognostic value of ambulatory blood pressure monitoring in refractory hypertension: a prospective study. Hypertension. 1998;31:712–8.
113. Schillaci G, Battista F, Pucci G. Nocturnal blood pressure dipping: systolic, diastolic or both? J Hypertens. 2014;32:699–700.
114. Bjorklund K, Lind L, Zethelius B, Andren LH. Isolated ambulatory hypertension predicts cardiovascular morbidity in elderly men. Circulation. 2003;107:1297–302.
115. Bobrie G, Chatellier G, Genes N, et al. Cardiovascular prognosis of "masked hypertension" detected by blood pressure self-measurement in elderly treated hypertensive patients. JAMA. 2004;291:1342–9.

116. Fagard RH, Van Den Broeke C, De Cort P. Prognostic significance of blood pressure measured in the office, at home and during ambulatory monitoring in older patients in general practice. J Hum Hypertens. 2005;19:801–7.
117. Ohkubo T, Kikuya M, Metoki H, et al. Prognosis of "masked" hypertension and "white-coat" hypertension detected by 24-h ambulatory blood pressure monitoring 10-year follow-up from the Ohasama study. J Am Coll Cardiol. 2005;46:508–15.
118. Mancia G, Facchetti R, Bombelli M, Grassi G, Sega R. Long-term risk of mortality associated with selective and combined elevation in office, home, and ambulatory blood pressure. Hypertension. 2006;47:846–53.

Chapter 10
Ambulatory Blood Pressure and Stroke

Philip B. Gorelick, Muhammad U. Farooq, and Jiangyong Min

Introduction

Raised blood pressure is the most important modifiable risk factor for stroke and has been referred to by some experts as the 'crown jewel' of stroke prevention [1–4]. Stroke, one of the most modifiable noncommunicable diseases, is well-suited for prevention as it has a high prevalence of disease, proven therapies to reduce stroke risk, a high frequency of disability, a substantial economic burden, and a number of modifiable risk factors [1]. In relation to the latter point, hypertension serves as the major nexus for stroke prevention. Stroke ranks as the second leading cause of death in the world and the fifth leading cause of death in the United States. Worldwide, there are an estimated 16 million first strokes and 5.7 million stroke deaths [5]. Furthermore, the annual absolute number of strokes, stroke survivors, related deaths, and disability-adjusted life years lost are on the rise; there has been a call to action to prevent and treat modifiable risks for cardiovascular disease such as hypertension [5]. Low- and middle-income countries are especially vulnerable to stroke occurrence and have been affected disproportionately.

Given the importance of elevated blood pressure in stroke causality, accurate measurement of blood pressure is critical [6–12]. Although ambulatory blood pressure monitoring (ABPM) may not be available in clinical practice in many places in the

P.B. Gorelick, M.D., M.P.H. (✉)
Mercy Health Hauenstein Neurosciences,
220 Cherry Street SE Room H 3037, Grand Rapids, MI 49503, USA

Department Translational Science & Molecular Medicine, Michigan State University, College of Human Medicine, Grand Rapids, MI, USA
e-mail: pgorelic@mercyhealth.com

M.U. Farooq, M.D. • J. Min, M.D., Ph.D.
Division of Stroke and Vascular Neurology, Mercy Health Hauenstein Neurosciences, 200 Jefferson Street SE, Grand Rapids, MI, USA
e-mail: farooqmu@mercyhealth.com; jiangyong.min@mercyhealth.com

© Springer International Publishing Switzerland 2016
W.B. White (ed.), *Blood Pressure Monitoring in Cardiovascular Medicine and Therapeutics*, Clinical Hypertension and Vascular Diseases,
DOI 10.1007/978-3-319-22771-9_10

world, it has been noted that additional costs associated with ABPM are counterbalanced by cost savings according to better targeted treatment [13]. Furthermore, use of ABPM to determine the presence of raised blood pressure is becoming or will become standard practice in developed countries around the globe. ABPM serves as the most accurate means to measure blood pressure, and as discussed in this textbook, may be useful in the evaluation of blood pressure variability, white coat hypertension, nocturnal hypertension, drug-resistant hypertension, efficacy of drug treatment over a 24-h time period, symptomatic hypotension, episodic hypertension, and masked hypertension. As we will soon explore in more detail, ABPM provides insights into stroke risk determination and targeted blood pressure management.

In this chapter, we review the following topics: background information regarding the relationship of hypertension to stroke, select studies from the authors' files on ABPM and stroke risk and how ABPM may inform management of blood pressure for stroke prevention and treatment, first and recurrent stroke prevention guidelines in the United States and the status of integration of ABPM into stroke risk assessment and blood pressure management.

Background Information: The Relationship of Hypertension to Stroke

In a review of major overviews of prospective cohort studies and meta-analysis of more than 40 randomized controlled trials of blood pressure lowering including over 188,000 persons and 6800 stroke events, Lawes and colleagues reported the following main findings: (1) In cohort studies, for each 10 mmHg lower systolic blood pressure (SBP), there was a decrease in stroke risk of about one third in persons aged 60–79 years; (2) The association was continuous down to at least blood pressure levels of 115/75 mmHg and across sexes, regions, stroke subtypes, and for stroke mortality and nonfatal stroke events; (3) The proportional association was age-dependent, but held true even among those who were 80 years of age; (4) In randomized controlled trials, a 10 mmHg reduction of SBP was associated with stroke risk reduction of about 1/3 (subjects were about 70 years of age when an event occurred); and (5) The benefit of blood pressure lowering was greater for larger blood pressure reductions; however, relative benefits were similar according to the type of blood pressure lowering medication, baseline blood pressure level, and past history of cardiovascular disease [14]. Furthermore, based on a meta-analysis of individual patient data, blood pressure lowering provides similar relative protection at all levels of baseline cardiovascular risk; however, there is greater absolute risk reduction as baseline risk increases [15]. The main findings from the Lawes and colleagues study are summarized in Table 10.1.

Besides a substantial observational epidemiological database of studies linking hypertension to stroke and numerous clinical trials that show the benefit of blood

Table 10.1 Main findings from epidemiological observational studies and randomized controlled trials on the relationship of stroke and blood pressure [14]

Observational studies
1. For each 10 mmHg lower SBP equates to approximately 1/3 less stroke in 60–79 year olds
2. The association is continuous down to at least blood pressure levels of 115/75 mmHg and holds across sexes, regions, stroke subtypes, for stroke mortality and nonfatal stroke events, and by age up to 80 years
Randomized controlled trials
1. A 10 mmHg SBP reduction was associated with a 1/3 reduction of stroke (mean age of participants at the time of event: approximately 70 years)
2. Larger blood pressure sreductions were associated with greater reduction of stroke
3. The association held for baseline blood pressure level, type of antihypertensive medication, and cardiovascular risk profile

pressure reduction on stroke incidence or recurrence, population attributable risk (PAR) calculations place hypertension as the single factor explaining the highest percentage of stroke risk. Estimates of the percentage of stroke explained by hypertension are in the 25 % to almost 50 % range [16, 17]. In the INTERSTROKE Study whereby participants from 22 countries from different geographic regions were enrolled in a large case–control study, it was shown that ten risk factors were associated with 90 % of stroke risk [18]. In this study, the PAR for hypertension in relation to stroke was 34.6 %. Overall, the relative risk or estimate of relative risk of hypertension for stroke is in the 3–8 range [19].

During the past decades, we have witnessed a major public health advance—a substantial decline in stroke mortality in the United States. An American Heart Association/American Stroke Association (AHA/ASA) expert panel concluded that the decline in stroke mortality was attributable to a combination of interventions and programs to reduce stroke risk. Furthermore, the panelists concluded that a key factor in the reduction of the stroke mortality over time was control of blood pressure [20].

Whereas all forms of raised blood pressure place one at risk for stroke, SBP has become a main target for stroke and cardiovascular disease prevention. SBP generally rises with age, whereas diastolic blood pressure increases until about age 50–55 years and falls thereafter when cardiovascular risk begins to heighten. As most persons with high blood pressure are 50 years of age or older, the importance of SBP as a cause of stroke and other cardiovascular disease is emphasized [21].

Blood pressure control in the United States has improved substantially over time [20]. It is now estimated that up to almost two thirds of persons with high blood pressure have blood pressure at or below the 140/90 mmHg level [21]. Despite this fact, blood pressure control in a number of past clinical trials of recurrent stroke prevention has fallen short of the mark [22, 23, 24]. In contradistinction, concerted efforts to control blood pressure and related risk factors in more recent recurrent stroke prevention clinical trials have yielded substantial benefits in relation to stroke reduction [25–27].

Table 10.2 Epidemiological basics of hypertension in relation to stroke and hypertension alone in the United States [19, 28]

Population attributable risk: ~25–50 %
Relative risk or estimate of relative risk: 3–8
Prevalence of hypertension in the United States: ~29 %
Lifetime risk of developing hypertension for individuals normotensive at age 55 years: 90 %
Prevalence of hypertension among persons ≥65 years: >2/3

Table 10.2 summarizes epidemiological facts about hypertension in relation to stroke and facts about hypertension in the United States [19, 28].

Ambulatory Blood Pressure Monitoring and Stroke: Review of Select Studies

Blood pressure measurement outside the outpatient office or hospital setting may include self-monitoring and ABPM. In the former case, the patient uses a blood pressure measurement devise and chooses to take and record their blood pressure at various times during the day. In the latter case, an ambulatory blood pressure monitor is deployed and blood pressure is automatically measured and recorded at set time intervals. Home or self-monitoring of blood pressure is reviewed in detail in this textbook in Chap. 2 and ABPM in Chap. 4. As a prelude to our discussion of ABPM and stroke, we first discuss select studies from the authors' files on blood pressure variability and stroke based on non-ABPM measures. We have chosen to emphasize blood pressure variability as it may have a substantial impact on stroke risk and brain morphology and function.

Studies of Blood Pressure Variability According to Non-ambulatory Blood Pressure Monitoring Measures

The concept that blood pressure variability measurements add information about stroke risk has been available since at least the early 1990s based on observations by the Swedish Trial in Old Patients (STOP) investigators that blood pressure lowering therapy decreased stroke risk more than expected compared to mean blood pressure lowering alone [29]. Interest in the topic was substantially rekindled and studied by Rothwell and colleagues in a series of publications in 2010 [30–33]. The Rothwell and colleagues' studies and review may be summarized as follows: (1) visit-to-visit SBP variability, beyond mean blood pressure, independently predicts stroke; (2) independent of mean SBP, calcium-channel blockers and diuretics, drugs that reduce visit-to-visit blood pressure variability provide the best stroke prevention, whereas non-selective beta blockers are least effective; and (3) visit-to-visit blood pressure variability accounts for the difference in treatment effect for stroke prevention in select clinical trials [29].

Therefore, in relation to stroke prevention, Rothwell and colleagues make a substantial argument that drugs that reduce blood pressure variability may be more beneficial than those that do not [30–33]. Instability or variation of blood pressure is not well-tolerated by the brain [34]. Consequences of long-term blood pressure variability may include brain atrophy, subcortical ischemic lesions, and cognitive impairment. Rothwell and colleagues replicated key prior findings in an observational study of home blood pressure monitoring, which showed that after transient ischemic attack or minor stroke, calcium channel blockers and diuretics decreased blood pressure variability and maximum home SBP [35]. The results were largely driven by improvement of morning blood pressure readings. Limitations of the Rothwell and colleagues conclusions are discussed elsewhere by Carlberg and Lindholm [29].

Table 10.3 summarizes additional select studies relating to blood pressure variability and non-ABPM measures [36–42].

Table 10.3 Select stroke study results on non-ABPM and blood pressure variability

Study	Results
Acute/Subacute stroke	
1. Harper et al. [36]	There is a marked fall in blood pressure in the first week after acute stroke (22/12 mmHg [SBP/DBP]) and a similar pattern if patients were treated with blood pressure-lowering agents
2. Kang et al. [37]	Variability of blood pressure (not average blood pressure) is associated with poorer functional ischemic stroke outcome at 3 months
3. Ko et al. [38]	Blood pressure variability measures are associated with hemorrhagic transformation independent of mean SBP in ischemic stroke patients
Nonacute/subacute stroke	
1. Yadav et al. [39]	In a genome-wide analysis of blood pressure variability, the NLGN1 locus is significantly associated with blood pressure variability but not ischemic stroke or its subtypes
2. Fukuhara et al. [40]	White-coat, masked, and sustained hypertension are associated with carotid artery stenosis in a Japanese population
3. Nagai et al. [41]	Exaggerated visit-to-visit blood pressure fluctuations are indicators of carotid artery atherosclerosis and stiffness independent of average blood pressure
4. Cuffe et al. [42]	Single measurements of 'normal' or 'low' blood pressure underestimate the prevalence of hypertension in transient ischemic attack and minor stroke patients

DBP diastolic blood pressure, *SBP* systolic blood pressure

Studies of ABPM and Stroke

Interest in circadian patterns of blood pressure variation has led to the study of daytime and night time variations in blood pressure. For example, at most individuals experience a dip in blood pressure by about 10–20 % which may be followed by a morning surge of blood pressure between the hours of 6 AM and 12 noon [43]. The morning surge has been associated with an increased risk of cardiovascular events such as stroke. A number of factors may contribute to the morning surge of blood pressure and include sympathetic nervous system and renin–angiotensin system activity, increases in platelet aggregation, plasminogen activator inhibition, mechanical flow abnormalities, ubiquitin–proteasome system, oxidative stress, plasma cortisol, older age, African-American race/ethnicity, and other factors [43]. In addition, external stimuli may underlie blood pressure surges. Previously, we reported cold weather-induced brain hemorrhage and hypothesized that a sudden surge in blood pressure induced by extreme cold weather could trigger intraparenchymal brain hemorrhage [44].

In relation to blood pressure regulation, it has been observed that night time may be a high risk period for ischemic brain injury, but an opportunity for interventional blood pressure management [45]. Night time is a period when normal blood pressure dipping, non-dipping, or extreme (exaggerated) blood pressure dipping may occur. Non-dipping and extreme dipping of blood pressure have been linked to ischemic brain injury. It has been shown, for example, that the frequency of white matter lesions on MRI head study may be more common in persons who have elevated nocturnal blood pressure on ABPM [46]. By targeting the underlying mechanism (e.g., sympathetic nervous system, renin–angiotensin system) with properly timed (evening) and appropriate type of antihypertensive, one may be able to avert such brain injury [47, 48].

When considering nighttime blood pressure, one must take into account sleep disturbances such as sleep-disordered breathing. For example, in one study short sleep duration was associated with incident stroke in hypertensive persons with silent cerebral infarcts [49]. Treatment of an emerging risk for stroke obstructive sleep apnea (OSA), with continuous positive airway pressure (CPAP), may lead to better blood pressure control, especially when there is resistant hypertension [50].

One should keep in mind that certain groups of patients may be at a higher risk of blood pressure variability. Long-term blood pressure variability may be exaggerated in Blacks, diabetics, and those with cardiovascular disease [51].

A number of ABPM studies that relate specifically to stroke or stroke surrogate markers will now be discussed. Substantial interest in blood pressure and stroke in Asia has led to a number of ABPM studies originating from these regions. Kario and colleagues have been leaders in the field. We now review key select studies or reviews on ABPM and stroke from this investigative group who studied elderly Japanese persons with hypertension, some of whom were enrolled in the Jichi Medical School ABPM Study.

Key findings from the Kario and colleagues' studies of ABPM are summarized [52–61]: (1) Japanese patients with hypertension who are extreme dippers at nighttime may be at higher risk of silent cerebral infarcts and clinical strokes during sleep due to either hypotension during night time hours or an exaggerated morning blood pressure surge, whereas reverse dipping may heighten risk of intracranial hemorrhage; (2) among hypertensive patients, hyperinsulinemia is associated with lacunar-type silent cerebral infarcts in the subcortical white matter, and hemostatic abnormalities are associated with multiple silent cerebral infarcts, especially those observed in the basal ganglia; (3) a higher morning blood pressure surge is associated with stroke risk independent of ambulatory and nocturnal falls in blood pressure, and the morning surge of blood pressure is associated with alpha-adrenergic activity and advanced silent hypertensive brain disease; (4) sleep pulse pressure and awake mean blood pressure are predictors of stroke after adjusting for stroke events; (5) hypertension in the morning is the strongest predictor of future stroke events; (6) in the International Collaborative Study of Prognostic Utility of ABPM, the amount of blood pressure dipping was a significant inverse predictor of stroke but not of cardiac events; (7) high-sensitivity C-reactive protein is associated with clinical stroke in addition to silent cerebral infarcts in elderly persons with hypertension; (8) the degree of morning blood pressure surge is associated with an increase of morning platelet aggregation activity; and (9) After adjustment for 24-h SBP, prothrombin fragments $1+2$ are positively associated with white matter hyperintensities.

We now review findings from additional ABPM studies of stroke. Nakamura, Oita, and Yamaguchi utilized a portable blood pressure monitor in 81 patients with chronic ischemic cerebrovascular disease and classified the subjects into two groups according to levels of diurnal and nocturnal blood pressure [62]. The main finding was that nocturnal blood pressure dipping in patients treated with blood pressure lowering medication might accelerate the risk of ischemic brain disease. Tomii and colleagues analyzed 24-h ABPM in 104 acute ischemic stroke patients on the second and eighth hospital days to assess global outcome according to the modified Rankin Scale score at 3 months [63]. Overall, mean values of systolic and diastolic blood pressure, pulse pressure, and heart rate based on the first ABPM determination and heart rate based on the second ABPM determination were inversely associated with functional independence and mean values of systolic and diastolic blood pressure on the first determination of ABPM and mean heart rate on the second ABPM determination were positively associated with poor global outcome.

In a case–control study, Zhang and colleagues enrolled 76 patients with transient ischemic attack or minor stroke and 82 controls from a normal population to determine whether circadian blood pressure differed when using 24-h ABPM and short-term measurement of heart rate variability [64]. As might be expected, a history of hypertension was more common among cases than controls (72.4 % vs. 48.8 %); however, circadian blood pressure patterns and heart rate variability were similarly distributed among patients and controls. Thus, the main findings of no differences between cases and controls for circadian blood pressure patterns were contrary to other studies of acute or subacute stroke patients.

Klarenbeek and colleagues carried out 24-h ABPM in 122 first-ever lacunar stroke patients to determine possible associations between ABPM and total burden of cerebral small vessel disease on brain magnetic resonance imaging (MRI) [65]. Markers of cerebral small vessel disease on MRI included asymptomatic lacunar infarcts, white matter lesions, cerebral microbleeds, and enlarged perivascular spaces. The authors reported that after adjustment for age and sex, higher 24-h systolic and diastolic ABPM measures at night or daytime were significantly associated with an increasing burden of cerebral small vessel disease.

Finally, based on 24-h ABPM results, Aznaouridis and colleagues explored the predictive value of an Ambulatory Systolic-Diastolic Pressure Regression Index (ASDPRI) from meta-analyses of seven longitudinal studies [66]. The predictive value of the ASDPRI was determined for future outcome events including cardiovascular ones, stroke, and all-cause mortality. An increase of 1 standard deviation of the ASDPRI was associated with an adjusted increase of risk of total cardiovascular events and stroke by 15 % and 30 %, respectively. Furthermore, the ASDPRI was a better predictor of stroke than total cardiovascular events, and furthermore, it predicted stroke better in non-hypertensives than hypertensives.

Table 10.4 summarizes key findings from additional select studies on stroke and ABPM [67–73].

There is a growing literature in relation to cognition, white matter lesions and other subcortical small vessel cerebrovascular disease, and ABPM, which is beyond the scope of this chapter. For further information on this topic, the reader is referred to several authoritative references [74, 75].

Table 10.4 Additional select studies of stroke and ambulatory blood pressure monitoring

Author	Results
1. Ohkubo et al. [67]	In the Ohasama study, ABPM is linearly associated with stroke risk, is more robust in predicting stroke than screening blood pressure, and daytime blood pressure better predicts stroke risk than nighttime blood pressure
2. Verdecchia et al. [68]	24-h pulse pressure is the main predictor of cardiac events, whereas 24-h mean blood pressure is the main predictor of cerebrovascular events
3. Stergiou et al. [69]	Abrupt change in physical activity may be a major determinant of the 2-peak diurnal variation of blood pressure and may act as a trigger factor for stroke
4. Vemmos et al. [70]	Different factors (see parentheses) correlate with higher 24-h blood pressure by stroke subtype: large artery atherosclerosis (history of hypertension, stroke severity); cardioembolic stroke (history of hypertension, stroke severity, hemorrhagic transformation, and brain edema); lacunar infarction (history of hypertension [but coronary artery disease with lower 24-h blood pressure]); infarct of undetermined cause (history of hypertension, stroke severity); and intracerebral hemorrhage (history of hypertension, cerebral edema)
5. Inoue et al. [71]	In the Ohasama study, 24-h systolic ambulatory blood pressure is the primary measure to importance for determining risk
6. Li et al. [72]	In the International Database on Ambulatory Blood Pressure in relation to cardiovascular outcome, morning blood pressure surge above the 90th percentile predicts most types of cardiovascular events
7. Skalidi et al. [73]	In a time-rate model for 24-h ABPM in acute stroke, increased systolic blood pressure values are associated with formation of brain edema

First and Recurrent Stroke Prevention Guidelines and Ambulatory Blood Pressure Monitoring

AHA/ASA First Stroke Prevention Guidelines

In the 2014 AHA/ASA guidance statement on primary stroke prevention, the following pertinent acknowledgements about blood pressure are discussed: (1) intra-individual variability of blood pressure may confer risk of stroke beyond mean blood pressure determination alone; (2) calcium channel blockers may be beneficial to reduce blood pressure variability, but such is not observed with beta blockers; and (3) measurement of nocturnal blood pressure (e.g., reverse or extreme dipping) and the ratio of nighttime to daytime blood pressure may provide useful information beyond mean 24-h blood pressure determination [28]. Furthermore, additional study is called for about possible stroke risk reduction by reduction of intra-individual blood pressure variability and nocturnal blood pressure [28].

Table 10.5 lists key 2014 AHA/ASA guideline recommendations for management of blood pressure to prevent a first stroke [28].

AHA/ASA Recurrent Stroke Prevention Guidelines

The 2014 AHA/ASA guideline on prevention of recurrent stroke is silent on the issue of ABPM [76]. However, the document does refer to blood pressure management in the AHA/ASA first stroke prevention guidance statement [28].

Table 10.6 lists key 2014 AHA/ASA guideline recommendations for managing blood pressure to prevent recurrent stroke [76].

Table 10.5 Key guideline recommendations for management of blood pressure to prevent a first stroke according to the American Heart Association/American Stroke Association [28]

1. Regular blood pressure screening[a]
2. Appropriate treatment including lifestyle modification and pharmacological treatment[a]
3. Annual screening of blood pressure and lifestyle modification for those with pre-hypertension (systolic blood pressure = 120–139 mmHg or diastolic blood pressure = 80–89 mmHg)[a]
4. Blood pressure target for those with hypertension: <140/90 mmHg[a]
5. It is more important to reach the blood pressure target (see 4 above) than is the choice of a specific blood pressure-lowering agent. Treatment should be individualized based on patient characteristics and tolerance to medication[a]
6. Self-measurement of blood pressure improves control[a]

[a]Class I, level of evidence A

Table 10.6 Key guideline recommendations for management of blood pressure to prevent a recurrent stroke according to the American Heart Association/American Stroke Association [76]

1. Initiate blood pressure therapy after the first several days, if blood pressure is $\geq$140 mmHg systolic or $\geq$90 mmHg diastolic[a]
2. Administration of blood pressure lowering therapy is of uncertain value, if blood pressure is <140 mmHg systolic and <90 mmHg diastolic[b]
3. Resumption of blood pressure lowering therapy is indicated beyond the first several days of acute stroke[c]
4. Blood pressure targets: it is reasonable to achieve the following goal: <140/90 mmHg[d]; and a systolic blood pressure <130 mmHg for patients with a recent lacunar infarction[e]
5. Lifestyle modifications are reasonable (e.g., salt restriction, weight loss, diet rich in fruits and vegetables, low-fat dairy products, regular aerobic exercise, and limited alcohol use)[f]
6. The optimal blood pressure lowering drug regimen is uncertain; however, diuretics or a combination of diuretics and an angiotensin-converting enzyme inhibitor is deemed useful[c]

[a]Class I, level of evidence B
[b]Class IIb, level of evidence C
[c]Class I, level of evidence A
[d]Class IIa, level of evidence B
[e]Class IIb, level of evidence B
[f]Class IIa, level of evidence C

Conclusion

Raised blood pressure is the most important modifiable risk factor for stroke. Accurate measurement of blood pressure is important. ABPM has been shown to be the best method to confirm elevated office blood pressure measurements and is considered to be a cost-effective approach. Raised systolic ambulatory blood pressure has been consistently and significantly associated with an increased risk of stroke. These findings and others have led the US Preventive Services Task Force to recommend ABPM as the reference standard for confirmation of the diagnosis of hypertension in a draft document on high blood pressure screening in adults [77].

As discussed in this chapter, ABPM is associated with or predicts a number of stroke-related structural brain changes such as white matter lesions and cerebral small vessel disease burden, silent strokes, hemorrhagic transformation of acute ischemic stroke and other acute brain changes, and functional alterations including poorer global outcome after acute stroke and cognitive impairment and is a major risk predictor for stroke beyond standard blood pressure measures. ABPM has an important future in stroke prevention, informing stroke prevention and treatment guidelines, and in future stroke prevention and treatment research.

References

1. Gorelick PB, Farooq MU, Min J. Population-based approaches for reducing stroke risk. Expert Rev Cardiovasc Ther (early online, 1–8 (2014). 10.1586/14779072.2015.987128. Accessed 29 November 2014 from informahealth.com.
2. Gorelick PB, Goldstein L, Ovbiagele B. New guidelines to reduce risk of atherosclerotic cardiovascular disease. Implications for stroke prevention in 2014. Stroke. 2014;45:945–7.
3. Gorelick PB, Farooq MU. Stroke: an emphasis on guidelines. Lancet Neurol. 2015;14(1):2–3.
4. Gorelick PB. Blood pressure and the prevention of cognitive impairment. JAMA Neurol. 2014;71:1211–3.
5. Feigin VL, Forouzanfar MH, Krishnamurthi R, et al. Global and regional burden of stroke during 1990-2010: findings from the Global Burden of Disease Study 2010. Lancet. 2014;383:245–55.
6. Pickering TG, Shimbo D, Haas D. Ambulatory blood-pressure monitoring. N Engl J Med. 2006;354:2368–74.
7. Weir MR. In the clinic: hypertension. Ann Intern Med. 2014;2:ITC2–14.
8. Clement DL, De Buyzere ML, De Bacquer DA, et al. Prognostic value of ambulatory blood-pressure recordings in patients with treated hypertension. N Engl J Med. 2003;348:2407–15.
9. Boggia J, Li Y, Thijs L, et al. Prognostic accuracy of day versus night ambulatory blood pressure: a cohort study. Lancet. 2007;370:1219–29.
10. Pickering TG, White WB, on behalf of the American Society of Hypertension Writing Group. ASH Position Article: when and how to use self (home) and ambulatory blood pressure monitoring. J Am Soc Hypertens. 2010;4:56–61.
11. Powers BJ, Olsen MK, Smith VA, Woolson RF, Bosworth HB, Oddone EZ. Measuring blood pressure for decision making and quality reporting: where and how many measures? Ann Intern Med. 2011;154:781–8.
12. Pickering TG, Miller NH, Ogedegbe G, Krakoff LR, Artinian NT, Goff D. Call to action on use and reimbursement for home blood pressure monitoring: executive summary. A joint scientific statement from the American Heart Association, American Society of Hypertension, and Preventive Cardiovascular Nurses Association. J Clin Hypertens. 2008;10:467–86.
13. Lovibond K, Jowett S, Barton P, Caufiled M, Heneghan C, Hobbs FDR, et al. Cost-effectiveness of options for the diagnosis of high blood pressure in primary care: a modelling study. Lancet. 2011;378:1219–30.
14. Lawes CMM, Bennett DA, Feigin VL, Rogers A. Blood pressure and stroke. An overview of published reviews. Stroke. 2004;35:1024–33.
15. The Blood Pressure Lowering Treatment Trialists' Collaboration. Blood pressure-lowering treatment based on cardiovascular risk: a meta-analysis of individual patient data. Lancet. 2014;384:591–8.
16. Gorelick PB. Stroke prevention. An opportunity for efficient utilization of health care resources during the coming decade. Stroke. 1994;25:220–4.
17. Gorelick PB. The future of stroke prevention by risk factor modification. In: Fisher M (ed). Handbook of clinical neurology; 94 (3rd series) Stroke Part III. Amsterdam: Elsevier; 2009; p. 1262–76
18. O'Donnell MJ, Xavier D, Lui L, et al. Risk factors for ischemic and intracerebral hemorrhagic stroke in 22 countries (the INTERSTROKE study): a case-control study. Lancet. 2010;376:112–23.
19. Goldstein LB, Bushnell CD, Adams RJ, et al. Guidelines for the primary prevention of stroke. A guideline for healthcare professionals from the American Heart Association/American Stroke Association. Stroke. 2011;42:517–84.
20. Lackland DT, Roccella EJ, Deutsch AF, et al. Factors influencing the decline in stroke mortality. A statement from the American Heart Association/American Stroke Association. Stroke. 2014;45:315–53.

21. More Americans getting high blood pressure under control: CDC. http://www.nlm.nih.gov/ medlineplus/news/fullstory_144572.html (accessed 2/19/14).
22. Gorelick PB. Burden of stroke and risk factors. In: Bornstein NM, editor. Stroke. Practical Guide for Clinicians. Basel: Karger; 2009. p. 9–23.
23. Towfighi A, Markovic D, Ovbiagele B. Consistency of blood pressure control after ischemic stroke. Stroke. 2014;45:1313–7.
24. Ruland S, Raman R, Chaturvedi S, Leurgans S, Gorelick PB. Awareness, treatment and control of vascular risk factors in African Americans with stroke. Neurology. 2003;60:64–8.
25. The SPS3 Study Group. Blood-pressure targets in patients with recent lacunar stroke: the SPS3 randomized trial. Lancet. 2013;382:507–15.
26. Progress Collaborative Group. Randomized trial of a perindopril-based blood-pressure-lowering regimen among 6105 individuals with previous stroke or transient ischemic attack. Lancet. 2001;358:1033–41.
27. Chimowitz MI, Lynn MJ, Derdeyn CP, Turan TN, Fiorella D, Lande BF, et al. Stenting versus aggressive medical therapy for intracranial arterial stenosis. N Engl J Med. 2011;365:993–1003.
28. Meschia JF, Bushnell C, Boden-Albala B, Braun LT, Bravata DM, Chaturvedi S, et al. Guidelines for the primary prevention of stroke. A statement for healthcare professionals from the American Heart Association/American Stroke Association. Stroke 2014;45. Accessed 29 October 2014. doi:10.1161/STR.0000000000000046/-/DCI.
29. Carlberg B, Lindholm LH. Stroke and blood-pressure variation: new permutations on an old theme. Lancet. 2010;375:867–9.
30. Rothwell PM. Limitations of the usual blood-pressure hypothesis and importance of variability, instability, and episodic hypertension. Lancet. 2010;375:938–48.
31. Rothwell PM, Howard SC, Dolan E, O'Brien E, Dobson JE, Dahlof B, Sever PS, Poulter NR. Prognostic significance of visit-to-visit variability, maximum systolic blood pressure, and episodic hypertension. Lancet. 2010;375:895–905.
32. Webb AJS, Fischer U, Mehta Z, Rothwell PM. Effects of anti-hypertensive-drug class on inter-individual variation in blood pressure and risk of stroke: a systematic review and meta-analysis. Lancet. 2010;375:905–15.
33. Rothwell PM, Howard SC, Dolan E, et al. Effects of beta blockers and calcium-channel blockers on within-individual variability in blood pressure and risk of stroke. Lancet Neurol. 2010;9:469–80.
34. Gorelick PB. Reducing blood pressure variability to prevent stroke? Lancet Neurol. 2010;9:448–9.
35. Webb AJS, Wilson M, Lovett N, Paul N, Fischer U, Rothwell PM. Response of day-to-day home blood pressure variability by antihypertensive drug class after transient ischemic attack or nondisabling stroke. Stroke. 2014;45:2967–73.
36. Harper G, Castleden CM, Potter JF. Factors affecting changes in blood pressure after acute stroke. Stroke. 1994;25:1726–9.
37. Kang J, Ko Y, Park JH, et al. Effect of blood pressure on 3-month functional outcome in the subacute stage of ischemic stroke. Neurology. 2012;79:2018–24.
38. Ko Y, Park JH, Yang H, et al. The significance of blood pressure variability for the development of hemorrhagic transformation in acute ischemic stroke. Stroke. 2010;41:2512–8.
39. Yadav S, Cotlarciuc I, Munroe PB, et al. Genome-wide analysis of blood pressure variability and ischemic stroke. Stroke. 2013;44:2703–9.
40. Fukuhara M, Arima H, Ninomiya T, et al. White-coat and masked hypertension are associated with carotid atherosclerosis in a general population. The Hisayama Study. Stroke. 2013;44:1512–7.
41. Nagai M, Hoshide S, Ishikawa J, Shimada K, Kario K. Visit-to-visit blood pressure variations: new independent determinants for carotid artery measures in the elderly at high risk of cardiovascular disease. J Am Soc Hypertens. 2011;5:184–92.

42. Cuffe RL, Howard SC, Algra A, Warlow CP, Rothwell PM. Medium-term variability of blood pressure and potential underdiagnosis of hypertension in patients with previous transient ischemic attack of minor stroke. Stroke. 2006;37:2776–83.
43. Patel PV, Wong JL, Aroroa R. The morning blood pressure surge: therapeutic implications. J Clin Hypertens. 2008;10:140–5.
44. Caplan LR, Neely S, Gorelick PB. Cold-related intracerebral hemorrhage. Arch Neurol. 1984;41:227.
45. White WB. The riskiest time of the brain. Could the nighttime be the right time for intervention? Hypertension. 2007;49:1215–6.
46. Schwartz GL, Bailey KR, Mosley T, et al. Association of ambulatory blood pressure with ischemic brain injury. Hypertension. 2007;49:1228–34.
47. Kario K, White WB. Early morning hypertension: what does it contribute to overall cardiovascular risk assessment? J Am Soc Hypertens. 2008;2:397–402.
48. Kario K. Proposal of RAS-diuretic vs. RAS-calcium antagonist strategies in high-risk hypertension: insight from the 24-hour ambulatory blood pressure profile and central pressure. J Am Soc Hypertens. 2010;4:215–8.
49. Eguchi K, Hoshide S, Ishikawa S, Shimada K, Kario K. Short sleep duration is an independent predictor of stroke events in elderly hypertensive patients. J Am Soc Hypertens. 2010;4:255–62.
50. Martinez-Garcia M-A, Capote F, Campos-Rodriguez F, et al. Effect of CPAP on blood pressure in patients with obstructive sleep apnea and resistant hypertension. The HIPARCO randomized clinical trial. JAMA. 2013;310:2407–15.
51. Berenson GS, Chen W, DasMahapatra P, et al. Stimulus response of blood pressure in black and white young individuals helps explain racial divergence in adult cardiovascular disease: The Bogalusa Heart Study. J Am Soc Hypertens. 2011;5:230–8.
52. Kario K, Pickering TG, Matsuo T, Hoshide S, Schwartz JE, Shimada K. Stroke prognosis and abnormal nocturnal blood pressure falls in older hypertensives. Hypertension. 2001;38:852–7.
53. Kario K, Matsuo T, Kobayashi H, Hoshide S, Shimada K. Hyperinsulinemia and hemostatic abnormalities are associated with silent lacunar cerebral infarcts in elderly hypertensive subjects. J Am Coll Cardiol. 2001;37:871–7.
54. Kario K, Pickering TG, Umeda Y, et al. Morning surge in blood pressure as a predictor of silent and clinical cerebrovascular disease in elderly hypertensives. Circulation. 2003;107:1401–6.
55. Kario K, Pickering TG, Hoshide S, et al. Morning blood pressure surge and hypertensive cerebrovascular disease: role of the alpha adrenergic sympathetic nervous system. Am J Hypertens. 2004;17:668–75.
56. Kario K, Ishikawa J, Eguchi K, et al. Sleep pulse pressure and awake mean pressure as independent predictors for stroke in older hypertensive patients. Am J Hypertens. 2004;17:439–45.
57. Kario K, Ishikawa J, Pickering TG, et al. Morning hypertension: the strongest independent risk factor for stroke in elderly hypertensive patients. Hypertens Res. 2006;29:581–7.
58. Pickering T, Schwartz J, Verdecchia P, et al. Prediction of strokes versus cardiac events by ambulatory monitoring of blood pressure: results from an international database. Blood Press Monit. 2007;12:397–9.
59. Ishikawa J, Tamura Y, Hoshide S, et al. Low-grade inflammation is a risk factor for clinical stroke events in addition to silent cerebral infarcts in Japanese older hypertensives: the Jichi Medical School ABPM Study, wave 1. Stroke. 2007;38:911–7.
60. Kario K, Yano Y, Matsuo T, Hoshide S, Asada Y, Shimada K. Morning blood pressure surge, morning platelet aggregation, and silent cerebral infarction in older Japanese hypertensive patients. J Hypertens. 2011;29:2433–9.
61. Nagai M, Hoshide S, Kario K. Association of prothrombotic status with markers of cerebral small vessel disease in elderly hypertensive patients. Am J Hypertens. 2012;25:1088–94.

62. Nakamura K, Oita J, Yamaguchi T. Nocturnal blood pressure dip in stroke survivors. A pilot study. Stroke. 1995;26:1373–8.
63. Tomii Y, Toyoda K, Suzuki R, et al. Effects of 24-hour blood pressure and heart rate recorded with ambulatory blood pressure monitoring on recovery from acute ischemic stroke. Stroke. 2011;42:3511–7.
64. Zhang WW, Cadilhac DA, Churilov L, Donnan GA, O'Callaghan C, Dewey HM. Does abnormal circadian blood pressure pattern really matter in patients with transient ischemic attack or minor stroke? Stroke. 2014;45:865–7.
65. Klarenbeek P, van Oostenbrugge RJ, Rouhl RPW, Knottnerus ILH, Staals J. Ambulatory blood pressure in patients with lacunar stroke. Association with total MRI burden of cerebral small vessel disease. Stroke. 2013;44:2995–9.
66. Aznaouridis K, Vlachopoulos C, Protogerou A, Stefanadis C. Ambulatory systolic-diastolic pressure regression index as a predictor of clinical events. A meta-analysis of longitudinal studies. Stroke. 2012;43:733–9.
67. Ohkubo T, Hozawa A, Nagai K, et al. Prediction of stroke by ambulatory blood pressure monitoring versus screening blood pressure measurements in a general population: the Ohasama study. J Hypertens. 2000;18:847–54.
68. Verdecchia P, Schillaci G, Reboldi G, Franklin SS, Porcellati C. Different prognostic impact of 24-hour mean blood pressure and pulse pressure on stroke and coronary artery disease in essential hypertension. Circulation. 2001;103:2579–84.
69. Stergiou GS, Vemmos KN, Pliarchopoulou KM, Synetos AG, Roussias LG, Mountokalakis TD. Parallel morning and evening surge in stroke onset, blood pressure, and physical activity. Stroke. 2002;33:1480–6.
70. Vemmos KN, Spengos K, Tsivgoulis G, et al. Factors influencing acute blood pressure values in stroke subtypes. J Hum Hypertens. 2004;18:253–9.
71. Inoue R, Ohkubo T, Kikuya M, et al. Stroke risk in systolic and combined systolic and diastolic hypertension determined using ambulatory blood pressure. The Ohasama study. Am J Hypertens. 2007;20:1125–31.
72. Li Y, Thijs L, Hansen TW, et al. Prognostic value of the morning blood pressure surge in 5645 subjects from 8 populations. Hypertension. 2010;55:1040–8.
73. Skalidi SJ, Manios ED, Stamatelopoulos KS, et al. Brain edema formation is associated with the time rate of blood pressure variation in acute stroke patients. Blood Press Monit. 2013;18:203–7.
74. White WB, Wolfson L, Wakefield DB, et al. Average daily blood pressure, not office blood pressure, is associated with progression of cerebrovascular disease and cognitive decline in older people. Circulation. 2011;124:2312–9.
75. Mok V, Gorelick PB, Chen C. Risk factors as possible targets of prevention of small vessel disease. In: Pantoni L, Gorelick PB, editors. Cerebral small vessel disease. Cambridge: Cambridge University Press; 2014. p. 311–22.
76. Kernan WN, Ovbiagele B, Black HR, et al. Guidelines for the prevention of stroke in patients with stroke and transient ischemic attack. A guideline for healthcare professionals from the American Heart Association/American Stroke Association. Stroke. 2014;45:2160–236.
77. US Preventive Services Task Force. Draft recommendation statement: high blood pressure in adults: screening.   http://www.uspreventiveservicestaskforce.org?Page/Document/RecommendationStatementDraft/hypertension-in-adults-screening-and-home-monitoring#Pod2. Accessed 27 December 2014

Part III
Ambulatory Blood Pressure Monitoring in Special Populations

Chapter 11
Ambulatory Blood Pressure Monitoring in Older Persons

Vinay Gulati and William B. White

Introduction

Ambulatory blood pressure monitoring (ABPM) has facilitated a comprehensive understanding of the physiology of blood pressure (BP) variation in older people. Management of hypertension has undergone important changes with the increasing acceptance of ABPM, a practice supported by extensive clinical and epidemiological research. As discussed in several chapters in this book, the utility of ABPM includes detection of white coat and masked hypertension, determination of nocturnal dipping patterns, and management of blood pressure control in subjects on complex antihypertensive drug regimens [1]. Geriatric patients comprise a distinct subgroup and may derive unique benefits with the use of ABPM.

Magnitude of the Problem

The prevalence of hypertension increases markedly with age. More than 50 % of people aged 60–69 years and about 75 % of people more than 70 years of age are reported to have hypertension [2]. The prevalence may be as high as 90 % in people older than 80 years [3]. Normotensive people at 55–65 years of age who survive to age 80–85 have approximately 90 % lifetime risk of developing hypertension as

V. Gulati, M.D.
Division of Cardiology, Hartford Hospital, Hartford, CT, USA

W.B. White, M.D. (✉)
Calhoun Cardiology Center, University of Connecticut School of Medicine,
263 Farmington Avenue, Farmington, CT 06030-3940, USA
e-mail: wwhite@uchc.edu

© Springer International Publishing Switzerland 2016
W.B. White (ed.), *Blood Pressure Monitoring in Cardiovascular Medicine and Therapeutics*, Clinical Hypertension and Vascular Diseases,
DOI 10.1007/978-3-319-22771-9_11

reported by the Framingham heart Study [4]. The presence of isolated systolic hypertension (ISH) with an increase in pulse pressure is commonly seen from middle age onwards [5]. Treatment of hypertension in the elderly has shown significant cardiac and cerebrovascular benefits as reported in several studies including the Systolic Hypertension in the Elderly Program (SHEP), the Systolic Hypertension in China (Syst-China) trial, the Systolic Hypertension in Europe trial (Syst-Eur), and the Hypertension in the Very Elderly Trial (HYVET) (the latter study in patients >80 years of age) [6–9].

Most of the studies have used office BP to detect hypertension. However, ABPM reflects actual BP values more reliably than office BP readings in the elderly [10]. Using ABPM to detect hypertension may alter the prevalence since white coat hypertension is more commonly reported in older individuals. A cross-sectional study conducted among 1047 individuals 60 years and older in Spain reported 68.8 % hypertensive patients based on clinical BP (≥140/90 mmHg or current BP medication use) and 62.1 % based on 24-h ABPM (≥130/80 mmHg or current BP medication use) [11]. Even though regular aerobic activity is known to decrease systolic and diastolic BP values, a rising trend of BP is observed in the elderly regardless of the level of physical activity. A recent study by Maselli et al. in subjects >65 years old who exercised regularly showed an increase in the mean 24-h BP and an increase in the prevalence of hypertension detected by ABPM from 50 to 65 % over a period of 3.5 years [12].

Changing Cardiovascular Physiology with Advancing Age

Many physiological changes occur as age advances. Increased stiffness of the arteries leads to reduction in the compliance causing increase in pulse pressure. Increased afterload due to less compliant aorta results in generation of higher systolic pressure and left ventricular hypertrophy (LVH) [13]. Cardiac Output declines with ageing. Left ventricular hypertrophy leads to diastolic dysfunction with reduction in left ventricular filling. Decrease in renal plasma flow stimulates the renin–angiotensin system promoting renal tubular sodium and water retention and increase in BP [14]. Sodium sensitivity increases with age [15]. Reduction in the beta-2 receptors and interplay of renin–angiotensin system, sympathetic nervous system, natriuretic factors, and endothelial dysfunction increase peripheral resistance. This, along with higher pulse pressure, leads to isolated systolic hypertension (ISH). The frequency of ISH varies in individuals due to complex interaction of these factors. Isolated systolic hypertension is more common in patients over the age of 60, and systolic blood pressure (SBP) is a better predictor of cardiovascular risk when compared to diastolic blood pressure (DBP) [16]. Decrease in the baroreceptor and chemoreceptor reactivity, decreased responsiveness to beta-adrenergic receptor stimulation, and decline in sodium conservation predispose older individuals to orthostatic and postprandial hypotension [17].

Ausculatory Gap

Clinical assessment of systolic BP in older individuals can be confounded by an auscultatory gap. It is the disappearance of the korotkoff sounds between the systolic BP and diastolic BP. Auscultatory gap is associated with increased arterial stiffness and carotid atherosclerosis, which is more commonly seen in older population and may be a surrogate marker of cardiovascular morbidity [18]. Not recognizing an auscultatory gap can result in an underestimation of systolic BP or an overestimation of diastolic BP.

Pseudohypertension

Pseudohypertension is more common in the elderly and should be suspected in patients with persistently elevated blood pressure measurements who develop hypotensive symptoms on drug therapy [19]. It is a result of increased arterial wall stiffness from advanced arteriosclerosis. The noninvasively measured BP is overestimated, as the BP cuff is unable to measure the true intraluminal BP. The prevalence of pseudohypertension in the elderly is very variable, ranging from 1.7 to as high as 70 % with most of the studies having difference in the selection of individuals studied [20]. Osler's sign may be used to screen potential patients with pseudohypertension, though it lacks reliability and has poor predictive value. The sign is positive if the brachial or radial artery is still palpable after the BP cuff has been inflated over systolic pressure. Among the 3387 persons older than 59 years screened for the Systolic Hypertension in the Elderly Program (SHEP) study, Osler maneuver was present in only 7.2 % subjects, most of them being men, hypertensive, and with a history of stroke [21]. The Osler maneuver may be positive in one third of hospitalized elderly patients [22].

Contrasting Ambulatory BP Monitoring to Home BP Measurement

Both ambulatory and home BP play a complementary role in guiding clinical decisions towards management of hypertension [23]. A comparable degree of association between markers of hypertensive end organ damage such as left ventricular hypertrophy, albuminuria, and carotid intimal-medial thickness is seen with home BP and 24-h BP [24]. However, ambulatory BP monitoring is superior to home BP monitoring due to the number of readings that can be obtained throughout a 24-h period, including times of sleep and physical activities. It reflects various aspects of BP profile that may go undetected by other types of BP measurements such as circadian BP variability, the morning surge of BP, and nocturnal dipping [25]. Compared to clinic (or office) BP, both ambulatory and home BP have shown to be a better predictor of future CV events [26]. The PAMELA study showed incremental increase in cardiovascular mortality with a rise in ambulatory BP, followed by home BP and then office BP [27].

What Are Normal Values of ABPM in the Elderly?

Defining normal values for ABPM in the very old population is complex as it involves both daytime and nighttime measurements with paucity of studies including population with extremes of age. Current recommendations for ambulatory BP measurements in adults provide values derived from outcome-driven thresholds [28]. The International Database of Ambulatory blood pressure in relation to Cardiovascular Outcome (IDACO) performed 24-h ABP monitoring in 5682 participants with mean age 59 years. In multivariate analyses, ABP thresholds were determined yielding 10-year cardiovascular risks similar to those associated with optimal (120/80 mmHg), normal (130/85 mmHg), and high (140/90 mmHg) blood pressure on office measurement. Over a median period of 9.7 years, systolic/diastolic thresholds for ambulatory hypertension were 131.0/79.4 mmHg, 138.2/86.4 mmHg, and 119.5/70.8 mmHg for 24 h, daytime, and nighttime, respectively [29].

Ambulatory BP normality studied in random population aged 65–74 years of age in Italy reported upper limit of normality for 24-h average BP (calculated as the value corresponding to 140/90 mmHg clinic BP) of about 120 mmHg systolic and 76 mmHg diastolic [30].

It is unclear if these threshold values are applicable across the whole age range. In a cross-sectional study of community-dwelling elderly subjects, 24-h ambulatory blood pressure monitoring was performed in 75 "young elderly," aged 60–79 years, and 81 "old elderly" aged 80 years and older. Mean conventional blood pressure, daytime blood pressure and night-time blood pressure were found to be 149/81 mmHg, 138/82 mmHg, and 119/69 mmHg, respectively, in the "young elderly" and 162/82 mmHg, 147/83 mmHg, and 133/71 mmHg, respectively, in the "old elderly" ($p<0.01$ for SBP). The night:day SBP ratio was significantly higher in the 'old' elderly compared with the 'young' elderly (0.90 vs. 0.86, respectively; $p<0.01$). The study showed age-related rise in SBP associated with advanced old age [31].

Current consensus values for ambulatory BP measurements in adults propose reference threshold of 135/85 mmHg for daytime, 120/70 mmHg for nighttime, and 130/80 mmHg for 24-h SBP/DBP means for diagnosis of hypertension [32, 33]. However, whether these values hold good for elderly population of 65 years of age and above is still an unresolved matter.

Reproducibility of Ambulatory Blood Pressure Measurements

Ambulatory blood pressure (BP) measurements have superior reproducibility compared to repeated clinic (or office) BP measurements in short- and long-term studies [34]. This has been observed in a number of trials that focused on younger middle-aged population [35]. Campbell et al. studied the reproducibility of clinic and ambulatory BP in a population between the ages of 75 and 90 years (mean = 82 years) with the subjects getting BP measured 2 years apart under similar conditions [36].

There were minimal mean changes in office, 24-h, and awake and sleep mean BP values between baseline and 2 years later. However, the standard deviation of the differences (SDDs) between visits was higher for office BP compared with the 24-h BP (17.8/9.0 mmHg vs. 11.7/5.9 mmHg, $p<0.01$ for both systolic and diastolic BP). The SDD for 24-h BP was also lower than the SDDs for the awake and sleep BP ($p<0.05$) (Table 11.1). The limits of agreement for the clinic systolic BP were larger

Table 11.1 Clinic and ambulatory blood pressures at two study periods in older persons ($n=72$)

BP parameter (mmHg)	Initial study (mean BP)	Two-year study (mean BP)	Changes between study periods	P-value between study periods	Standard deviation of the differences	Repeatability coefficient (RC)
Clinic systolic	136	136	0.02	0.990	17.8*	35.5*
Clinic diastolic	71	68	−2.9	**0.008**	9.0*	18.0*
Clinic PP	65	68	2.9	0.080	14	28
24 h systolic	130	131	1.1	0.433	11.7	23.3
24 h diastolic	66	67	0.2	0.814	6.0	12.0
24 h PP	63	64	0.92	0.270	7.1	14.2
Awake systolic	132	132	0.5	0.754	12.7**	25.5**
Awake diastolic	68	68	0.04	0.956	6.4**	12.8**
Awake PP	63	64	0.50	0.599	8.0	16.0
Sleep systolic	122	125	3.2	0.052	13.7**	27.5**
Sleep diastolic	60	60	0.72	0.441	7.8	15.6
Sleep PP	62	64	2.5	**0.016**	8.7	17.4
Pre-awake systolic	126	129	4.3	**0.036**	16.7	33.4
Pre-awake diastolic	62	63	1.6	0.191	9.9	19.9
Pre-awake PP	64	66	2.7	0.065	12.0	24
Post-awake systolic	134	138	4.3	0.066	19.4	38.9
Post-awake diastolic	72	71	−0.44	0.726	10.4	20.9
Post-awake PP	62	67	4.7	**0.011**	15.4	30.8

Adapted from Campbell et al. [36] with permission
PP pulse pressure, bolded typeface are significant *p*-values
*$p<0.01$ compared to clinic BP; **$p<0.05$ compared to 24-h BP

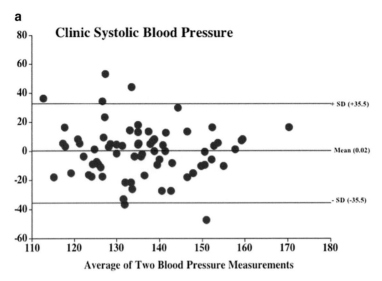

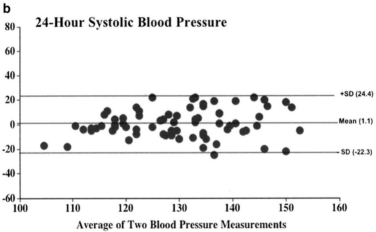

Fig. 11.1 Limits of agreement for the office systolic BP in a very elderly cohort taken 2 years apart (**a**) and for systolic BP taken by 24-h BP monitoring (**b**) using the methods of Bland–Altman (Adapted from Campbell et al. [36] with permission)

than for the 24-h ambulatory systolic BP in this population. The upper and lower limits of agreement in systolic BPs were 35.5 and −35.5 mmHg for the clinic pressure and 24.5 mmHg and -22.3 mmHg for the 24-h BPs, respectively (Fig. 11.1).

Due to the improved reproducibility of ambulatory BP (versus office BP) in older people, the sample size required in clinical trials will be much smaller if 24-h BP is the primary efficacy end point rather than the office BP [37]. Table 11.2 shows sample size calculations for a very elderly population being evaluated in a clinical interventional trial across a variety of estimated mean effects [36]. As shown in the Table, a much larger study population would be required to detect an effect of an intervention on clinic BP versus systolic BP or pulse pressure using 24-h BP.

Table 11.2 Sample size estimation based on utility of clinic and ambulatory BP components in a clinical trial of very elderly subjects

Number of subjects required per group for systolic BP (SBP) change from baseline					
Effect size for SBP (mmHg)	Clinic BP	24 h SBP	Awake SBP	Sleep SBP	Early morning SBP
3	553	239	281	327	656
4	311	135	158	184	370
5	199	86	101	118	236
7	102	44	52	60	121
9	62	27	31	36	73

Number of subjects required per group for pulse pressure change from baseline					
Effect size for pulse pressure (mmHg)	Clinic pulse pressure	24 h pulse pressure	Awake pulse pressure	Sleep pulse pressure	Early morning pulse pressure
3	342	88	112	132	414
4	192	50	63	74	233
5	123	32	40	48	149
7	63	16	20	24	76
9	38	10	12	15	46

Adapted from Campbell et al. [36] with permission

Prognostic Value of ABPM in the Elderly

Prospective cohort studies in adults have shown 24-h BP measurements to be a more robust predictor of cardiovascular risk due to hypertension than BP measured in doctor's office [38, 39]. The superiority of ambulatory BP over conventional office BP in predicting cardiovascular outcome was reported in a meta-analysis of more than 7000 participants studied over a median period of 9.5 years [40]. However, there are few studies on subjects older than 65 years of age and even less in persons greater than 80 years of age.

In a prospective cohort study in hypertensive patients older than 65 years that had a mean follow-up period of 6.7 years [41], ABPM was shown to be a better predictor of cardiovascular mortality than clinic BP measurement with nocturnal BP values demonstrating more important relations with outcomes than the diurnal BP. After adjusting for the clinic BP values, for each 10-mmHg increase in diurnal SBP and nocturnal SBP, the relative risk of cardiovascular death rose by 10 % and 18 %, respectively. A sub-study of the Syst-Eur trial compared the prognostic significance of conventional and ambulatory BP measurement in patients >60 years of age with isolated systolic hypertension [42]. This analysis demonstrated that ambulatory systolic BP was a significant predictor of cardiovascular risk over and above conventional clinic-derived BP. Furthermore, the ability of ABPM to predict cardiovascular events is observed in patients with hypertension who also have type 2 diabetes mellitus [43]. Isolated ambulatory hypertension in presence of normal office blood pressure confers poor cardiovascular prognosis in the elderly [44].

In addition to cardiovascular disease, ambulatory BP is also a better predictor of renal and cerebrovascular disease in older people with hypertension [45]. The 24-h systolic BP plays an important role in predicting the progression of subcortical white matter hyperintensity (WMH) volume burden associated with functional decline in mobility and impairment of cognitive function in older people [46]. White and co-workers studied the importance of ambulatory BP on the progression of small vessel disease of the brain in a prospective cohort of persons between 75 and 89 years of age [47]. Ambulatory and clinic BP monitoring, magnetic resonance imaging (MRI), mobility studies, and neuropsychological testing were performed at baseline and after 24 months on the 72 subjects who completed all aspects of the study. The relationships among the changes in clinic and ambulatory BP and changes in WMH, mobility, and cognitive measures were assessed at 24 months. Changes in ambulatory systolic BP, but not clinic systolic BP, were associated with increases in WMH volume as well as with impairment of several measures of mobility and cognition. Similar associations were observed for 24-h systolic BP, awake systolic BP, and sleep systolic BP, but not for the surge between the sleep and awake time at the 24-month time point. Loess scatter plots of 24-h systolic BP and WMH demonstrated higher WMH at higher levels of 24-h systolic BP and larger changes in 24-h systolic BP over time. Larger increases in WMH were also observed with increases in 24-h systolic BP (Fig. 11.2). In contrast, similar relations between the clinic systolic or change in clinic systolic BP and changes in WMH at 24 months were not observed (Fig. 11.3).

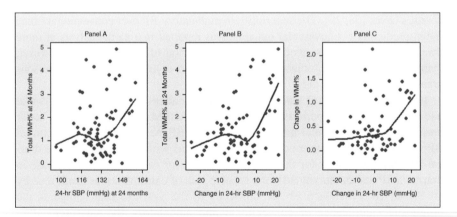

Fig. 11.2 White matter hyperintensity (WMH) and ambulatory blood pressure (BP) in a cohort of older people (*from* [47] *with permission*). Locally weighted smoother plots of 24-h average systolic BP (SBP) and WMH lesions (as percent of total intracranial volume). (**a**) 24-h SBP versus WMH (%); (**b**) change in 24-h SBP and total WMH at 24 months and (**c**) change in 24-h SBP and change in WMH (%) at 24 months

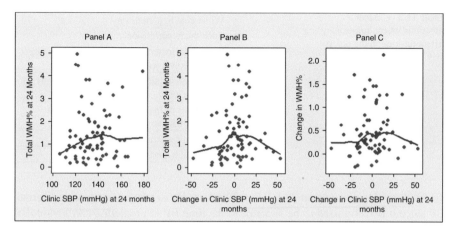

Fig. 11.3 White matter hyperintensity (WMH) and clinic blood pressure (BP) in a cohort of older people (*from* [47] *with permission*). Locally weighted smoother plots of clinic systolic BP (SBP) and WMH lesions (as percent of total intracranial volume are shown. (**a**) Clinic SBP and total WMH (%) at 24 months; (**b**) change in clinic SBP and change in WMH (%) at 24 months and (**c**) change in 24 h SBP and change in WMH (%) at 24 months

Practical Applications of ABPM in Older Population

The feasibility of technical success of ABPM in the elderly is comparable to that seen in younger population, with similar adverse effects of sleep disturbance and mild pain and bruising during cuff inflation [48]. Extreme variations of blood pressure with intermittent periods of high and low BP are often observed with ABPM in older people [49]. As age progresses, certain patterns of blood pressure are more frequent and these are important to recognize from the point of view of clinical management [28]. White coat hypertension is more common in older versus younger population. The increases in 24-h systolic BP in elderly are associated with higher pulse pressure and higher prevalence of isolated systolic hypertension. Exaggerated BP variability and early morning BP surge is also more frequent than in younger and middle-aged patients. The circadian variation in BP is often disrupted with non-dipping pattern observed in the nighttime. Postural and postprandial hypotension are also more common in the elderly. Table 11.3 outlines some of the clinical situations where ambulatory BP monitoring may be useful in older people [50].

White Coat Hypertension

White coat hypertension in untreated patients or white coat effect in treated patients was originally defined as an elevated office BP $\geq$140 mmHg systolic and/or $\geq$90 mmHg diastolic with a mean awake ambulatory BP <135/85 mmHg in untreated individuals. Latest guidelines now propose this definition for patients with office BP

Table 11.3 Clinical situations where ambulatory BP monitoring in the elderly may be useful

- White coat hypertension
- Episodic hypertension
- Borderline hypertension with or without target organ involvement
- Evaluation of patients refractory to therapy for hypertension
- Symptoms of hypotension in patients on antihypertensive therapy
- Autonomic dysfunction
- Nocturnal hypertension

≥140/90 mmHg and a mean 24-h BP <130/80 mmHg to take into account nocturnal BP since it is recognized to be superior to daytime BP in predicting cardiovascular risk [28, 33]. Furthermore, the 24-h mean BP is a more reproducible value than the awake, daytime BP values [1, 28].

White coat hypertension/white coat effect is seen in 15–25 % of the elderly and is a more common syndrome in older versus younger people [51, 52]. Indeed, age is an independent factor influencing white coat hypertension [53] and even seen more frequently in centenarians [54]. Cross-sectional and prospective cohort studies have shown repeatedly that people with white coat hypertension have a better prognosis than those with sustained hypertension outside of the clinical environment [38, 39]. In some clinical outcome studies, patients with WCH may have a slightly increased, nonsignificant cardiovascular risk compared with normotensive individuals, though in most of the studies showing this effect, the ambulatory BP of the white coat hypertensive patients was higher than in normotensive individuals [55, 56]. A meta-analysis performed by the IDACO group showed that any increased risk of future cardiovascular event in a patient with white coat hypertension was very small and substantially lower than the risk seen with either persistent hypertension or masked hypertension [57].

Several guidelines recommend ABPM in patients suspected of having white coat hypertension [1, 2, 32]. In the US, this diagnosis (ICD-9-CM code 796.2, ICD-10-CM code R03.0) is a key indication for ambulatory BP monitoring recognized for coverage by the Centers for Medicare and Medicaid Services [58].

Isolated Systolic Hypertension

A gradual rise in systolic BP attributed to increased aortic stiffness is observed as age advances. Diastolic BP peaks and plateaus in the fifth–sixth decades of life and begins to decline thereafter [59]. The pulse wave velocity used to estimate arterial distensibility correlates well with ambulatory systolic BP and may be used as a surrogate to estimate aortic stiffness [60]. Epidemiologic studies have shown that isolated systolic hypertension is seen in more than 90 % of hypertensive patients >70 years of age with a higher prevalence in women than men [61]. The 24-h systolic BP is associated with more substantial adverse cardiovascular events and mortality than the ambulatory diastolic BP [62]. The Systolic Hypertension in the Elderly Program (SHEP), a randomized, double-blind, placebo-controlled trial on 4736 subjects >60 years of age, demonstrated that treatment of isolated systolic hypertension in older patients reduced all strokes, both fatal and nonfatal, by 36 %; all myocardial infarctions (MIs), both fatal and nonfatal, by 27 %; all coronary heart disease by 27 %; and all cardiovascular disease by 32 %. Total mortality was reduced by 13 % [6]. Ambulatory systolic BP is a better predictor of cardiovascular risk than office systolic BP. The cardiovascular risk conferred by a conventional systolic BP of 160 mmHg in the doctor's office is similar to that associated with a 24-h, daytime or nighttime systolic BP of 142 mmHg, 145 mmHg, or 132 mmHg, respectively [42]. In addition, the pulse pressure is an independent determinant of cardiovascular risk in older persons [63]. In the population-based Framingham Heart Study of 1924 subjects between 50 and 79 years of age, pulse pressure was superior to systolic or diastolic BP in predicting coronary artery disease risk [64]. Ambulatory pulse pressure has also been directly associated with cardiovascular risk [65].

Circadian Variation of Blood Pressure

The circadian pattern of blood pressure and heart rate observed in humans correlates with cardiovascular events, including both myocardial infarction and stroke [66]. Reduction of about 10–30 % of blood pressure is observed during sleep relative to the awake period in majority of normotensive and hypertensive people. This is followed by a rise in BP upon awakening which coincides with the transition from sleep to wakefulness [67].

A non-dipping pattern which is defined as a reduced or absent decline in sleep BP (generally less than 10 % decline) is seen in 25–35 % of hypertensive people and is more commonly seen in older people, both in men, women, and centenarian patients [68–71]. Increasing age is observed to be an independent marker of non-dipping after correction for confounding factors of diabetes, reduced glomerular filtration rate, low HDL-cholesterol, and elevated urinary albumin excretion [72]. This BP pattern is associated with increased target organ damage including left ventricular hypertrophy, albuminuria, and small vessel disease of the brain [25, 73, 74]. Cardiovascular prognosis is worse in elderly non-dippers with ISH than with dipper profiles [42]. Patients lacking a nocturnal decline in the BP are prone to developing congestive heart failure, myocardial infarction, stroke, and progression to end-stage renal failure. Increased incidence of fatal and non-fatal CV events is also observed in association with blunted decline in nocturnal BP [75–77].

Studies have shown poor reproducibility of the nocturnal dipping status [78, 79]. Absolute nocturnal BP values are more reproducible than the categories of dippers and non-dippers. The study observing reproducibility of ambulatory BP in elderly subjects by Campbell et al. found substantial variability in the dipping status over a period of 2 years [36]. Changes in hypertensive status based on absolute nocturnal systolic BP demonstrated improved reproducibility compared with categorical changes.

Reversal of the normal nocturnal decline in BP causes a "non-dipper/riser" pattern and an exaggerated rate of rise of BP upon awakening may create a "surge" pattern and early morning hypertension. In a recent cross-sectional study of 6147 hypertensive patients (2137 of whom were ≥60 year of age) evaluated by 48-h ABPM, the prevalence of non-dipping was significantly higher in older than younger patients (63.1 % vs. 41.1 %; $p<0.001$). A larger difference between age groups was observed in the prevalence of the riser BP pattern (19.9 % in older vs. 4.9 % in younger patients [80].

Larger increases in morning BP may be pathological and associated with higher rates of cardiovascular events [81, 82]. The most well-described example of this phenomenon was a prospective cohort study in 519 older (mean age 72 years) Japanese patients with systolic hypertension with 41 months of observed follow-up. For each 10 mmHg increase in baseline early morning systolic BP, the relative risk of stroke increased by 22 % [83]. The extent of the early-morning BP surge was defined as the difference between the average SBP during the 2 h after awakening minus the average systolic BP during the 1 h that included the lowest sleeping BP values. In the group of patients that had a surge of ≥55 mmHg (top decile of the population), the risk of multiple lacunar infarctions was approximately twofold higher after matching for age and the 24-h BP (57 % vs. 33 %; $p<0.001$) compared to the non-surge patients in whom the average morning increase in systolic BP was 9 mmHg.

Higher cardiovascular morbidity with nocturnal non-dipping and early morning BP rise in older patients with hypertension makes it desirable to monitor and control BP over 24 h [84]. Patients should be evaluated by ABPM to ensure proper evaluation of cardiovascular risk associated with variations of the 24-h BP pattern in order to formulate a therapeutic treatment plan accordingly.

Autonomic Dysregulation

Orthostatic hypotension due to age-associated reductions in baroreflex function and increases in venous insufficiency is more common in the elderly and confers high risk for cardiovascular events and falls [85, 86]. Other factors contributing to orthostasis in the older population is the higher prevalence of diabetes and the use of medications such as diuretics and alpha-1 adrenergic blockers. Orthostatic BP dysregulation due to aging also increases the prevalence of orthostatic hypertension [87]. Increases in orthostatic systolic BP can be as high as 20 mmHg or more. These patients have higher frequency of left ventricular hypertrophy, coronary artery disease, and cerebrovascular disease than elderly patients with hypertension with or without orthostatic hypotension [88].

Postprandial hypotension, defined as a decrease in systolic BP of more than 20 mmHg up to 1 h after eating without change in heart rate, is more frequently observed in older persons [89]. It is associated with higher incidence of falls, syncope, coronary events, stroke, and mortality in the elderly [90, 91].

Conclusions

Ambulatory BP monitoring provides insight into the relationships among BP, target organ involvement, and cardiovascular outcomes in older people. Use of ambulatory BP measurements in older people refines our ability to determine prognosis. The use of out-of-office measurement also helps to guide therapy, particularly in patients with well-recognized syndromes such as masked and white coat hypertension. Finally, clinical trials of antihypertensive therapies enhance the determination of efficacy (and safety) of drugs and devices in older persons.

References

1. Pickering TG, White WB. When and how to use self (home) and ambulatory blood pressure monitoring. J Am Soc Hypertens. 2010;4:56–61.
2. Chobanian AV, Bakris GL, Black HR, Joint National Committee on Prevention, Detection, Evaluation, and Treatment of High Blood Pressure, National Heart, Lung, and Blood Institute, National High Blood Pressure Education Program Coordinating Committee, et al. Seventh report of the Joint National Committee on prevention, detection, evaluation, and treatment of high blood pressure. Hypertension. 2003;42:1206–52.
3. Wang Y, Wang QJ. The prevalence of prehypertension and hypertension among US adults according to the new joint national committee guidelines: new challenges of the old problem. Arch Intern Med. 2004;164(19):2126–34.
4. Vasan RS, Beiser A, Seshadri S, et al. Residual lifetime risk for developing hypertension in middle-aged women and men: the Framingham Heart Study. JAMA. 2002;287(8):1003–10.
5. Franklin SS, Levy D. Aging, blood pressure, and heart failure: what are the connections? Hypertension. 2011;58(5):760–2.
6. Perry Jr HM, Davis BR, Price TR, et al. Effect of treating isolated systolic hypertension on the risk of developing various types and subtypes of stroke: the Systolic Hypertension in the Elderly Program (SHEP). JAMA. 2000;284(4):465–71.
7. Wang JG, Staessen JA, Gong L, Liu L. Chinese trial on isolated systolic hypertension in the elderly. Systolic Hypertension in China (Syst-China) Collaborative Group. Arch Intern Med. 2000;160(2):211–20.
8. Staessen JA, Fagard R, Thijs L, et al. Randomised double-blind comparison of placebo and active treatment for older patients with isolated systolic hypertension. The Systolic Hypertension in Europe (Syst-Eur) Trial Investigators. Lancet. 1997;350(9080):757–64.
9. Beckett NS, Peters R, Fletcher AE, HYVET Study Group, et al. Treatment of hypertension in patients 80 years of age or older. N Engl J Med. 2008;358(18):1887–98.
10. Parati G, Pickering TG. Home blood-pressure monitoring: US and European consensus. Lancet. 2009;373(9667):876–8.
11. Banegas JR, de la Cruz JJ, Graciani A, et al. Impact of ambulatory blood pressure monitoring on reclassification of hypertension prevalence and control in older people in Spain. J Clin Hypertens (Greenwich). 2015;17(6):453–61.
12. Maselli M, Giantin V, Franchin A, et al. Detection of blood pressure increments in active elderly individuals: the role of ambulatory blood pressure monitoring. Nutr Metab Cardiovasc Dis. 2014;24:914–20.
13. Cheitlin MD. Cardiovascular physiology-changes with aging. Am J Geriatr Cardiol. 2003;12(1):9–13.
14. Conti S, Cassis P, Benigni A. Aging and renin-angiotensin system. Hypertension. 2012; 60:878–83.

15. Stokes GS. Management of hypertension in the elderly patient. Clin Interv Aging. 2009; 4:379–89.
16. Franklin SS, Larson MG, Khan SA, et al. Does the relation of blood pressure to coronary heart disease risk change with aging? The Framingham Heart study. Circulation. 2001;103: 1245–9.
17. Pugh KG, Wei JY. Clinical implications of physiological changes in the aging heart. Drugs Aging. 2001;18(4):263–76.
18. Cavallini MC, Roman MJ, Blank SG, Pini R, Pickering TG, Devereux RB. Association of the auscultatory gap with vascular disease in hypertensive patients. Ann Intern Med. 1996; 124:877–83.
19. Pickering TG, Hall JE, Appel LJ, et al. Recommendations for blood pressure measurement in humans and experimental animals: part 1: blood pressure measurement in humans: a statement for professionals from the subcommittee of professional and public education of the American Heart Association Council on high blood pressure research. Circulation. 2005;111:697–716.
20. Zweifler AJ, Shahab ST. Pseudohypertension: a new assessment. J Hypertens. 1993;11:1–6.
21. Wright JC, Looney SW. Prevalence of positive Osler's manoeuver in 3387 persons screened for the Systolic Hypertension in the Elderly Program (SHEP). J Hum Hypertens. 1997; 11:285–9.
22. Belmin J, Visintin JM, Salvatore R, Sebban C, Moulias R. Osler's maneuver: absence of usefulness for the detection of pseudohypertension in an elderly population. Am J Med. 1995;98:42–9.
23. White WB, Gulati V. Managing hypertension with ambulatory blood pressure monitoring. Curr Cardiol Rep. 2015;17(2):2. doi:10.1007/s11886-014-0556-6.
24. Verdecchia P, Angeli F, Mazzotta G, Gentile G, Reboldi G. Home blood pressure measurements will not replace 24-hour ambulatory blood pressure monitoring. Hypertension. 2009;54:188–95.
25. Pickering TG, Shimbo D, Haas D. Ambulatory blood-pressure monitoring. N Engl J Med. 2006;354:2368–74.
26. Ohkubo T, Imai Y, Tsuji I, et al. Home blood pressure measurement has a stronger predictive power for mortality than does screening blood pressure measurement: a population-based observation in Ohasama, Japan. J Hypertens. 1998;16:971–5.
27. Sega R, Facchetti R, Bombelli M, et al. Prognostic value of ambulatory and home blood pressures compared with office blood pressure in the general population: follow-up results from the Pressioni Arteriose Monitorate e Loro Associazioni (PAMELA) study. Circulation. 2005;111:1777–83.
28. O'Brien E, Parati G, Stergiou G, et al. The European Society of Hypertension Working Group on Blood Pressure Monitoring. European Society of Hypertension position paper on ambulatory blood pressure monitoring. J Hypertens. 2013;31:1731–68.
29. Kikuya M, Hansen TW, Thijs L, et al. International database on ambulatory blood pressure monitoring in relation to Cardiovascular Outcomes Investigators. Diagnostic thresholds for ambulatory blood pressure monitoring based on 10-year cardiovascular risk. Circulation. 2007;24:2145–52.
30. Sega R, Cesana G, Milesi C, Grassi G, Zanchetti A, Mancia G. Ambulatory and home blood pressure normality in the elderly: data from the PAMELA population. Hypertension. 1997;30:1–6.
31. O'Sullivan C, Duggan J, Atkins N, O'Brien E. Twenty-four-hour ambulatory blood pressure in community-dwelling elderly men and women, aged 60-102 years. J Hypertens. 2003; 21(9):1641–7.
32. Mancia G, Fagard R, Narkiewicz K, Task Force Members, et al. 2013 ESH/ESC Guidelines for the management of arterial hypertension: the task force for the management of arterial hypertension of the European Society of Hypertension (ESH) and of the European Society of Cardiology (ESC). J Hypertens. 2013;31:1281–357.
33. O'Brien E, Parati G, Stergiou G, et al. Ambulatory blood pressure measurement: what is the international consensus? Hypertension. 2013;62:988–94.

34. James GD, Pickering TG, Yee LS, Harshfield GA, Riva S, Laragh JH. The reproducibility of average ambulatory, home and clinic pressures. Hypertension. 1988;11:545–9.
35. Mansoor GA, McCabe EJ, White WB. Long-term reproducibility of ambulatory blood pressure. J Hypertens. 1994;12:703–8.
36. Campbell P, Ghuman N, Wakefield D, Wolfson L, White WB. Long-term reproducibility of ambulatory blood pressure is superior to office blood pressure in the very elderly. J Hum Hypertens. 2010;24(11):749–54.
37. Conway J, Johnston J, Coats A, Somers V, Sleight P. The use of ambulatory blood pressure monitoring to improve the accuracy and reduce the numbers of subjects in clinical trials of antihypertensive agents. J Hypertens. 1988;6:111–6.
38. Clement DL, De Buyzere ML, De Bacquer DA, et al. Prognostic value of ambulatory blood-pressure recordings in patients with treated hypertension. N Engl J Med. 2003;348:2407–15.
39. Dolan E, Stanton A, Thijs L, et al. Superiority of ambulatory over clinic blood pressure measurement in predicting mortality: the Dublin outcome study. Hypertension. 2005;46:156–61.
40. Hansen TW, Kikuya M, Thijs L, et al. Prognostic superiority of daytime ambulatory over conventional blood pressure in four populations: a meta-analysis of 7,030 individuals. J Hypertens. 2007;25:1554e64.
41. Burr ML, Dolan E, O'Brien EW, et al. The value of ambulatory blood pressure in older adults: the Dublin outcome study. Age Ageing. 2008;37:201–6.
42. Staessen JA, Thijs L, Fagard R, et al. Predicting cardiovascular risk using conventional vs ambulatory blood pressure in older patients with systolic hypertension: Systolic Hypetension in Europe Trial Investigators. JAMA. 1999;282:539–46.
43. Eguchi K, Pickering TG, Hoshide S, et al. Ambulatory blood pressure is a better marker than clinic blood pressure in predicting cardiovascular events in patients with/without type 2 diabetes. Am J Hypertens. 2008;21:443–50.
44. Bjorklund K, Lind L, Zethelius B, Andren B, Lithell H. Isolated ambulatory hypertension predicts cardiovascular morbidity in elderly men. Circulation. 2003;107(9):1297–302.
45. Ghuman N, Campbell P, White WB. Role of ambulatory and home blood pressure recording in clinical practice. Curr Cardiol Rep. 2009;11:414–21.
46. Abraham HM, Wolfson L, Moscufo N, Guttmann CR, Kaplan RF, White WB. Cardiovascular risk factors and small vessel disease of the brain: blood pressure, white matter lesions, and functional decline in older persons. J Cereb Blood Flow Metab. 2015. doi: 10.1038/jcbfm.2015.121.
47. White WB, Wolfson L, Wakefield DB, et al. Average daily blood pressure, not office blood pressure, is associated with progression of cerebrovascular disease and cognitive decline in older people. Circulation. 2011;124(21):2312–9.
48. Trenkwalder P. Automated blood pressure measurement (ABPM) in the elderly. Z Kardiol. 1996;85 suppl 3:85–91.
49. Grodzicki T, Rajzer M, Fagard R, et al. Ambulatory blood pressure monitoring and postprandial hypotension in elderly patients with isolated systolic hypertension. Systolic Hypertension in Europe (SYST-EUR) Trial Investigators. J Hum Hypertens. 1998;12:161–5.
50. National High BP. Education Program Working Group report on ambulatory blood pressure monitoring. Arch Intern Med. 1990;150:2270–80.
51. Trenkwalder P, Plaschke M, Steffes-Tremer I, et al. "White-coat" hypertension and alerting reaction in elderly and very elderly hypertensive patients. Blood Press. 1993;2:262–71.
52. Manios ED, Koroboki EA, Tsivgoulis GK, et al. Factors influencing white-coat effect. Am J Hypertens. 2008;21:153–8.
53. Mansoor GA, McCabe EJ, White WB. Determinants of the white-coat effect in hypertensive subjects. J Hum Hypertens. 1996;10(2):87–92.
54. Jumabay M, Ozawa Y, Kawamura H, et al. White coat hypertension in centenarians. Am J Hypertens. 2005;18:1040–5.
55. Fagard RH, Cornelissen VA. Incidence of cardiovascular events in white-coat, masked and sustained hypertension versus true normotension: a meta-analysis. J Hypertens. 2007;25:2193–8.

56. Pierdomenico SD, Cuccurullo F. Prognostic value of white-coat and masked hypertension diagnosed by ambulatory monitoring in initially untreated subjects: an updated meta analysis. Am J Hypertens. 2011;24:52–8.
57. Franklin SS, Thijs L, Hansen TW, International Database on Ambulatory Blood Pressure in Relation to Cardiovascular Outcomes Investigators, et al. Significance of white-coat hypertension in older persons with isolated systolic hypertension: a meta-analysis using the International Database on Ambulatory Blood Pressure Monitoring in Relation to Cardiovascular Outcomes population. Hypertension. 2012;59:564–71.
58. Centers for Medicare & Medicaid Services. Medicare coverage policy – decisions. ABPM monitoring (#CAG-00067N). 2001. http://www.cms.gov/medicare-coverage-database/details/nca-decisionmemo.aspx.
59. Burt VL, Whelton P, Roccella EJ, et al. Prevalence of hypertension in the U.S. adult population: results from the Third National Health and Nutrition Examination Survey, 1988–1991. Hypertension. 1995;25:305–13.
60. Asmar RG, Brunel PC, Pannier BM, Lacolley PJ, Safar E. Arterial distensibility and ambulatory blood pressure monitoring in essential hypertension. Am J Cardiol. 1988;61(13):1066–70.
61. Franklin SS, Gustin W, Wong ND, et al. Hemodynamic patterns of age-related changes in blood pressure: the Framingham Heart Study. Circulation. 1997;96:308–15.
62. Fagard RH, Van Den Broeke C, De Cort P. Prognostic significance of blood pressure measured in the office, at home and during ambulatory monitoring in older patients in general practice. J Hum Hypertens. 2005;19:801–7.
63. Blacher J, Staessen JA, Girerd X, et al. Pulse pressure not mean pressure determines cardiovascular risk in older hypertensive patients. Arch Intern Med. 2000;160(8):1085–9.
64. Franklin SS, Khan SA, Wong ND, Larson MG, Levy D. Is pulse pressure useful in predicting risk for coronary heart disease? The Framingham Heart Study. Circulation. 1999;100(4):354–60.
65. Verdecchia P, Schillaci G, Reboldi G, Franklin SS, Porcellati C. Different prognostic impact of 24-h mean blood pressure and pulse pressure on stroke and coronary artery disease in essential hypertension. Circulation. 2001;103:2579–84.
66. White WB. Circadian variation of blood pressure: clinical relevance and implications for cardiovascular chronotherapeutics. Blood Press Monit. 1997;2:47–51.
67. White WB, Gulati V. Managing hypertension with ambulatory blood pressure monitoring. Curr Cardiol Rep. 2015;17:1–9.
68. Fotherby MD, Potter JF. Twenty-four-hour ambulatory blood pressure in old and very old subjects. J Hypertens. 1995;13(12):1742–6.
69. Bertinieri G, Grassi G, Rossi P, et al. 24-hour blood pressure profile in centenarians. J Hypertens. 2002;20(9):1765–9.
70. White WB, Mansoor GA, Tendler BE, Anwar YA. Nocturnal blood pressure epidemiology, determinants, and effects of antihypertensive therapy. Blood Press Monit. 1998;3:43–51.
71. Di Lorio A, Marini E, Lupinetti M, Zito M, Abate G. Blood pressure rhythm and prevalence of vascular events in hypertensive subjects. Age Ageing. 1999;28:23–8.
72. Ayala DE, Moya A, Crespo JJ, on behalf of the Hygia Project Investigators, et al. Circadian pattern of ambulatory blood pressure in hypertensive patients with and without type 2 diabetes. Chronobiol Int. 2013;30:99–115.
73. Cuspidi C, Giudici V, Negri F, Sala C. Nocturnal nondipping and left ventricular hypertrophy in hypertension: an updated review. Expert Rev Cardiovasc Ther. 2010;8:781–92.
74. Fan HQ, Li Y, Thijs L, et al. Prognostic value of isolated nocturnal hypertension on ambulatory measurement in 8711 individuals from 10 populations. J Hypertens. 2010;28:2036–45.
75. Boggia J, Li Y, Thijs L, et al. Prognostic accuracy of day versus night ambulatory blood pressure: a cohort study. Lancet. 2007;370:1219–29.
76. Brotman DJ, Davidson MB, Boumitri M, et al. Impaired diurnal blood pressure variation and all-cause mortality. Am J Hypertens. 2008;21:92–7.

77. Hermida RC, Ayala DE, Fernandez JR, et al. Sleep-time blood pressure: prognostic value and relevance as a therapeutic target for cardiovascular risk reduction. Chronobiol Int. 2013; 30:68–86.
78. Omboni S, Parati G, Palatini P, et al. Reproducibility and clinical value of nocturnal hypotension: prospective evidence from the SAMPLE study. J Hypertens. 1998;16:733–8.
79. Cuspidi C, Meani S, Valerio C, et al. Reproducibility of dipping/non-dipping pattern in untreated essential hypertensive patients: impact of sex and age. Blood Press Monit. 2007; 12:101–6.
80. Hermida RC, Ayala DE, Crespo JJ, et al. Influence of age and hypertension treatment- time on ambulatory blood pressure in hypertensive patients. Chronobiol Int. 2013;30:176–91.
81. Kario K, White WB. Early morning hypertension: what does it contribute to overall cardiovascular risk assessment? J Am Soc Hypertens. 2008;2:397–402.
82. White WB. Cardiovascular risk and therapeutic intervention for the early morning surge in blood pressure and heart rate. Blood Press Monit. 2001;6:63–72.
83. Kario K, Pickering TG, Umeda Y, et al. Morning surge in blood pressure as a predictor of silent and clinical cerebrovascular disease in elderly hypertensives: a prospective study. Circulation. 2003;107:1401–6.
84. White WB. Importance of blood pressure control over a 24-hour period. J Manag Care Pharm. 2007;13(suppl B):34–9.
85. Davis BR, Langford HG, Blaufox MD, et al. The association of postural changes in systolic blood pressure and mortality in persons with hypertension: the Hypertension Detection and Follow-up Program experience. Circulation. 1987;75:340–6.
86. Masaki KH, Schatz IJ, Burchfiel CM, et al. Orthostatic hypotension predicts mortality in elderly men: the Honolulu Heart Program. Circulation. 1998;98:2290–5.
87. Kario K, Eguchi K, Nakagawa Y, et al. Relationship between extreme dippers and orthostatic hypertension in elderly hypertensive patients. Hypertension. 1998;31:77–82.
88. Kario K, Eguchi K, Hoshide S, et al. U-curve relationship between orthostatic blood pressure change and silent cerebrovascular disease in elderly hypertensives: orthostatic hypertension as a new cardiovascular risk factor. J Am Coll Cardiol. 2002;40:133–41.
89. Mathias CJ. Postprandial hypotension: pathophysiological mechanisms and clinical implications in different disorders. Hypertension. 1991;18(5):694–704.
90. Aronow WS, Ahn C. Association of postprandial hypotension with incidence of falls, syncope, coronary events, stroke, and total mortality at 29 month follow-up in 499 older nursing home residents. J Am Geriatr Soc. 1997;45(9):1051–3.
91. Fisher AA, Davis MW, Srikusalanukul W, Budge MM. Postprandial hypotension predicts all-cause mortality in older, low-level care residents. J Am Geriatr Soc. 2005;53(8):1313–20.

Chapter 12
Ambulatory Blood Pressure Monitoring in Children and Adolescents

Ian Macumber and Joseph T. Flynn

Introduction

Hypertension in children is a significant and growing problem. A review of recent data from the National Health and Nutrition Survey (NHANES) [1] estimates that in 8–17-year old children there was a 2.3 % increase in the prevalence of prehypertension and a 1 % increase in the prevalence of hypertension from 1963 to 2002, putting the overall prevalences at 4 % and 10 %, respectively. Since pediatric hypertension has been closely linked with childhood obesity [2], this trend can be expected to continue as the childhood obesity epidemic worsens.

This increased prevalence of pediatric hypertension is concerning, as there is substantial evidence that elevated blood pressure (BP) in children is associated with both childhood and future target-organ damage [2]. High childhood BP has been shown to increase arterial stiffnessand left ventricular hypertrophy (LVH) [2] and carotid intima-media thickness (cIMT) [3], a predictor of atherosclerosis in adults. In addition, it has been shown that hypertension can affect cognition in children, potentially by decreasing reactivity of the cerebral vasculature [4]. Children with hypertension are likely to remain hypertensive as they reach adulthood [5] and childhood hypertension strongly correlates with the risk of end-organ damage in adulthood, such as increased cIMT and LVH [6].

Given the significant implications of childhood hypertension, it is important to have an accurate method for evaluating BP in pediatric populations. BP measured in the clinic/office setting, otherwise known as casual blood pressure (cBP), have traditionally been the first step taken to evaluate patients for potential hypertension. However, this technique has multiple pitfalls including, inherent inaccuracy of automated machines used in physician offices, poor technique for auscultatory BP, and

I. Macumber, M.D. • J.T. Flynn, M.D., M.S. (✉)
Division of Nephrology, Seattle Children's Hospital, Seattle, WA 98105, USA
e-mail: joseph.flynn@seattlechildrens.org

© Springer International Publishing Switzerland 2016   227
W.B. White (ed.), *Blood Pressure Monitoring in Cardiovascular Medicine and Therapeutics*, Clinical Hypertension and Vascular Diseases,
DOI 10.1007/978-3-319-22771-9_12

the white coat effect [7]. Intermittent home BPs taken by parents or caretakers also are problematic because few home BP devices are validated in children and there is a lack of normative data for home BP in children [7].

Thus, ambulatory blood pressure monitoring (ABPM) has been increasingly advocated as a tool for diagnosis and management of childhood hypertension. As discussed elsewhere in this text, ABPM has the advantage of eliminating observer bias and improper technique [8] and is a cost-effective way of evaluating BP in children [9, 10]. It has been shown to be better than casual BP at predicting left ventricular mass (LVM), arterial stiffness, and increased cIMT in children [2]. There are also hypertensive states that require ABPM for diagnosis, such as masked hypertension and white coat hypertension.

However, there are some shortcomings to using ABPM in children. It is not recommended for children under 5 years of age, as most children will not tolerate wearing the device for 24 h. The normative data that is most often used needs to be expanded across different ethnicities. Further study also needs to be done in youth correlating ABPM results and target organ damage. Despite these limitations, ABPM has become increasingly recommended for evaluating BP in children and its use continues to increase.

Methodology

Equipment

Available devices for pediatric ABPM currently utilize one of two techniques for BP detection: oscillometric or auscultatory. While most devices will use one or the other, there are some that offer both [11]. Both the oscillometric and auscultatory methods have advantages and limitations. The oscillometric devices are most commonly used in pediatrics due to their ease of use and fewer erroneous readings compared to auscultatory devices. However, oscillometric ABPM devices are susceptible to the same potential errors as oscillometric devices used for casual BP readings and have lower accuracy ratings than the auscultatory devices. Systolic and diastolic BPs are not measured directly, but are back-calculated from the mean arterial pressure (MAP). The formulas for these calculations are proprietary and are not standardized [2]. Auscultatory devices use Korotkoff sounds to measure BP and although both the American Heart Association [2] and the National High Blood Pressure Education Program Working Group [12] recommend using the fifth Korotkoff sound to determine diastolic BP in children rather than the fourth Korotkoff sound, current devices may use either one [11]. There are also currently no normative data available for auscultatory ABPM in children and adolescents. It is important to remember that there are currently monitors on the market that have not been validated. A complete listing of devices that have been validated by the accepted criteria such as the British Hypertension Society standard can be obtained at www.dableducational.org.

Nursing Implications

Nurses and other staff that will be involved in ABPM should be properly trained for placement of ABPM and patient education. Following a standardized approach will help ensure valid BP readings and maintain functionality of equipment. Staff will need to be responsible for upkeep of equipment, including at least yearly calibration, cleaning of hardware, and laundering of cloth BP cuff covers. In addition, a careful history of contraindications to ABPM should be taken prior to placement of the device. These include severe clotting disorders and rhythm disturbances. It should be noted, however, that vein thrombosis secondary to ABPM has not been reported in children.

Appropriate cuff size is essential for accurate BP measurements and published guidelines should be followed closely [12]. The BP cuff should have an inflatable bladder that is at least 40 % of the arm circumference at a point midway between the olecranon and the acromion and the cuff bladder should cover 80–100 % of the arm circumference [12]. Not all cuffs will be able to fit patients to those criteria. In that case, it is recommended to use a larger cuff size rather than a smaller cuff size, as smaller cuff sizes overestimate BP readings to a greater extent than larger cuff sizes diminish them. It is recommended that the ABPM cuff is placed on the child's nondominant arm so that school work and other daily activities are not affected by the monitoring. However, if there is a significant BP discrepancy between the two arms, the arm with the higher BP should be used, even if it is the dominant arm. There are medical exceptions to the recommendation of using the nondominant arm, such as if the child has had arterial surgery or dialysis access on the nondominant side. The ambulatory BP readings should be compared with clinic BP readings obtained using the same technique of measurement. Cuff placement should be adjusted or device recalibrated if the average of three values is greater than 5 mmHg different [2].

Patient education is also very important for successful completion of the study. Patients and parents should be instructed to keep the arm still during all readings, how to stop a reading if there is excessive pain, and to keep monitor from getting wet [2]. A diary should be provided to the patient to record sleep and awake times, time of medication administrations (especially antihypertensives), times of heavy activities or other stressful events, and any adverse events or symptoms such a dizziness or syncope.

Editing and Analysis Periods

Ideally, the ABPM device should be programmed to record BP measurements every 20 min while awake and every 30 min during sleep. Less frequent readings increase the chances of missing data and could compromise the quality of the ABPM study. At least one valid reading per hour is required for an ABPM study to be considered adequate. Manual editing of BP readings should be kept to a minimum and the software should be programmed to exclude invalid readings. Automated exclusion is generally preferred to manual inspection of the BP readings. Current recommendations for pediatric ABPM are to exclude SBP's >220 mmHg and 60 mmHg, DBP >120 and <35 mmHg, heart rate >180 and <40 beats per minute, and pulse pressure >120 or <40 mmHg [2]. These differ from the adult exclusion criteria, which have higher SBP and DBP limits and lower heart rate limits [13].

The time periods of most interest are the awake period, sleep period, and the entire 24-h period. The definition of the sleep and awake periods can be predetermined or can be adjusted based on the patient's sleep diary. While using the sleep diary to adjust awake and sleep periods is labor-intensive, it has been shown that using predetermined time periods can lead to significant misclassification and misinterpretation of ABPM data [14] and therefore it is recommended that providers use sleep diaries to determine patients' wake–sleep periods.

Interpretation

Normative Data

There is a distinct lack of robust normative data for pediatric ABPM. Although large-scale ABPM studies in healthy children have been conducted using both ausculatory and oscillometric devices, the only "normative" data that have found widespread use are the oscillometric values published by the German Working Group on Pediatric Hypertension [15], from original data gathered by Soergel at al. [16]. These BP percentiles are presented in Table 12.1, categorized by sex, age, and height. While this is currently the best data available, it has some significant limitations. It is unclear how generalizable the data are, as only Caucasian children from Central Europe were included in the study. There were few short children included in the analysis, making it harder to apply the values to children with impaired growth, such as those with chronic kidney disease. There was very little variability in DBP, which is not the case for resting casual DBP. The DBP values were also rather high, with the awake 90th percentile around 80–81 mmHg and the awake 95th percentile around 82–84 mmHg, regardless of sex or height [15]. While some of these problems may be related to the oscillometric technique, which is known to be less accurate for DBP, they do call into question the utility of these values. Clearly, further studies involving larger, more diverse groups of children and perhaps utilizing both the oscillometric and auscultatory technique are needed to generate better normative ABPM values for children and adolescents.

Definition of Hypertension

In 2014, the American Heart Association (AHA) updated their scientific statement regarding ABPM in children and adolescents [2]. This statement reinforced previous definitions of prehypertension and hypertension defined in the 2008 AHA

Table 12.1 Normative data for ABPM in children and adolescents

Normal values for ambulatory blood pressure (mmHg) for boys by height

	Height (cm)													
	120	125	130	135	140	145	150	155	160	165	170	175	180	185
24-h DSBP														
BP percentile 50th	104.5	105.3	106.2	107.2	108.3	109.5	110.9	112.5	114.2	116.1	118.0	119.7	121.5	123.2
75th	109.2	110.1	111.1	112.1	113.3	114.6	116.1	117.7	119.5	121.4	123.2	125.0	126.6	128.2
90th	113.8	114.8	115.9	116.9	118.2	119.5	121.0	122.6	124.4	126.3	128.1	129.8	131.3	132.8
95th	116.8	117.8	118.9	120.0	121.2	122.5	124.0	125.7	127.4	129.3	131.1	132.6	134.1	135.5
99th	122.9	123.9	125.0	126.1	127.3	128.6	130.1	131.7	133.4	135.2	136.8	138.2	139.4	140.5
Day-time SBP														
BP percentile 50th	110.8	111.1	111.5	112.0	112.7	113.7	115.1	116.8	118.6	120.6	122.6	124.4	126.2	128.0
75th	116.2	116.5	116.9	117.4	118.0	119.0	120.4	122.1	124.2	126.4	128.4	130.3	132.2	134.1
90th	121.7	121.9	122.2	122.5	123.0	123.9	125.3	127.1	129.4	131.9	134.1	136.1	138.0	139.9
95th	125.2	125.3	125.5	125.7	126.0	126.9	128.3	130.2	132.7	135.3	137.6	139.6	141.6	143.5
99th	132.6	132.4	132.2	132.0	132.1	132.8	134.2	136.3	139.1	142.2	144.7	146.8	148.6	150.5
Night-time SBP														
BP percentile 50th	93.6	94.6	95.6	96.7	97.9	99.0	100.1	101.3	102.6	104.1	105.6	107.2	108.7	110.2
75th	98.6	99.8	101.0	102.3	103.6	104.7	105.9	107.1	108.4	109.9	111.5	113.1	114.6	116.1
90th	103.3	104.8	106.3	107.8	109.3	110.6	111.8	113.0	114.3	115.7	117.2	118.8	120.3	121.8
95th	106.3	107.9	109.7	111.4	113.0	114.4	115.7	116.8	118.1	119.4	120.9	122.4	123.9	125.3
99th	112.1	114.2	116.5	118.7	120.8	122.5	123.8	124.9	126.0	127.1	128.4	129.6	131.0	132.2
24-h DBP														

(continued)

Table 12.1 (continued)

Normal values for ambulatory blood pressure (mmHg) for boys by height

		Height (cm)													
		120	125	130	135	140	145	150	155	160	165	170	175	180	185
BP percentile	50th	65.6	65.9	66.1	66.4	66.6	66.9	67.1	67.2	67.3	67.5	67.6	67.8	68.0	68.2
	75th	69.7	69.9	70.2	70.4	70.6	70.8	71.0	71.1	71.2	71.3	71.5	71.7	71.8	71.9
	90th	73.9	74.1	74.2	74.4	74.5	74.7	74.8	74.8	74.9	75.1	75.3	75.4	75.5	75.6
	95th	76.7	76.8	76.9	76.9	77.0	77.1	77.1	77.2	77.3	77.5	77.7	77.8	77.9	78.0
	99th	82.7	82.5	82.3	82.1	81.9	81.8	81.8	81.8	81.9	82.2	82.5	82.7	82.9	83.0
Day-time DBP															
BP percentile	50th	72.3	72.3	72.2	72.1	72.1	72.1	72.1	72.1	72.2	72.3	72.6	72.8	73.1	73.4
	75th	76.5	76.4	76.3	76.2	76.0	76.0	75.9	75.9	76.0	76.2	76.5	76.8	77.2	77.5
	90th	80.2	80.1	79.9	79.7	79.5	79.4	79.3	79.3	79.4	79.7	80.0	80.5	80.9	81.3
	95th	82.4	82.2	82.0	81.8	81.5	81.4	81.2	81.2	81.3	81.7	82.1	82.6	83.1	83.6
	99th	86.5	86.2	85.9	85.6	85.2	85.0	84.8	84.8	85.0	85.4	86.0	86.6	87.3	87.9
Night-time DBP															
BP percentile	50th	54.3	54.8	55.1	55.5	55.8	56.0	56.2	56.2	56.3	56.5	56.7	56.9	57.1	57.3
	75th	57.6	58.2	58.8	59.2	59.6	59.9	60.1	60.2	60.2	60.3	60.5	60.6	60.8	60.9
	90th	60.7	61.4	62.1	62.7	63.2	63.5	63.7	63.8	63.8	63.9	63.9	64.0	64.1	64.2
	95th	62.6	63.4	64.2	64.8	65.4	65.8	66.0	66.0	66.0	66.0	66.1	66.1	66.1	66.2
	99th	66.2	67.2	68.2	69.0	69.7	70.1	70.4	70.4	70.3	70.3	70.2	70.1	70.0	69.9
24-h MAP															
BP percentile	50th	77.5	78.1	78.7	79.3	79.9	80.5	81.1	81.7	82.3	83.1	83.9	84.7	85.5	86.3
	75th	81.8	82.4	83.0	83.5	84.1	84.6	85.2	85.9	86.6	87.3	88.1	89.0	89.8	90.7
	90th	86.3	86.7	87.2	87.6	88.0	88.5	89.1	89.7	90.3	91.1	91.9	92.7	93.5	94.3
	95th	89.3	89.6	89.9	90.2	90.5	90.9	91.4	91.9	92.6	93.3	94.0	94.8	95.6	96.4
	99th	95.9	95.7	95.5	95.4	95.4	95.6	95.9	96.3	96.7	97.4	98.0	98.7	99.4	100.1

Normal values for ambulatory blood pressure (mmHg) for boys by height

Height (cm)	120	125	130	135	140	145	150	155	160	165	170	175	180	185
Day-time MAP														
BP percentile 50th	83.8	84.1	84.3	84.5	84.7	85.0	85.4	85.8	86.4	87.1	88.0	89.0	90.0	91.0
75th	88.5	88.7	88.9	89.0	89.1	89.4	89.6	90.1	90.7	91.6	92.6	93.7	94.9	96.1
90th	92.9	93.0	93.1	93.1	93.1	93.2	93.4	93.8	94.5	95.4	96.5	97.7	99.0	100.3
95th	95.6	95.6	95.6	95.5	95.5	95.5	95.7	96.0	96.7	97.7	98.8	100.1	101.4	102.8
99th	101.0	100.7	100.5	100.2	99.9	99.7	99.8	100.1	100.8	101.7	102.9	104.3	105.7	107.1
Night-time MAP														
BP percentile 50th	66.8	67.6	68.3	69.0	69.6	70.1	70.6	71.2	71.9	72.7	73.6	74.5	75.4	76.2
75th	71.0	71.9	72.7	73.4	73.9	74.4	74.9	75.4	76.0	76.8	77.6	78.3	79.1	79.8
90th	75.9	76.6	77.3	77.9	78.3	78.6	78.9	79.2	79.7	80.3	80.9	81.5	82.1	82.7
95th	79.5	80.0	80.5	80.9	81.2	81.3	81.4	81.5	81.9	82.3	82.8	83.3	83.8	84.3
99th	88.4	88.1	87.8	87.6	87.2	86.7	86.3	86.0	86.0	86.1	86.3	86.5	86.8	87.0

Normal values for ambulatory blood pressure (mmHg) for girls by height

Height (cm)	120	125	130	135	140	145	150	155	160	165	170	175
24-h SBP												
BP percentile 50th	104.0	105.0	106.0	106.8	107.6	108.7	109.9	111.2	112.4	113.7	115.0	116.4
75th	108.2	109.3	110.3	111.2	112.1	113.2	114.6	115.9	117.0	118.0	119.2	120.4
90th	112.0	113.2	114.3	115.3	116.2	117.4	118.7	120.0	121.0	121.8	122.8	123.8
95th	114.3	115.6	116.7	117.7	118.7	119.9	121.2	122.5	123.3	124.1	124.9	125.8
99th	118.8	120.1	121.3	122.4	123.4	124.6	126.0	127.1	127.7	128.2	128.8	129.3
Day-time SBP												

(continued)

Table 12.1 (continued)

Normal values for ambulatory blood pressure (mmHg) for girls by height

		Height (cm)											
	BP percentile	120	125	130	135	140	145	150	155	160	165	170	175
24-h SBP	50th	110.0	110.5	111.0	111.6	112.2	113.1	114.3	115.6	117.0	118.3	119.8	121.2
	75th	114.4	115.0	115.7	116.3	117.0	118.1	119.4	120.7	121.9	123.1	124.2	125.3
	90th	118.2	119.0	119.7	120.4	121.3	122.5	123.9	125.2	126.4	127.3	128.1	128.9
	95th	120.4	121.3	122.1	122.9	123.8	125.1	126.5	127.9	129.1	129.8	130.5	131.0
	99th	124.5	125.5	126.4	127.4	128.5	129.9	131.5	133.0	134.0	134.5	134.8	135.0
Night-time SBP	50th	95.0	95.7	96.4	96.9	97.5	98.1	98.9	100.0	101.1	102.2	103.4	104.6
	75th	99.4	100.3	101.2	101.9	102.6	103.4	104.4	105.5	106.4	107.3	108.2	109.2
	90th	103.3	104.4	105.5	106.5	107.5	108.5	109.5	110.5	111.2	111.8	112.4	113.1
	95th	105.6	106.9	108.1	109.3	110.4	111.6	112.7	113.6	114.1	114.4	114.8	115.3
	99th	109.8	111.5	113.1	114.7	116.2	117.7	118.9	119.5	119.6	119.4	119.3	119.4
	50th	65.9	65.9	66.0	66.1	66.2	66.3	66.5	66.7	67.0	67.4	68.0	68.6
	75th	68.6	68.9	69.2	69.5	69.8	70.1	70.4	70.6	70.7	71.0	71.3	71.6
	90th	70.9	71.4	71.9	72.4	72.9	73.4	73.8	74.0	74.1	74.2	74.4	74.5
	95th	72.2	72.8	73.4	74.1	74.7	75.3	75.7	76.0	76.1	76.2	76.2	76.2
	99th	74.6	75.3	76.2	77.1	77.9	78.7	79.3	79.7	79.9	79.9	79.9	79.7
Day-time DBP	50th	73.2	72.8	72.4	72.1	71.8	71.7	71.8	72.0	72.4	73.1	73.9	74.8
	75th	76.9	76.6	76.4	76.2	76.1	76.1	76.1	76.2	76.4	76.8	77.3	77.8
	90th	80.1	79.9	79.8	79.8	79.7	79.8	79.9	79.9	79.9	80.0	80.2	80.5
	95th	81.9	81.8	81.8	81.8	81.9	82.0	82.0	82.0	82.0	81.9	82.0	82.0
	99th	85.3	85.3	85.4	85.6	85.8	85.9	86.0	85.9	85.7	85.4	85.2	84.9

Normal values for ambulatory blood pressure (mmHg) for girls by height

		Height (cm)											
		120	125	130	135	140	145	150	155	160	165	170	175
		24-h SBP											
		Night-time DBP											
BP percentile	50th	55.4	55.3	55.1	54.8	54.6	54.4	54.3	54.4	54.6	54.9	55.1	55.4
	75th	59.5	59.5	59.4	59.3	59.1	58.9	58.8	58.7	58.8	58.9	61.0	59.3
	90th	63.1	63.3	63.4	63.4	63.3	63.1	63.0	62.9	62.9	62.9	66.9	63.1
	95th	65.2	65.5	65.7	65.8	65.8	65.7	65.6	65.5	65.5	65.5	70.8	65.5
	99th	69.1	69.6	70.1	70.4	70.6	70.8	70.8	70.7	70.7	70.6	79.0	70.4
		24-h MAP											
BP percentile	50th	77.2	77.8	78.3	78.7	79.2	79.7	80.2	80.8	81.5	82.3	83.1	84.0
	75th	80.6	81.2	81.8	82.4	82.9	83.5	84.1	84.7	85.3	85.9	86.6	87.4
	90th	83.6	84.2	84.9	85.5	86.1	86.7	87.3	87.9	88.4	88.9	89.5	90.1
	95th	85.3	86.0	86.7	87.4	88.0	88.6	89.2	89.7	90.2	90.6	91.1	91.7
	99th	88.5	89.2	89.9	90.6	91.3	91.9	92.5	93.0	93.3	93.6	94.0	94.5
		Day-time MAP											
BP percentile	50th	83.3	83.7	84.0	84.1	84.3	84.5	84.9	85.5	86.2	87.0	88.0	88.9
	75th	87.4	87.9	88.2	88.5	88.7	88.9	89.3	89.8	90.3	90.9	91.6	92.2
	90th	90.9	91.5	91.9	92.2	92.4	92.7	93.0	93.4	93.7	94.1	94.5	94.9
	95th	92.9	93.6	94.0	94.4	94.6	94.9	95.1	95.4	95.6	95.8	96.1	96.4
	99th	96.6	97.4	97.9	98.3	98.6	98.8	99.0	99.0	99.0	99.0	99.0	99.1
		Night-time MAP											

(continued)

Table 12.1 (continued)

Normal values for ambulatory blood pressure (mmHg) for girls by height

		Height (cm)											
		120	125	130	135	140	145	150	155	160	165	170	175
	24-h SBP												
BP percentile	50th	68.0	68.2	68.4	68.5	68.7	69.0	69.3	69.8	70.4	71.2	72.0	72.8
	75th	72.6	72.7	72.9	73.0	73.2	73.5	73.9	74.3	74.8	75.4	76.1	76.9
	90th	76.8	76.9	77.0	77.2	77.4	77.7	78.0	78.3	78.6	79.1	79.6	80.3
	95th	79.5	79.4	79.6	79.7	79.9	80.2	80.4	80.6	80.8	81.2	81.6	82.2
	99th	84.6	84.4	84.5	84.6	84.8	85.0	85.0	85.0	85.0	85.0	85.3	85.6

Normal values for ambulatory blood pressure (mmHg) for boys by age

		Age (years)											
		5	6	7	8	9	10	11	12	13	14	15	16
	24-h SBP												
BP percentile	50th	104.6	105.5	106.3	107.0	107.7	108.8	110.4	112.6	115.1	117.8	120.6	123.4
	75th	109.0	110.0	111.0	111.9	112.8	114.1	115.9	118.2	120.9	123.7	126.5	129.4
	90th	113.4	114.7	115.8	116.8	117.9	119.2	121.2	123.7	126.4	129.3	132.1	134.9
	95th	116.4	117.7	118.9	120.0	121.1	122.5	124.6	127.1	129.9	132.7	135.5	138.2
	99th	122.7	124.1	125.4	126.6	127.7	129.2	131.4	134.0	136.9	139.5	142.0	144.5
	Day-time SBP												
BP percentile	50th	111.1	111.5	111.9	112.2	112.6	113.4	114.9	117.0	119.5	122.3	125.3	128.2
	75th	115.7	116.3	116.8	117.3	117.9	118.8	120.5	122.9	125.6	128.5	131.5	134.6
	90th	120.1	120.9	121.6	122.2	122.9	124.0	125.9	128.4	131.2	134.2	137.3	140.4
	95th	122.9	123.8	124.6	125.3	126.1	127.3	129.3	131.8	134.7	137.7	140.8	143.9
	99th	128.5	129.6	130.6	131.5	132.3	133.7	135.8	138.6	141.5	144.4	147.4	150.4
	Night-time SBP												

Normal values for ambulatory blood pressure (mmHg) for boys by age

		Age (years)											
	BP percentile	5	6	7	8	9	10	11	12	13	14	15	16
	50th	95.0	95.5	96.1	96.7	97.3	98.1	99.4	101.2	103.4	105.8	108.3	110.9
	75th	99.2	100.2	101.1	102.0	102.9	103.9	105.3	107.1	109.3	111.9	114.4	116.9
	90th	103.4	104.9	106.2	107.5	108.5	109.6	111.0	112.8	115.0	117.5	120.0	122.5
	95th	106.3	108.0	109.6	111.0	112.1	113.2	114.6	116.3	118.6	121.0	123.4	125.9
	99th	112.3	114.6	116.7	118.4	119.6	120.7	121.9	123.4	125.5	127.8	130.1	132.3
24-h DBP	BP percentile												
	50th	65.3	65.7	66.1	66.3	66.5	66.6	66.9	67.2	67.4	67.7	68.1	68.6
	75th	68.8	69.3	69.6	69.9	70.0	70.2	70.5	70.8	71.0	71.4	71.8	72.3
	90th	72.2	72.6	73.0	73.2	73.3	73.4	73.7	74.0	74.3	74.6	75.1	75.6
	95th	74.4	74.8	75.1	75.2	75.3	75.4	75.7	75.9	76.2	76.6	77.0	77.5
	99th	78.9	79.0	79.1	79.1	79.1	79.1	79.3	79.6	79.9	80.2	80.7	81.3
Day-time DBP	BP percentile												
	50th	72.2	72.4	72.5	72.5	72.3	72.1	72.0	72.0	72.2	72.5	73.0	73.5
	75th	75.9	76.1	76.3	76.4	76.2	76.0	76.0	76.0	76.2	76.5	77.0	77.6
	90th	79.1	79.3	79.7	79.8	79.7	79.5	79.5	79.5	79.7	80.0	80.6	81.3
	95th	81.0	81.3	81.6	81.8	81.7	81.5	81.5	81.6	81.7	82.1	82.8	83.5
	99th	84.5	84.8	85.2	85.5	85.4	85.3	85.3	85.4	85.6	86.1	86.8	87.7
Night-time DBP	BP percentile												
	50th	55.0	55.3	55.5	55.7	55.8	55.8	55.9	56.0	56.3	56.5	56.8	57.1
	75th	58.5	59.1	59.5	59.8	60.0	60.0	60.0	60.1	60.3	60.5	60.7	60.9
	90th	62.3	63.2	63.8	64.2	64.3	64.2	64.1	64.1	64.1	64.2	64.3	64.3
	95th	65.1	66.1	66.8	67.1	67.1	66.9	66.7	66.5	66.5	66.5	66.4	66.4
	99th	71.6	72.7	73.5	73.5	73.2	72.6	71.9	71.4	71.1	70.8	70.6	70.3

(continued)

Table 12.1 (continued)

Normal values for ambulatory blood pressure (mmHg) for boys by age

		Age (years)											
		5	6	7	8	9	10	11	12	13	14	15	16
BP percentile	**24-h MAP**												
	50th	77.4	77.9	78.7	79.3	79.7	80.2	80.8	81.7	82.7	83.8	85.1	86.4
	75th	81.4	81.9	82.7	83.4	83.8	84.3	85.0	85.9	86.9	88.0	89.3	90.5
	90th	85.5	86.0	86.8	87.4	87.9	88.3	88.9	89.7	90.6	91.6	92.7	93.9
	95th	88.3	88.7	89.5	90.0	90.4	90.8	91.3	91.9	92.7	93.7	94.7	95.7
	99th	94.3	94.6	95.1	95.4	95.6	95.7	95.8	96.2	96.7	97.3	98.1	98.9
BP percentile	**Day-time MAP**												
	50th	83.5	84.1	84.5	84.8	84.9	85.0	85.3	85.9	86.8	88.0	89.4	90.8
	75th	87.5	88.2	88.8	89.2	89.4	89.5	89.9	90.6	91.5	92.7	94.2	95.7
	90th	91.3	92.1	92.8	93.3	93.5	93.7	94.0	94.7	95.6	96.8	98.3	99.8
	95th	93.6	94.5	95.3	95.8	96.1	96.2	96.5	97.1	98.0	99.2	100.6	102.1
	99th	98.2	99.2	100.1	100.7	101.0	101.0	101.2	101.6	102.4	103.4	104.7	106.1
BP percentile	**Night-time MAP**												
	50th	66.7	67.7	68.6	69.2	69.7	70.0	70.5	71.2	72.1	73.1	74.0	74.9
	75th	70.5	71.7	72.8	73.5	74.1	74.5	75.0	75.6	76.4	77.2	78.0	78.6
	90th	74.7	76.0	77.2	78.1	78.6	78.9	79.3	79.7	80.3	80.8	81.3	81.7
	95th	77.6	79.0	80.2	81.1	81.6	81.8	82.0	82.3	82.6	82.9	83.2	83.4
	99th	84.1	85.7	86.9	87.6	87.8	87.7	87.4	87.1	86.9	86.8	86.6	86.4

Normal values for ambulatory blood pressure (mmHg) for girls by age

	Age (years)											
	5	6	7	8	9	10	11	12	13	14	15	16
24-h SBP												

Normal values for ambulatory blood pressure (mmHg) for girls by age

BP percentile	Age (years)											
	5	6	7	8	9	10	11	12	13	14	15	16
50th	102.8	104.1	105.3	106.5	107.6	108.7	109.7	110.7	111.8	112.8	113.8	114.8
75th	107.8	109.1	110.4	111.5	112.6	113.6	114.7	115.7	116.7	117.6	118.4	119.2
90th	112.3	113.7	115.0	116.1	117.2	118.2	119.2	120.2	121.2	121.9	122.6	123.2
95th	114.9	116.4	117.7	118.9	120.0	121.1	122.1	123.0	123.9	124.5	125.0	125.6
99th	119.9	121.5	123.0	124.3	125.5	126.5	127.5	128.4	129.0	129.5	129.7	130.0
Day-time SBP												
BP percentile												
50th	108.4	109.5	110.6	111.5	112.4	113.3	114.2	115.3	116.4	117.5	118.6	119.6
75th	113.8	114.9	115.9	116.8	117.6	118.5	119.5	120.6	121.7	122.6	123.5	124.3
90th	118.3	119.5	120.6	121.5	122.4	123.3	124.3	125.3	126.4	127.2	127.9	128.5
95th	120.9	122.2	123.3	124.3	125.2	126.2	127.2	128.2	129.2	129.9	130.4	130.9
99th	125.6	127.1	128.4	129.6	130.6	131.7	132.7	133.7	134.5	135.0	135.2	135.4
Night-time SBP												
BP percentile												
50th	94.8	95.6	96.2	96.8	97.5	98.2	99.0	99.7	100.5	101.3	102.0	102.9
75th	100.2	101.1	101.8	102.5	103.2	104.0	104.7	105.2	105.8	106.3	106.8	107.3
90th	105.3	106.3	107.2	108.0	108.8	109.5	110.1	110.4	110.7	110.9	111.0	111.2
95th	108.4	109.6	110.6	111.5	112.3	113.0	113.5	113.6	113.7	113.6	113.5	113.5
99th	114.5	116.0	117.3	118.4	119.3	119.9	120.1	119.8	119.4	118.8	118.2	117.8
24-h DBP												
BP percentile												
50th	65.5	65.6	65.8	65.9	66.0	66.2	66.4	66.6	67.0	67.2	67.5	67.7
75th	68.9	69.1	69.2	69.3	69.5	69.8	70.0	70.4	70.8	71.1	71.2	71.4
90th	72.1	72.2	72.3	72.4	72.6	72.9	73.2	73.7	74.1	74.4	74.6	74.7
95th	74.0	74.1	74.2	74.2	74.4	74.7	75.1	75.6	76.1	76.4	76.6	76.7
99th	77.6	77.6	77.6	77.6	77.7	78.0	78.4	79.1	79.7	80.1	80.4	80.5

(continued)

Table 12.1 (continued)

Normal values for ambulatory blood pressure (mmHg) for girls by age

BP percentile	Age (years)											
	5	6	7	8	9	10	11	12	13	14	15	16
Day-time DBP												
50th	72.6	72.6	72.4	72.2	72.0	71.8	71.8	72.1	72.4	72.8	73.2	73.5
75th	76.7	76.6	76.5	76.3	76.0	75.9	75.9	76.2	76.5	76.8	77.0	77.2
90th	80.2	80.2	80.0	79.8	79.5	79.3	79.4	79.6	80.0	80.2	80.3	80.3
95th	82.3	82.2	82.1	81.8	81.5	81.3	81.4	81.6	82.0	82.2	82.2	82.1
99th	86.1	86.0	85.8	85.5	85.2	85.0	85.0	85.3	85.6	85.7	85.6	85.4
Night-time DBP												
50th	56.4	55.9	55.5	55.1	54.8	54.6	54.3	54.2	54.3	54.5	54.9	55.3
75th	61.1	60.6	60.1	59.7	59.4	59.2	58.9	58.7	58.7	58.7	58.8	59.1
90th	65.6	65.1	64.6	64.1	63.8	63.7	63.4	63.1	62.9	62.8	62.8	62.8
95th	68.5	67.9	67.4	66.9	66.6	66.5	66.2	65.9	65.6	65.4	65.3	65.2
99th	74.2	73.6	72.9	72.4	72.2	72.0	71.8	71.4	71.1	70.7	70.3	70.0
24-h MAP												
50th	77.5	78.0	78.4	78.8	79.2	79.6	80.2	80.9	81.5	82.2	82.7	83.0
75th	81.2	81.7	82.1	82.5	82.9	83.3	84.0	84.7	85.4	86.0	86.5	86.8
90th	84.6	85.0	85.4	85.7	86.1	86.5	87.1	87.9	88.6	89.2	89.7	89.9
95th	86.6	87.0	87.3	87.6	87.9	88.3	88.9	89.7	90.5	91.0	91.5	91.7
99th	90.5	90.8	90.9	91.0	91.2	91.6	92.2	93.0	93.7	94.2	94.6	94.8
Day-time MAP												

Normal values for ambulatory blood pressure (mmHg) for girls by age

	Age (years)											
BP percentile	5	6	7	8	9	10	11	12	13	14	15	16
50th	83.7	83.9	84.0	84.1	84.2	84.4	84.7	85.2	85.9	86.5	87.1	87.7
75th	88.2	88.3	88.4	88.4	88.4	88.5	88.9	89.4	90.1	90.8	91.4	91.9
90th	92.2	92.2	92.2	92.1	92.0	92.1	92.4	93.0	93.6	94.3	94.8	95.4
95th	94.6	94.5	94.4	94.2	94.1	94.2	94.4	95.0	95.6	96.2	96.8	97.3
99th	99.0	98.7	98.5	98.2	97.9	97.9	98.1	98.6	99.2	99.7	100.2	100.7
Night-time MAP												
BP percentile												
50th	68.7	68.8	68.8	68.8	68.9	69.1	69.3	69.6	70.1	70.6	71.2	71.8
75th	73.0	73.1	73.1	73.2	73.4	73.6	73.8	74.1	74.5	74.9	75.4	75.9
90th	76.9	77.0	77.1	77.2	77.4	77.6	77.8	78.0	78.3	78.6	78.9	79.3
95th	79.2	79.4	79.6	79.7	79.8	80.1	80.2	80.3	80.5	80.7	80.9	81.2
99th	83.8	84.1	84.2	84.3	84.5	84.6	84.7	84.6	84.6	84.6	84.6	84.7

Table 12.2 Classification of BP in children and adolescents based on casual and ambulatory BP measurements

Classification	Office BP [1]	Mean Ambulatory SBP or DBP [2, 3]	SBP or DBP Load [3, 4] (%)
Normal BP	<90th percentile	<95th percentile	<25
White coat hypertension	≥95th percentile	<95th percentile	<25
Prehypertension	≥90th percentile or >120/80	<95th percentile	≥25
Masked hypertension	<95th percentile	>95th percentile	≥25
Ambulatory (sustained) hypertension	>95th percentile	>95th percentile	25–50
Severe ambulatory hypertension	>95th	>95th percentile	>50

[a]Based on the Fourth Report [12]
[b]Based on the pediatric ABPM values in Table 12.2
[c]For either the wake or sleep period of the study, or both
[d]For patients with elevated load but normal mean ABPM and office BP that is either normal (<90th percentile) or hypertensive (>95th percentile), no specific ABPM classification can be assigned based on current evidence and expert consensus. These "unclassified" patients should be evaluated on a case-by-case basis, taking into account the etiology of hypertension and the absence or presence of other cardiovascular risk factors

ABPM recommendations, as well as addressed concerns regarding those older recommendations.

The 2008 AHA statement suggested using the following classification for BP in pediatric patients based on office and ambulatory BP: normotensive, white coat hypertensive, masked hypertensive, prehypertensive, and ambulatory hypertensive [11]. The 2008 AHA statement also recommended including severe ambulatory hypertension and discussed issues with diastolic hypertension, nocturnal hypertension, mean arterial pressure, and uncategorized patients [11]. These recommendations are summarized in Table 12.2. It should be noted that classification of pediatric ambulatory BP differs from adult BP classification in a variety of ways: adult BP categories are defined by fixed BP levels and not BP percentiles, there is no prehypertension category in adults, and BP loads up to 30 % are considered normal While these differences largely reflect expert opinion, the AHA classification scheme has found widespread acceptance in both clinical and research use of ABPM in children and adolescents.

Prehypertension, Ambulatory Hypertension, and Severe Ambulatory Hypertension

In a child without any other major comorbidities, a mean ambulatory BP ≥90th percentile or >120/80 mmHg, and <95th percentile with elevated BP loads ≥25 % is considered prehypertensive. There is currently a lack of data regarding clinical outcomes in children with ABPM-diagnosed prehypertension, although, at least one study has found increased LVM and arterial stiffness in prehypertensive children compared to normotensive children [17], and experts in pediatric hypertension believe it represents a higher risk state.

Ambulatory hypertension is defined as mean SBP or DBP >95th percentile with a BP load of ≥25 and <50 %. Patients with BP loads >50 % are considered to have severe ambulatory hypertension. Sustained hypertension diagnosed by ABPM has been shown to correlate more strongly with LVM than casual BPs [18]. Pediatric hypertension based on ABPM values is also correlated with vascular damage such as increased carotid intimal-media thickness [19] and renal damage defined as increased prevalence of microalbuminemia [20]. Clinical outcomes in specific patient populations are discussed in further detail later in this chapter.

White Coat Hypertension and Masked Hypertension

White coat hypertension (WCH) is a condition in which casual BPs are ≥95th percentile, but ambulatory BP <95th percentile with less than 25 % BP load. Although home or self-measured BP can theoretically be used to help identify patients with WCH, in children this condition is best diagnosed with ABPM. WCH has higher prevalence in obese patients and in patients less than 12 years old [21] and while the overall pediatric prevalence is unknown, estimates have ranged from 10 to 60 % [22], with one recent retrospective study finding a prevalence of 30 % [23]. Patients with WCH have higher LVM [24] and increased risk of progressing to ambulatory hypertension than controls. At least one study found target-organ-damage prevalence similar to that in children with confirmed sustained hypertension [23]. These patients therefore require follow-up with repeat ABPM to monitor their status.

Masked hypertension is essentially the inverse of WCH, with casual BPs below the 95th percentile, but ambulatory BP greater than the 95th percentile with ≥25 % BP load on ABPM. The prevalence of this is unknown, but estimates have ranged as high as 9.7 % in pediatric patients referred for hypertension evaluation [24]. As casual BPs are normal, it is difficult to know when to evaluate for masked hypertension with ABPM. Masked hypertension may be suspected when multiple other care providers report hypertension, the patient has risk factors for hypertension such as renal disease or obesity, or when there is other evidence of potential hypertension based on elevations in LVMI. Masked hypertension has been associated with increased LVH in pediatric populations [11, 24], as well as increased risk of progression to sustained ambulatory hypertension [25]. As with WCH, ABPM is considered the gold standard for the evaluation of masked hypertension.

Isolated Diastolic Hypertension

The 2014 AHA statement recognized that some children have isolated diastolic hypertension and incorporated DBP into their ambulatory BP classification [2]. While the clinical significance of this is not entirely clear, it appears that diastolic hypertension may be associated with underlying secondary causes of hypertension [26] and the presence of it may signal the need for further workup to determine the cause of the hypertension. As alluded to earlier, there are some difficulties, however, in interpreting diastolic BPs using ABPM. Due to their ease of use, most ABPM machines used in pediatrics use the oscillometric technique, which has been shown to be less accurate measuring DBP than SBP [27]. However, as previously stated, it is thought that the normative data for DBP by Wühl et al. is high, and DBP readings above 95th percentile given from that data would certainly be considered hypertensive by most practitioners, especially in younger children.

Nocturnal Hypertension and 3Nocturnal Dipping

Isolated nocturnal hypertension has significant prognostic implications for patients with a variety of other medical conditions, which will be discussed in more detail later. In adults, it has been shown to be the single best BP parameter predictive of cardiovascular disease [28]. The clinical significance in otherwise healthy pediatric patients is not known, but given the significant effects in adults and in specific pediatric populations, the authors of the 2014 AHA statement recommend that isolated nocturnal hypertension be treated as masked hypertension [2].

Adequate nocturnal dipping is defined as a decrease from mean awake SBP and DBP of at least 10 % to sleep SBP and DBP. Inadequate nocturnal dipping is defined as decrease of less than 10 %. Much like with nocturnal hypertension, inadequate nocturnal dipping has been shown to have prognostic value for specific populations of pediatric patients, such as those with diabetes [29], although its clinical significance in nondiabetic children is unclear. There have been racial disparities seen with nocturnal dipping, with African Americans having higher sleep BPs and less nocturnal dipping than White children [30]. Recent unpublished data from our center also suggests that obese children have a higher prevalence of inadequate nocturnal dipping than lean children.

Mean Arterial Pressure

ABPM devices that use the oscillometric technique directly measure MAP and then back-calculate to generate the SBP and DBP values. These calculated values can vary significantly when compared to BPs obtained by manual auscultation [31]. The algorithms used to calculate SBP and DBP are specific to the manufacturer, and different devices therefore may give different results. In addition, MAP is a composite of both SBP and DBP, making it a simpler tool than using both. Because of this, some have questioned whether MAP may be more useful than SBP and DBP for diagnosing hypertension in pediatrics. One recent cross-sectional study compared diagnosis of hypertension using MAP as opposed to SBP and DBP [32]. Using a hypertension definition of ≥95th percentile for either MAP or SBP/DBP, the authors found that the

MAP criteria identified 19 % more hypertensive patients than the SBP/DBP criteria. However, there are few published data evaluating the prognostic value of MAP in pediatrics. In the ESCAPE trial, therapeutic interventions based on MAP were shown to improve outcomes in pediatric patients with CKD [33]. There are currently no other studies in pediatric populations evaluating clinical outcomes and MAP. More studies assessing intermediate and long-term clinical outcomes using MAP will need to be conducted before we can recommend using it instead of SBP and DBP.

Secondary Hypertension and Special Populations

Secondary Hypertension

Secondary hypertension refers to hypertension that is caused by an identifiable, underlying cause such as renal artery stenosis. It is much more common in children than in adults and is therefore always a consideration when a child or teen is being evaluated for elevated BP. There are certain signs that are potentially suggestive of secondary hypertension such as hypertension detected in very young children, patients with stage 2 hypertension, or in patients with clinical signs that indicate systemic conditions [7].

ABPM can also help differentiate between primary and secondary hypertension (see Fig. 12.1). Increased sleep SBP loads and increased awake and sleep DBP loads

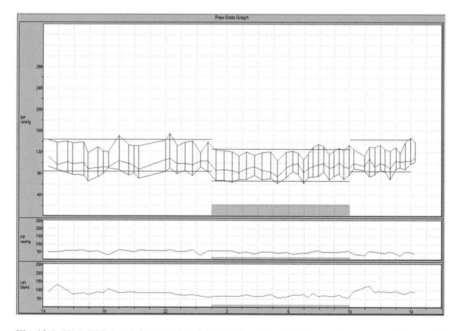

Fig. 12.1 High DBP Loads in secondary hypertension. The patient was a hypertensive16-year-old boy with one small scarred kidney. The awake DBP load was 45 % and the sleep DBP load was 86 %

are highly specific for a secondary etiology of hypertension [26]. Decreased nocturnal dipping has also been associated with secondary hypertension in children [34].
As more data are generated, ABPM may become a more reliable tool for identifying
secondary hypertension and may help guide diagnostic workup. Conditions in which
ABPM may be particularly helpful are summarized in Table 12.3.

While there are no BP targets devised specifically for the management of secondary hypertension, some experts recommend using the 90th percentile to define
secondary hypertension in relevant patients as opposed to the 95th percentile.
The following section covers specific etiologies of secondary hypertension and the
utility of ABPM in each condition.

Diabetes

The prevalence of hypertension in adolescent type 1 diabetics in the United States
is estimated to be between 22 and 29 % [35, 36]. The 2014 ISPAD Clinical Practice
Consensus Guideline states that hypertension is a major risk factor for both micro-
and macro-vascular complications in adolescent type 1 diabetic patients and recog-
nizes the role that ABPM has in managing hypertension in the pediatric diabetic
population [37]. It has been shown that early detection of diabetic nephropathy and
hypertension in diabetics significantly decreases the risk of progressing to end-stage
renal failure [37]. While hypertension is known to increase cardiovascular disease
in adults, there are currently few data in children on cardiovascular morbidity or
mortality in relation to hypertension. One recent study, however, found that elevated
BP loads detected on ABPM in children with type 1 diabetes were associated with

Table 12.3 Conditions in which ABPM may be particularly helpful

Condition	Relevance of ABPM	Benefit
Secondary hypertension	Elevated load, abnormal dipping variability	ABPM results may indicate higher likelihood for secondary causes
Diabetes mellitus (Types 1 and 2)	Elevated load, abnormal dipping variability	Tighter BP control may limit development of diabetic nephropathy, retinopathy
Chronic kidney disease	Prevalence of HTN, masked HTN	Tighter BP control may delay CKD progression
Dialysis	BP loads, Masked HTN	Better correlation with target organ damage than pre/post-dialysis BPs
Renal transplant	Masked HTN, abnormal circadian variation	Tighter BP control may delay graft loss
White coat and masked HTN	Can only be diagnosed on ABPM	Patient may not require extensive diagnostic testing
Treatment of patients with HTN	Response to interventions	Better BP control may improve outcome

increased B-type natriuretic peptide and abnormal tissue Doppler echocardiography indices, indicating early-stage cardiac dysfunction [38]. In adolescents, nocturnal hypertension is especially associated with the development of diabetic nephropathy and other signs of end-organ damage such as increased carotid intimal thickness [29, 39]. These patients also have estimated prevalence of 10 % and 32 % for masked hypertension and white coat hypertension, respectively. It is also estimated that between 24 and 42 % of type 1 diabetic children have non-dipping status [36].

Type 2 diabetes in youth has been consistently shown to run a greater risk of cardiovascular complications than type 1 diabetes including hypertension, microalbuminuria, diabetic nephropathy, and mortality [37, 40]. In fact, up to 50 % of children diagnosed with type 2 diabetes under the age of 18 will develop end-stage renal disease within 20 years of their diagnosis. However, there is conflicting evidence regarding the role of hypertension in the progression of kidney disease. While it is well-documented that hypertension increases progression of CKD in adult type 2 diabetics, one large pediatric study did not find any association with risk of renal disease and hypertension, and in fact found that prescription of renin angiotensin aldosterone inhibitors was a major risk factor for renal failure [41]. The Improving Renal Complications in Adolescents with Type 2 Diabetes Through Research (iCARE) Cohort Study [42] is a large, prospective cohort study that is currently examining a variety of risk factors for albuminuria and progression of CKD in adolescent type 2 diabetes patients, including hypertension diagnosed by ABPM, and hopefully will shed more light on the role of ABPM in the management of children with type 2 diabetes.

Chronic Kidney Disease

Hypertension in patients with chronic kidney disease (CKD)is recognized as a risk factor for worse cardiovascular outcomes as well as progression to end-stage renal disease. 24-h ABPM has proven to be superior to clinic BP measurements and at least equivalent to other home BP measurement methods for monitoring hypertension in children with CKD [43]. Increased BP variability in patients with CKD, thought to be due to sympathetic nervous system overactivity [44], has been shown to increase risk of end-organ damage and cardiovascular events. Recent evidence from the Chronic Kidney Disease in Children (CKiD) Study found that children with CKD and hypertension had significantly increased BP variability and significantly decreased heart rate variability compared to CKD patients without hypertension [45]. This is an important finding which suggests that treatment strategies to control sympathetic nervous system overactivity should be utilized in hypertensive children with CKD.

BP goals in children with CKD are still being evaluated. Citing data from the "Effect of Strict Blood Pressure Control and ACE Inhibition on the Progression of CRF in Pediatric Patients" (ESCAPE Trial) [46] from the European Society of Hypertension notes that strict BP control to 24-h MAP below the 50th percentile may increase 5-year renal survival [47]. Similar outcomes have been shown when

24-h BP mean by ABPM is kept below the 75th percentile, and renal survival is worse when 24-h ambulatory BP mean is greater than the 90th percentile. It should be noted, however, that ABPM may not be universally available, and clinicians may need to rely upon casual BP readings to make treatment decisions. The casual BP value that is equivalent to a 24-h MAP value is unknown, making it hard to translate the ESCAPE findings into clinical practice. Nonetheless, given the strength of the ESCAPE trial findings, it is recommended that caregivers aim for stricter BP control, at least less than the 90th percentile, when treating patients with CKD.

End-Stage Renal Disease and Dialysis

It is estimated that 40 % of mortality in children on maintenance hemodialysis in the United States is secondary to cardiovascular causes [48]. Given this, it is essential that BPs are accurately assessed and hypertension aggressively treated in this patient population. Many children on dialysis have their BPs assessed by pre- or post-dialysis recordings. However, these BP measurements may be inaccurate and have poor test–retest reliability [49]. ABPM has proven more sensitive and specific method and provides a more comprehensive BP profile than pre- and post-dialysis BPs for diagnosing hypertension and improves the predictability of BP as a risk factor for target organ damage [49]. Dialysis patients with elevated BP loads diagnosed by ABPM were more likely to have LVH and non-dipping status than patients without elevated BP loads. It has been recommended that ABPM become the standard for monitoring BPs in patients on dialysis [49]. More recent data suggests that 48-h ABPM may be even more effective than 24-h ABPM for diagnosing daytime and nighttime hypertension, decreased dipping, and assessing risks for elevated LVMI in intermittent hemodialysis patients [50].

Kidney Transplant

ABPM is a critical tool for assessing BPs in pediatric patients after renal transplantation (see Fig. 12.2). Ambulatory hypertension affects a significant percentage (potentially a majority) of pediatric patients who receive kidney transplants, and abnormalities on ABPM in these patients are associated with LVH and other target organ damage [8]. In addition, there is increased incidence of masked hypertension and abnormal circadian variation in BP, including sleep hypertension and blunted and reversed BP dipping, which requires ABPM for diagnosis [8]. Optimal BP treatment guided by repeat ABPM decreases target organ damage [51], increases stable graft function compared to those that remain hypertensive [52], and decreases proteinuria (a marker of chronic allograft nephropathy).

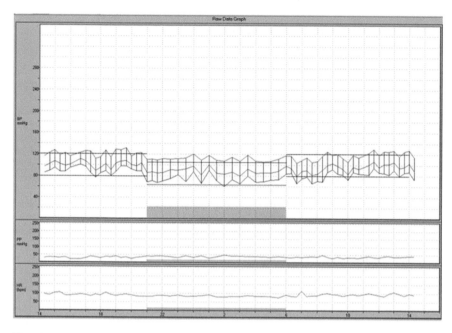

Fig. 12.2 Severe nocturnal hypertension in a renal transplant recipient. The patient was a 7-year-old boy 6 months following renal transplant. The sleep BP loads were 100 % for SBP and 95 % for DBP; SBP dipping was 6.7 % and DBP dipping was 14 %. He was also hypertensive while awake, although BP loads were not as high as while asleep

Conclusion

ABPM has proven to be an effective method of measuring BP in the pediatric population. It is better correlated with clinical outcomes such as left ventricular hypertrophy, eliminating observer bias and improper technique, and allowing for the diagnosis of white coat hypertension and masked hypertension. There are some shortcomings to using ABPM in children, such as generalizability of the available normative data, but as more data are gathered we expect that it will be an even more effective tool in the diagnosis and management of pediatric hypertension.

References

1. Din-Dzietham R, Liu Y, Bielo M-V, Shamsa F. High blood pressure trends in children and adolescents in national surveys, 1963 to 2002. Circulation. 2007;116(13):1488–96.
2. Flynn JT, Daniels SR, Hayman LL, et al. Update: ambulatory blood pressure monitoring in children and adolescents a scientific statement from the American Heart Association. Hypertension. 2014;63(5):1116–35.

3. Ayer JG, Harmer JA, Nakhla S, et al. HDL-cholesterol, blood pressure, and asymmetric dimethylarginine are significantly associated with arterial wall thickness in children. Arterioscler Thromb Vasc Biol. 2009;29(6):943–9.
4. Wong LJ, Kupferman JC, Prohovnik I, et al. Hypertension impairs vascular reactivity in the pediatric brain. Stroke. 2011;42(7):1834–8.
5. Chen X, Wang Y. Tracking of blood pressure from childhood to adulthood a systematic review and meta–regression analysis. Circulation. 2008;117(25):3171–80.
6. Juonala M, Magnussen CG, Venn A, et al. Influence of Age on associations between childhood risk factors and carotid intima-media thickness in adulthood clinical perspective the cardiovascular risk in young Finns study, the childhood determinants of adult health study, the Bogalusa heart study, and the Muscatine study for the International Childhood Cardiovascular Cohort (i3C) consortium. Circulation. 2010;122(24):2514–20.
7. Flynn JT, Urbina EM. Pediatric ambulatory blood pressure monitoring: indications and interpretations. J Clin Hypertens. 2012;14(6):372–82.
8. Flynn JT. Ambulatory blood pressure monitoring should be routinely performed after pediatric renal transplantation. Pediatr Transplant. 2012;16(6):533–6.
9. Swartz SJ, Srivaths PR, Croix B, Feig DI. Cost-effectiveness of ambulatory blood pressure monitoring in the initial evaluation of hypertension in children. Pediatrics. 2008;122(6):1177–81.
10. Davis ML, Ferguson MA, Zachariah JP. Clinical predictors and impact of ambulatory blood pressure monitoring in pediatric hypertension referrals. J Am Soc Hypertens; 2014;8(9):660–7.
11. Urbina E, Alpert B, Flynn J, et al. Ambulatory blood pressure monitoring in children and adolescents: recommendations for standard assessment a scientific statement from the American Heart Association Atherosclerosis, Hypertension, and Obesity in Youth Committee of the council on cardiovascular disease in the young and the council for high blood pressure research. Hypertension. 2008;52(3):433–51.
12. National High Blood Pressure Education Program. The fourth report on the diagnosis, evaluation, and treatment of high blood pressure in children and adolescents: US Department of Health and Human Services, National Institutes of Health, National Heart, Lung, and Blood Institute, National Hight Blood Pressure Education Program; 2005.
13. Winnicki M, Canali C, Mormino P, Palatini P. Ambulatory blood pressure monitoring editing criteria: is standardization needed? Am J Hypertens. 1997;10(4):419–27.
14. Jones HE, Sinha MD. The definition of daytime and nighttime influences the interpretation of ABPM in children. Pediatr Nephrol. 2011;26(5):775–81.
15. Wühl E, Witte K, Soergel M, Mehls O, Schaefer F. Hypertension GWGoP. Distribution of 24-h ambulatory blood pressure in children: normalized reference values and role of body dimensions. J Hypertens. 2002;20(10):1995–2007.
16. Soergel M, Kirschstein M, Busch C, et al. Oscillometric twenty-four-hour ambulatory blood pressure values in healthy children and adolescents: a multicenter trial including 1141 subjects. J Pediatr. 1997;130(2):178–84.
17. Urbina EM, Khoury PR, McCoy C, Daniels SR, Kimball TR, Dolan LM. Cardiac and vascular consequences of pre-hypertension in youth. J Clin Hypertens. 2011;13(5):332–42.
18. Sorof JM, Cardwell G, Franco K, Portman RJ. Ambulatory blood pressure and left ventricular mass index in hypertensive children. Hypertension. 2002;39(4):903–8.
19. Lande MB, Carson NL, Roy J, Meagher CC. Effects of childhood primary hypertension on carotid intima media thickness a matched controlled study. Hypertension. 2006;48(1):40–4.
20. Seeman T, Pohl M, Palyzova D, John U. Microalbuminuria in children with primary and white-coat hypertension. Pediatr Nephrol. 2012;27(3):461–7.
21. Stergiou GS, Rarra VC, Yiannes NG. Changing relationship between home and office blood pressure with increasing age in children: the Arsakeion School study. Am J Hypertens. 2008;21(1):41–6.

22. Stabouli S, Kotsis V, Zakopoulos N. Ambulatory blood pressure monitoring and target organ damage in pediatrics. J Hypertens. 2007;25(10):1979–86.
23. Litwin M, Niemirska A, Ruzicka M, Feber J. White coat hypertension in children: not rare and not benign? J Am Soc Hypertens. 2009;3(6):416–23.
24. Stabouli S, Kotsis V, Toumanidis S, Papamichael C, Constantopoulos A, Zakopoulos N. White-coat and masked hypertension in children: association with target-organ damage. Pediatr Nephrol. 2005;20(8):1151–5.
25. Lurbe E, Torro I, Alvarez V, et al. Prevalence, persistence, and clinical significance of masked hypertension in youth. Hypertension. 2005;45(4):493–8.
26. Flynn JT. Differentiation between primary and secondary hypertension in children using ambulatory blood pressure monitoring. Pediatrics. 2002;110(1):89–93.
27. Skirton H, Chamberlain W, Lawson C, Ryan H, Young E. A systematic review of variability and reliability of manual and automated blood pressure readings. J Clin Nurs. 2011;20(5-6):602–14.
28. Hansen TW, Li Y, Boggia J, Thijs L, Richart T, Staessen JA. Predictive role of the nighttime blood pressure. Hypertension. 2011;57(1):3–10.
29. Lurbe E, Redon J, Kesani A, et al. Increase in nocturnal blood pressure and progression to microalbuminuria in type 1 diabetes. N Engl J Med. 2002;347(11):797–805.
30. Harshfield GA, Barbeau P, Richey PA, Alpert BS. Racial differences in the influence of body size on ambulatory blood pressure in youths. Blood Press Monit. 2000;5(2):59–63.
31. Amoore JN. Oscillometric sphygmomanometers: a critical appraisal of current technology. Blood Press Monit. 2012;17(2):80–8.
32. Šuláková T, Feber J. Should mean arterial pressure be included in the definition of ambulatory hypertension in children? Pediatr Nephrol. 2013;28(7):1105–12.
33. Wuehl E, Trivelli A, Picca S, et al. Strict blood-pressure control and progression of renal failure in children. N Engl J Med. 2009;361(17):1639–50.
34. Seeman T, Palyzová D, Dušek J, Janda J. Reduced nocturnal blood pressure dip and sustained nighttime hypertension are specific markers of secondary hypertension. J Pediatr. 2005;147(3):366–71.
35. Duncan GE, Li SM, Zhou X-H. Prevalence and trends of a metabolic syndrome phenotype among US adolescents, 1999–2000. Diabetes Care. 2004;27(10):2438–43.
36. Šuláková T, Janda J, Černá J, et al. Arterial HTN in children with T1DM—frequent and not easy to diagnose. Pediatr Diabetes. 2009;10(7):441–8.
37. Donaghue KC, Wadwa RP, Dimeglio LA, et al. Microvascular and macrovascular complications in children and adolescents. Pediatr Diabetes. 2014;15 Suppl 20:257–69.
38. Kır M, Cetin B, Demir K, et al. Can ambulatory blood pressure monitoring detect early diastolic dysfunction in children with type 1 diabetes mellitus: correlations with B-type natriuretic peptide and tissue Doppler findings. Pediatr Diabetes. 2014.
39. Lee SH, Kim JH, Kang MJ, Lee YA, Yang SW, Shin CH. Implications of nocturnal hypertension in children and adolescents with type 1 diabetes. Diabetes Care. 2011;34(10):2180–5.
40. Ettinger LM, Freeman K, DiMartino-Nardi JR, Flynn JT. Microalbuminuria and abnormal ambulatory blood pressure in adolescents with type 2 diabetes mellitus. J Pediatr. 2005;147(1):67–73.
41. Dart AB, Sellers EA, Martens PJ, Rigatto C, Brownell MD, Dean HJ. High burden of kidney disease in youth-onset type 2 diabetes. Diabetes Care. 2012;35(6):1265–71.
42. Dart AB, Wicklow BA, Sellers EA, et al. The improving renal complications in adolescents with type 2 diabetes through the research (iCARE) Cohort Study: rationale and protocol. Can J Diabetes. 2014;38(5):349–55.
43. Wühl E, Hadtstein C, Mehls O, Schaefer F. Home, clinic, and ambulatory blood pressure monitoring in children with chronic renal failure. Pediatr Res. 2004;55(3):492–7.
44. Flynn J, Woroniecki R. Pathophysiology of hypertension. In: Avner ED, Harmon WE, Niaudet P, editors. Pediatric nephrology. Philadelphia: Lippincott Williams & Wilkins; 2004. p. 1154–77.

45. Barletta G-M, Flynn J, Mitsnefes M, et al. Heart rate and blood pressure variability in children with chronic kidney disease: a report from the CKiD study. Pediatr Nephrol. 2014;29(6):1059–65.
46. Wühl E, Mehls O, Schaefer F, (eds.) (2008). Nephroprotection by intensified blood pressure control: final results of the ESCAPE-trial. Journal of Hypertension. Lippincott Williams & Wilkins: Philadelphia.
47. Lurbe E, Cifkova R, Cruickshank JK, et al. Management of high blood pressure in children and adolescents: recommendations of the European Society of Hypertension. J Hypertens. 2009;27(9):1719–42.
48. Lilien MR, Groothoff JW. Cardiovascular disease in children with CKD or ESRD. Nat Rev Nephrol. 2009;5(4):229–35.
49. Chaudhuri A, Sutherland SM, Begin B, et al. Role of twenty-four-hour ambulatory blood pressure monitoring in children on dialysis. Clin J Am Soc Nephrol. 2011;6(4):870–6.
50. Haskin O, Wong CJ, McCabe L, Begin B, Sutherland SM, Chaudhuri A. 44-h ambulatory blood pressure monitoring: revealing the true burden of hypertension in pediatric hemodialysis patients. Pediatr Nephrol. 2014;30(4):653–60.
51. Balzano R, Lindblad YT, Vavilis G, Jogestrand T, Berg UB, Krmar RT. Use of annual ABPM, and repeated carotid scan and echocardiography to monitor cardiovascular health over nine yr in pediatric and young adult renal transplant recipients. Pediatr Transplant. 2011;15(6):635–41.
52. Seeman T, Šimková E, Kreisinger J, et al. Improved control of hypertension in children after renal transplantation: Results of a two-year Interventional Trial. Pediatr Transplant. 2007;11(5):491–7.

Chapter 13
Ambulatory Blood Pressure Monitoring in Special Populations: During Pregnancy

Ramón C. Hermida and Diana E. Ayala

Introduction

Hypertensive complications in pregnancy are associated with increased risk of both adverse fetal/neonatal outcomes, including preterm birth, intrauterine growth retardation (IUGR), and perinatal death, as well as maternal outcomes, including acute renal or hepatic failure, antepartum and postpartum hemorrhage, and even death [1–3]. Hypertensive complications in pregnancy range from hypertension alone (gestational hypertension [GH]) through proteinuria and multiorgan dysfunction (preeclampsia [PE]) to seizures (eclampsia) [4]. Reported rates of GH and PE vary substantially, ranging from 4 to 15 % and 2 to 5 %, respectively [5–7]. However, these rates might well underestimate actual ones [8], since the rather large variation in reported prevalence is likely due to under-ascertainment and/or misclassification of GH and PE [8–10]. Furthermore, since the majority of cases of GH and PE are typically diagnosed at term, the increasing trend of early elective delivery contributes to additional underestimation of their prevalence [11].

Many of the physiologic changes of PE are essentially a reversal of those that accompany a healthy pregnancy, i.e., absence of normal increase in plasma volume, elevation of blood pressure (BP), increase of peripheral vascular resistance, and

R.C. Hermida, Ph.D. (✉) • D.E. Ayala, M.D., M.P.H., Ph.D.
Bioengineering and Chronobiology Laboratories, Atlantic Research Center for Information and Communication Technologies (AtlantTIC), University of Vigo, Vigo (Pontevedra) 36310, Spain
e-mail: rhermida@uvigo.es

© Springer International Publishing Switzerland 2016
W.B. White (ed.), *Blood Pressure Monitoring in Cardiovascular Medicine and Therapeutics*, Clinical Hypertension and Vascular Diseases,
DOI 10.1007/978-3-319-22771-9_13

decrease (insufficiency) of aldosterone concentration [12]. Even though the exact cause of PE is unknown, several mechanisms have been suggested, including enhanced sensitivity to vasopressors, abnormal maternal immunologic reaction, and imbalance of vasoactive prostaglandin (thromboxane A_2 and prostacyclin) concentrations, resulting in small arteries vasoconstriction, platelet activation, and uteroplacental insufficiency [12–15]. Maternal risk factors for GH and PE include nulliparity, advanced age, multiple births, diabetes, chronic hypertension, obesity, previous or family history of PE, different father and/or ≥ 10 years since last pregnancy, renal disease, and circulating antiphospholipid antibodies [3, 5, 6, 16–18]. Decreased risk of GH and PE has been associated with placenta previa, summer births, daily low-dose aspirin (particularly when ingested daily at bedtime and commencing early in pregnancy) and calcium supplementation, and BP-lowering and glucose-lowering medications to control, respectively, hypertension and diabetes [3, 16, 19–24].

Several clinical, biochemical, and biophysical tests have been applied to predict development of GH or PE later in pregnancy, but with inconsistent and usually rather low specificity and sensitivity [25]. Because an elevated BP after 20-week gestation is common to the definition of both GH and PE [4, 26], several studies [27–30] have assessed if these complications may be predicted on the basis of office cuff BP measured during conventional antenatal visits. Clinic BP values, however, have several shortcomings: they are representative of only a very small fraction of the 24-h BP profile, usually under circumstances that may have pressor effect, and the technique is fraught with potential errors, including instrument defects and poor examiner technique [31]. Not surprisingly, several investigators have found office BP measurements to be neither diagnostic nor sufficiently predictive of the development of hypertension in pregnancy [8, 9, 32–35], showing both disappointing sensitivity, as low as 9 % [36], and positive predictive value, as low as 8 % [29]. Nonetheless, the diagnosis of GH continues to rely on conventional clinic BP measurements that are interpreted relative to fix threshold values, i.e., 140/90 mmHg for systolic (SBP)/diastolic BP (DBP) after 20-week gestation [4, 26]. These reference thresholds for clinic BP measurements, the same one used to diagnose essential hypertension in nongravid women [37], are applied independently of gestational age at the time of BP measurement.

Ambulatory BP monitoring (ABPM) has been suggested as a logical approach to overcoming many of the shortcomings and uncertainties associated with clinical BP measurement in pregnancy [8, 9, 33, 34, 38–40]. Indeed, multiple studies have evaluated the potential prognostic value of ABPM for the early detection of GH and PE [40–53]. However, many ABPM-based studies evidence the same kind of methodological deficiency as clinic BP-based ones: most investigators reporting on the potential prognostic value of ABPM failed to take into account gestational age at the time of measurement on their findings [41, 42, 45, 49, 50], thus disregarding the predictable changes in BP level that occur throughout gestation.

Predictable BP Trends during Gestation in Healthy and Complicated Pregnancies

Noninvasive around-the-clock ABPM investigations have documented predictable differences in ambulatory BP between clinically healthy and hypertensive pregnant women during the course of gestation [38, 54, 55]. Hermida et al. [55] conducted a prospective ABPM study on 403 (207 nullipara) untreated Spanish pregnant women. Among them, 235 remained normotensive, 128 developed GH, and 40 developed PE. The SBP and DBP of each pregnant woman were automatically assessed every 20 min between 07:00 and 23:00 h and every 30 min during the night for 48 consecutive hours at the time of recruitment (usually within the first trimester of pregnancy), and thereafter every 4 weeks until delivery. A 48-h, instead of the most common 24-h, monitoring was chosen to improve reproducibility of results, as previously demonstrated both in nonpregnant [56] and pregnant women [57].

In normotensive pregnancies, ambulatory BP steadily decreases until the middle of gestation and then increases only slightly until delivery (Fig. 13.1, top). In contrast, women who develop GH or PE exhibit a stable SBP and DBP during the first half of pregnancy and thereafter a continuous linear and significantly greater increase until delivery (Fig. 13.1, bottom) [55]. According to these findings, the ABPM-derived 48-h SBP/DBP means during the first trimester of pregnancy already differ significantly between women who will remain normotensive throughout pregnancy and those who will later develop hypertensive complications. At the 14th week of gestation, the 48-h SBP/DBP means of women who developed GH or PE were significantly greater—115/67 mmHg—than of those who had a healthy normotensive pregnancy—103/60 mmHg. Differences in the 48-h SBP/DBP means between healthy and complicated pregnancies can be observed, therefore, quite before the actual clinical diagnosis of GH or PE is made, typically in the third trimester of pregnancy. The results of this study on women systematically sampled by 48-h ABPM throughout gestation not only confirm the predictable gestation-stage-dependent BP variation, but provide proper information to establish both around-the-clock and gestational-age-dependent reference limits for SBP and DBP [58], essential for the early identification of women at risk for developing hypertensive complications later in pregnancy [8, 9, 33, 34, 38, 59].

Circadian BP Patterns in Normotensive and Hypertensive Pregnant Women

An importantadvantage of around-the-clock ABPM is thorough description and quantification of the mostly predictable 24-h BP variation that results from the interrelationship of various internal and external time-of-day influences: (1) rest/activity-associated changes in behavior (including activity routine and level, meal timings

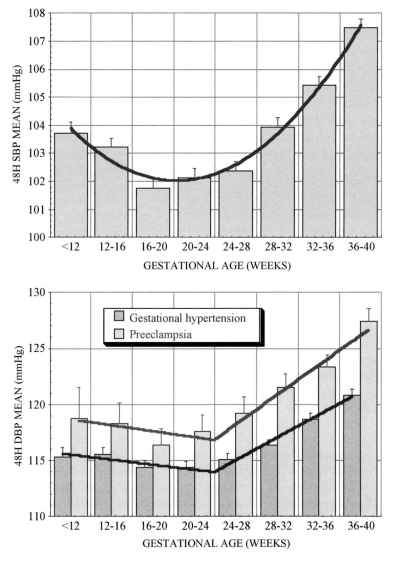

Fig. 13.1 Variation of the 48-h SBP mean throughout gestation in normotensive pregnancies (*top*; 1408 ABPM profiles of 48-h duration obtained from 235 women) and women who developed either GH (*bottom*; 800 ABPM profiles from 128 women) or PE (*bottom*; 222 ABPM profiles from 40 women). Updated from [55]

and content, mental stress, and posture); (2) day–night divergence in ambient temperature, humidity, and noise; and (3) circadian (~24 h) rhythms in neuroendocrine, endothelial, BP-modulating peptide, and hemodynamic parameters, e.g., plasma noradrenaline and adrenaline (autonomic nervous system), atrial natriuretic and calcitonin gene-related peptides, and renin, angiotensin, and aldosterone (renin-angiotensin-aldosterone system) [60–62]. Such 24-h BP variability also characterizes clinically healthy pregnant women and those who develop GH or PE [9, 36, 38, 63–66]. Many reports indicate alteration in the 24-h BP pattern during gestation can be used either to predict PE or to assess its severity [8, 9, 33, 34, 66]. However, few studies have reported on the normal 24-h BP pattern in uncomplicated pregnancies [47, 50, 67], most of them without comparison to complicated pregnancies, an issue only occasionally addressed [9, 36, 38, 49, 63–65]. By the use of ABPM, several authors have found reduced BP decline during sleep in women with PE [9, 38, 63–65], whereas others even reported a reversed circadian BP pattern towards higher sleep-time than awake-time mean BP associated with PE [66, 68, 69]. A major limitation of most of the latter studies is that they have usually been conducted during the last stages of pregnancy. Moreover, they were not specifically designed to assess if ABPM might, indeed, be used to predict GH and PE.

Normal 24-h BP values in pregnancy have been established by several ABPM trials, including one involving a primigravid population of 98 women sampled at five different gestational ages [47], and a second one involving 235 normotensive pregnant women systematically sampled every 4 weeks from early in the first trimester of pregnancy until delivery, as described in the previous section, and that also provided comparison with the 24-h BP pattern of complicated pregnancies [38, 58, 65]. Figure 13.2 presents the 24-h pattern of SBP (left) and DBP (right) assessed by 48-h ABPM per trimester of pregnancy for clinically healthy normotensive women and those who developed GH or PE. BP data were pooled over an idealized single 24-h span to simplify graphic presentations.

A statistically significant increased 48-h SBP/DBP mean was documented in pregnancies complicated with GH or PE compared to uncomplicated pregnancies in all three trimesters (p always <0.001). Differences in the hourly BP means between normotensive and hypertensive women were also statistically significant at all circadian times and in each trimester of gestation, even after correcting for multiple testing (Fig. 13.2). No differences ($p > 0.108$) were detected during the first trimester of pregnancy in the 48-h SBP/DBP means between women who later developed GH versus PE. The 48-h SBP/DBP means of normotensive pregnant women were statistically *lower* in the second as compared to the first trimester ($p < 0.001$) in keeping with the documented trends of BP variation with increasing gestational age (Fig. 13.1). In the second trimester, there was statistically significant difference in the 48-h SBP/DBP means ($p = 0.002/0.038$) between the two groups of women who subsequently developed GH and PE [65]. Panel C of Fig. 13.2, for women sampled by 48-h ABPM during their third trimester of pregnancy, shows larger between-groups differences than those documented for the first and second trimesters of pregnancy (panels A and B of Fig. 13.2, respectively). BP slightly increased from the second to the third trimester in normotensive pregnancies, up to values equivalent to those obtained in the first trimester for the same women. In women who developed GH or PE, BP increased greatly from the second to the third trimester, the increase in BP being greater for women who developed PE versus GH (Fig. 13.1). Accordingly, during the third trimester, the difference in 48-h SBP/DBP means between the GH and PE groups was statistically significant ($p < 0.001$).

Panel A

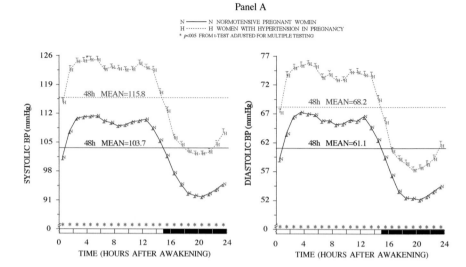

Panel B

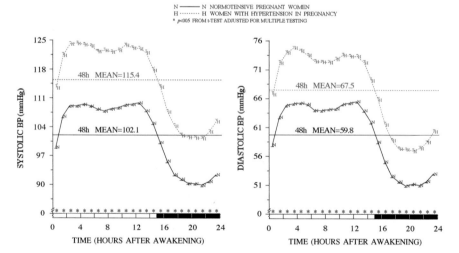

Fig. 13.2 24-h pattern of SBP (*left*) and DBP (*right*) of normotensive pregnancies (*continuous line*) and women who developed GH or PE (*dashed line*) sampled by 48-h ABPM. Each graph shows hourly means and standard errors of data for each group of pregnant women. *Dark shading* along *lower horizontal axis* of graphs denotes the average hours of nighttime sleep across the sample. *Panel A*: Women evaluated during the first trimester of pregnancy (<14 weeks gestation). *Panel B*: Women evaluated during the second trimester of pregnancy (14–27 weeks gestation). *Panel C*: Women evaluated during the third trimester of pregnancy (≥27 weeks gestation). Updated from [65]

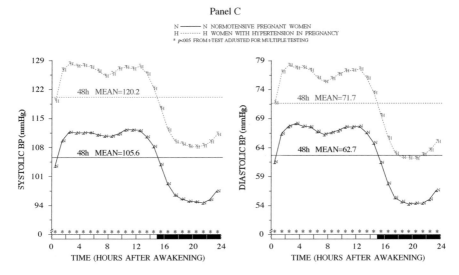

Fig. 13.2   (continued)

The results depicted in Fig. 13.2 indicate statistically significant differences in ambulatory BP between healthy and complicated pregnancies that are detectable as early as the first trimester of pregnancy; nonetheless, at this stage of gestation, both SBP and DBP for women with a later diagnosis of GH and PE were still well within the currently accepted, but as discussed below, outdated, normal physiologic BP range [65]. Despite this available information, the diagnosis of hypertension in pregnancy based on ABPM [51] has frequently relied on the very same reference thresholds established for the diagnosis of essential hypertension, i.e., 130/80 mmHg for the 24-h SBP/DBP means [37]. These reference thresholds have several shortcomings for use in pregnancy, as documented in the following section.

24-h BP Patterns in Men, Nonpregnant Women, and Pregnant Women

Apart from the predictable changes in BP with gestational age (Fig. 13.1), epidemiologic studies report significant sex differences in BP and heart rate [59, 70–73]. Typically, men exhibit lower heart rate and higher BP than women, the differences being larger for SBP than DBP [39, 71]. These differences become apparent during adolescence and remain significant until 55–60 years of age [74]. Results from a recent large long-term prospective study on cardiovascular and cerebrovascular morbidity and mortality of subjects evaluated by periodic, at least annually, 48-h ABPM reveal the outcome-based 48 h SBP/DBP reference thresholds for the diagnosis of hypertension to be 10/5 mmHg lower for women than men [72].

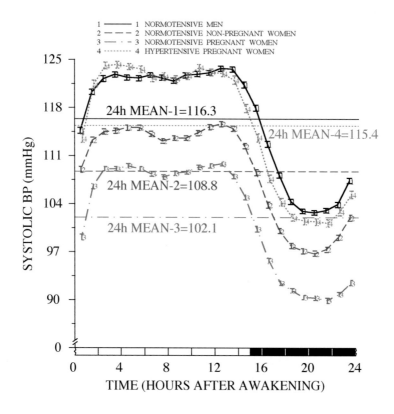

Fig. 13.3 24-h SBP pattern of clinically healthy normotensive men (Group 1: 643 individuals) and normotensive nonpregnant women (Group 2: 504 individuals), normotensive pregnant women (Group 3: 546 ABPM profiles from 235 women), and women who developed GH or PE (Group 4: 412 ABPM profiles from 168 women) sampled by 48-h ABPM during the second trimester of pregnancy (14–27 weeks gestation). Each graph shows hourly means and standard errors of data for each group of subjects. *Dark shading* along *lower horizontal* axis of graphs denotes the average hours of nighttime sleep across the subject sample. Updated from [38]

The sex differences in BP regulation are illustrated in Fig. 13.3, which presents, first, the 24-h SBP pattern of 643 clinically healthy young-adult men and 504 non-pregnant normotensive women, 18–40 years of age [71]. Data of these 1147 normo-tensive subjects, matched by age, ethnicity, and, to the extent possible, body weight and height to the population of pregnant women that provided data for Figs. 13.1 and 13.2, were obtained using the same sampling scheme, i.e., ABPM performed every 20 min from 07:00 to 23:00 h and every 30 min during the night for 48 con-secutive hours. Figure 13.3 also illustrates the 24-h BP pattern of normotensive pregnant women and those who developed GH or PE evaluated by 48-h ABPM during the second trimester of gestation. Figure 13.3 documents: (1) ambulatory SBP is significantly higher in young-adult normotensive men than similarly aged nonpregnant normotensive women ($p < 0.001$); (2) as previously demonstrated [65], ambulatory SBP during the second trimester of gestation is significantly diminished in women having normotensive pregnancies compared to ones later complicated with GH or PE ($p<0.001$), although these differences between healthy and complicated pregnancies can already be observed during the first trimester of pregnancy (Fig. 13.2, panel A); (3) ambulatory SBP is significantly lower in normotensive pregnant women than in normotensive nonpregnant women ($p<0.001$), as a consequence of the diminished BP during the second trimester of gestation in healthy pregnancies (Figs. 13.1 and 13.2); (4) ambulatory SBP is significantly higher in women who developed GH or PE evaluated during the second trimester of gestation than in normotensive women, either pregnant or nonpregnant ($p<0.001$); and (5) ambulatory SBP is fully equivalent in clinically healthy normotensive men and in pregnant women who developed GH or PE when sampled during the second trimester of pregnancy ($p=0.187$).

Although Fig. 13.3, as an example, presents data from pregnant women sampled during their second trimester of gestation, the conclusions are similar for the same women sampled by 48-h ABPM before 14 weeks gestation, i.e., during the first trimester [36, 38, 64, 65]. These significant differences in ambulatory BP that are expressed several months before the diagnosis of GH or PE cannot be established by clinic BP measurements until very late in pregnancy, well within the third trimester. Of additional significant clinical relevance is the finding that the detected 48-h SBP/DBP means, which differ between healthy and complicated pregnancies by ~12/7 mmHg, still fall below the threshold limits currently accepted for the diagnosis of hypertension in pregnancy [4, 26]. Until recently [39], knowledge of the diminished BP of nongravid women as compared to men plus the decrease in BP during the second half of gestation in normotensive pregnant women was not taken into account when establishing reference BP thresholds for the diagnosis of hypertension in pregnancy, whether based either on unreliable clinic BP measurements [4, 26] or the more reproducible ambulatory ones [37]. The unfortunate consequence of reliance upon the currently accepted thresholds established for clinic BP and ABPM measurements is high risk of misdiagnosis, i.e., gestational normotension when, in actuality, it should be GH.

24-h BP Mean for Diagnosis of Hypertension in Pregnancy

In chronic essential hypertension, the correlation between BP level and target organ damage, cardiovascular disease risk, and long-term prognosis is greater for ABPM than clinic BP measurement [75–77]. Accordingly, several investigators have attempted to extrapolate these advantages of ABPM to the diagnosis of hypertension in pregnancy and prediction of pregnancy outcome. As in essential hypertension, the most common approach for diagnosing hypertension in pregnancy has been reliance on the ABPM-derived 24-h BP mean. However, previous studies have reported inconsistent 24-h BP mean threshold reference values for the diagnosis of GH that only occasionally have been tested prospectively [42, 78]. Moreover, there is considerable controversy regarding the comparative prognostic value of the awake versus asleep BP means for the prediction of complications in pregnancy [43, 44, 47, 49].

A large number of studies have addressed the utility of the 24-h BP mean to predict GH and/or PE, often with significant deficiencies and limitations [38]. For example, Kyle et al. [49] investigated the usefulness of the second trimester 24-h BP mean as a screening test for predicting the development of hypertension later in pregnancy. They reported the awake SBP mean was elevated at 18 and 28 weeks gestation in women who subsequently developed "preeclampsia," defined by them as women with an increase in clinic DBP of ≥25 mmHg during gestation or clinic DBP ≥90 mmHg, independent of SBP or proteinuria, which differs greatly from how it is currently defined [4, 26]. The first criterion—a fixed increase in clinic SBP/DBP throughout gestation—has been eliminated from the current definition of GH [26], and the second criterion, totally disregarding SBP and proteinuria for the proper definition of PE, is inaccurate and thus of very low prognostic value [8, 9, 33, 40, 51]. Despite the significant difference in BP detected between the compared groups, the best predictive BP parameter of the study by Kyle et al. [49] was mean arterial BP ≥85 mmHg at 28 weeks gestation, providing sensitivity of 65 %, specificity of 81 %, and positive predictive value of 31 % for the improperly defined "preeclampsia." Daytime and nighttime BP means were of similar predictive value.

Penny et al. [51] used a threshold value of 135/85 mmHg for the 24-h SBP/DBP means to assess the ability of ABPM to predict development of severe hypertension (clinic SBP/DBP measurements ≥160/110 mmHg), proteinuria, birth weight < third percentile for gestational age, preterm delivery, and admission of the newborn to the neonatal intensive care unit. The authors justified their conceptual approach on the invalid claim that the 135/85 mmHg thresholds for the 24-h SBP/DBP means, greater than the ones of 130/80 mmHg currently used for non-pregnant women [37], are comparable to the 140/90 mmHg thresholds commonly used for clinic SBP/DBP. Moreover, as described above, such threshold values established independent of gestational age ignore the reported predictable BP changes that occur throughout pregnancy (Fig. 13.1). Despite all these major limitations, the authors concluded that a 24-h BP mean >135/85 mmHg in the second half of pregnancy is a significantly better predictor than conventional office BP values ≥140/90 mmHg for the development of cuff-substantiated severe hypertension.

Bellomo et al. [42] also evaluated the prognostic value of ABPM in pregnancy using reference thresholds of 125/74 mmHg, 128/78 mmHg, and 121/70 mmHg for the 24 h, awake, and asleep SBP/DBP means, respectively, in women sampled on just one occasion during their third trimester of pregnancy. These investigators reported that the 24-h BP mean is superior to clinic BP measurements obtained at the same time during the third trimester of gestation for prediction of pregnancy outcome.

Brown et al. [43] reported 70 % sensitivity to predict later detection of either GH or PE by clinic BP defined by the thresholds of ≥140/90 mmHg, when using a fixed non-varying by gestational age cutoff value of 62 mmHg for the asleep DBP mean obtained from ABPM done between 18- and 30-week gestation. They also suggested fixed threshold values of 115 mmHg for the 24-h SBP mean and 106 mmHg for the asleep SBP mean were predictive of later GH or PE, but again with relatively low sensitivities, 77 % and 54 %, respectively. In actuality, this research study describes the potential ability of the highly reproducible ABPM to predict the poorly reproducible clinic BP ≥140/90 mmHg threshold later in pregnancy.

Higgins et al. [48] applied the same questionable approach of investigating ABPM as a potential predictor of future clinic BP measurements in pregnancy. They studied 1048 women evaluated by 24-h ABPM at 18–24 weeks gestation. The best overall predictor for PE was the 24-h DBP mean, which when using a fixed cutoff threshold value of 71 mmHg provided a test with sensitivity of only 22 % and positive predictive value of only 15%.

The illustrative examples presented above highlight the limitation of relying solely on the ABPM-derived 24-h or even awake or asleep SBP/DBP means determined early in pregnancy to predict later development of GH or PE defined exclusively in terms of clinic BP and the thresholds of ≥140/90 mmHg. ABPM is unquestionably of higher prognostic value than conventional clinic BP measurements. However, due to poor results from the diagnostic test based only on the basis of the 24-h BP mean—namely the identification by ABPM of women who might or might not show elevated clinic BP later in pregnancy—the most extended, in our opinion wrong and unjustified, conclusion in the obstetric field so far is that ABPM is not a suitable tool for the early identification of GH or PE, and therefore should not be used in pregnancy [48].

The findings of studies entailing a different approach of utilizing ABPM-derived data by Hermida & Ayala [32], in contrast, clearly substantiate the ability of ABPM to predict early in pregnancy the risk of GH and PE. They performed a study on 113 pregnant women sampled for 48 h every 4 weeks from the first obstetric examination until delivery, thus providing 759 ABPM profiles in total, to assess the sensitivity and specificity of the 48-h BP mean per trimester of pregnancy in identifying hypertensive complications. This was accomplished by comparing distributions of the 48-h BP mean values of both healthy and complicated pregnancies, without assuming an a priori threshold for the diagnosis of GH based on mean BP [32]. Sensitivity ranged from 32 % for DBP in the second trimester to 84 % for SBP in the third trimester. Specificity, however, was as low as 7 % for the first trimester DBP. Results from this study revealed the threshold values for the 48-h SBP/DBP means that would eventually provide the highest combined sensitivity and specificity in the diagnosis of hypertension in pregnancy are: 111/66 mmHg in the first trimester of pregnancy, 110/65 mmHg in the second trimester, and 114/69 mmHg in the third trimester (Table 13.1). The corresponding threshold values in each of the three trimesters of pregnancy for the awake SBP/DBP means were 115/70, 115/69, and 118/72 mmHg; and 99/58, 98/56, and 104/60 mmHg for the asleep SBP/DBP means, respectively (Table 13.1 [32]). These apparently low values, reflecting the predictable changes in BP during gestation in normotensive pregnant women plus the expected diminished BP in pregnant as compared to nonpregnant women (Fig. 13.3), are fully equivalent to those proposed by other independent investigators to define normal ABPM values in pregnancy [47, 79].

In the attempt to validate prospectively these results, Hermida & Ayala calculated the sensitivity and specificity of the 48-h, awake, and asleep BP means for the early identification of hypertension in pregnancy using the reference threshold values provided above (and also in Table 13.1) when analyzing data described in Figs. 13.1 and 13.2 [78]. As an illustrative example, Fig. 13.4 represents the frequency histo-

Table 13.1 Diagnostic SBP/DBP thresholds (mmHg) for diagnosis of GH and PE based on ABPM for pregnant women as a function of gestational age[a]

ABPM characteristic	First trimester (<14 weeks gestation)	Second trimester (14–27 weeks gestation)	Third trimester (≥27 weeks gestation)
48 h mean			
SBP	111	110	114
DBP	66	65	69
Awake mean			
SBP	115	115	118
DBP	70	69	72
Asleep mean			
SBP	99	98	104
DBP	58	56	60

[a]Data from [77, 78]. Alternatively, hypertension in pregnancy might be defined as a hyperbaric index (HBI) ≥15 mmHg×h independent of pregnancy stage (see text). The HBI is defined as total area during the entire 24-h period of any given subject's BP above a time-varying threshold defined by a tolerance interval calculated as a function of gestational age [33, 34]

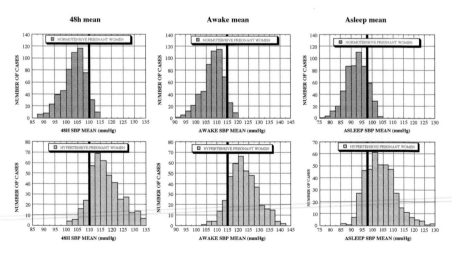

Fig. 13.4 Frequency distribution of 48-h (*left*), awake (*center*), and asleep SBP mean (*right*) from normotensive (*top*; 546 ABPM profiles from 235 women) and hypertensive pregnant women (*bottom*; 412 ABPM profiles from 168 women) sampled by 48-h ABPM during the second trimester of pregnancy (14–27 weeks gestation). The tested reference thresholds of 110, 115, and 98 mmHg for the 48-h, awake, and asleep SBP mean, respectively, are represented as *thick vertical lines* in each graph. Updated from [78]

grams with the distributions of the 48-h (left), awake (center), and asleep SBP means (right) calculated from the 958 ABPM profiles of 48 h duration obtained from the participating pregnant women in their second trimester of pregnancy. Comparison of the histograms of the normotensive (top) and hypertensive pregnancies (bottom) does not reveal clear separation between the two populations for any of the three mean BP values investigated. However, testing prospectively the previously established second trimester thresholds (110, 115, and 98 mmHg for the 48-h, awake, and asleep SBP mean, respectively [32]) reveals relatively small overlap between healthy and complicated pregnant women. Only 40 out of the 546 (7.3 %) BP profiles representative of normotensive pregnant women in the second trimester of gestation have a 48-h SBP mean >110 mmHg, while 362 out of the 412 (87.9 %) profiles representative of those who later developed GH or PE show a 48-h SBP mean above this threshold. Results are similar for the awake SBP mean (Fig. 13.4, center), although the overlap between the distributions of values of normotensive and hypertensive women is slightly higher for the asleep SBP mean (Fig. 13.4, right). Results further indicate a slightly larger overlap of BP mean values between normotensive and hypertensive women during the first trimester, and a slightly smaller overlap of the data sampled during the third trimester. Thus, the sensitivity and specificity of the diagnosis of hypertension in pregnancy based on mean SBP values increase with gestational age. The sensitivity and specificity of the DBP means according to the threshold values listed in Table 13.1 are consistently lower than they are for the SBP means at all stages of pregnancy [78].

These findings on the prospective evaluation per trimester of the prognostic value in pregnancy of the mean BP values derived from ABPM were additionally compared to those obtained from clinic BP measurements on the same women. For data obtained during the second trimester, the total overlap between normotensive and hypertensive pregnancies was 97.7 and 98.2 % for clinic SBP and DBP, respectively. Women who later developed GH or PE had during the second trimester of pregnancy clinic SBP values as low as 100 mmHg, with only 33 out of a total of 412 SBP values (8 %) actually ≥140 mmHg. These findings thus indicate very poor sensitivity at all stages of gestation, mainly for clinic DBP. Specificity, on the contrary, was very high, as just a very small proportion of women in this study, including those with PE, showed conventional clinic BP values ≥140/90 mmHg, even during most of their third trimester of pregnancy.

The results of this prospective trial [78] corroborate, first, the advantages of ABPM over clinic BP values for the early identification of hypertension in pregnancy. Relative to the 130/80 mmHg reference thresholds for 24-h SBP/DBP means proposed for the general population [37], the thresholds listed in Table 13.1 as a function of gestational age reflect the previously documented [71] expected lower BP in women as compared to men, the expected further decrease in BP in gravid as compared to nongravid women [36, 38, 64, 65], and the predictable changes in BP as a function of gestational age [38, 54, 55]. Results presented in Fig. 13.4 corroborate prospectively that the diagnosis of hypertension in pregnancy based on mean BP values derived from ABPM should be established from thresholds much lower than those currently used in clinical practice [39]. Although the sensitivity and specificity in the diagnosis of hypertension can still be improved by the use of other indexes derived from ABPM (for example, by the tolerance-hyperbaric test subsequently discussed) [8, 9, 33, 34, 38], the results of rigorously conducted studies indicate the 48-h, awake, and asleep BP means (Fig. 13.4) provide a diagnostic test markedly superior to clinic BP measurements, rendering ABPM a more useful tool for the clinical evaluation and early identification of complications in pregnancy.

Early Identification of Hypertension in Pregnancy with the Tolerance-Hyperbaric Test

The differing 24-h BP pattern between healthy and complicated pregnancies at all gestational ages, as shown in Fig. 13.2 [36, 38, 63–65], suggests the diagnosis of hypertension in pregnancy might be improved without reliance only on 24-h SBP/DBP mean values that disregard information on 24-h BP variability [32], and the use for diagnosis of a time-specified reference limit [38, 58]. Once the time-varying threshold, given for instance by the upper limit of a time-qualified tolerance interval derived per each hour of the activity and sleep spans [58], is available, the hyperbaric index (HBI), as a determinant of entire 24-h BP excess, can be calculated as the total area of any given subject's BP above the threshold [8, 9, 33, 34, 59, 80]. The HBI as well as the duration of BP excess (percentage time of excess, defined as the percentage time during the 24 h when the BP of the test subject exceeds the upper limit of the tolerance interval) can then be used as nonparametric endpoints for assessing hypertension in pregnancy. This so-called tolerance-hyperbaric test, by which the diagnosis of hypertension is based on the HBI calculated with reference to a time-specified tolerance limit, has been shown to provide high sensitivity and specificity for the early identification of subsequent hypertension in pregnancy [33], thereby constituting a valuable approach for the prediction of pregnancy outcome [8, 9]. Because the conventional assessment of GH relies on office values ≥140/90 mmHg for SBP/DBP [4, 26], results based on the determination of BP excess have been usually expressed as a function of the maximum HBI, defined as the maximum of the three values of HBI determined for SBP, mean arterial BP, and DBP, respectively, for any given individual [9, 33, 34, 59, 80]. The prospective evaluation of the reproducibility of this ABPM-based test for early identification of complications in pregnancy was found to show a sensitivity of 93 % for women evaluated by ABPM during their first trimester of gestation [34]. Sensitivity improved with gestational age, as BP also increases steadily during the second half of gestation in women who develop hypertension in pregnancy (Fig. 13.1).

Beyond the studies summarized above, several other authors have reported consistent positive results when testing the ability of the HBI derived from ABPM to predict pregnancy outcome [81–84]. Benedetto et al. [81] performed 24-h ABPM at 8–16 and 20–25 weeks gestation in 104 women at risk of GH or PE. Best sensitivity and specificity were obtained between 20 and 25 weeks gestation with the 24-h mean and the HBI of SBP using as cut-off values 103 mmHg (sensitivity: 88 %; specificity: 75 %) and 10 mmHg×h (sensitivity: 70 %; specificity: 92 %), respectively. The authors concluded ABPM in pregnancy allows definition of objective cut-off values that can be particularly useful in routine clinical practice when the risk of developing GH or PE must be calculated for each individual woman. Shaginian [84] evaluated 34 apparently healthy pregnant women by 72-h ABPM finding elevated HBI for SBP in the first trimester of pregnancy for the 17 women who developed GH or PE during the second half of gestation compared to the 17 women who remained normotensive until delivery. On the contrary, Vollebregt et al. [85] reported limited accuracy of the HBI in predicting hypertension in pregnancy from a study of 101 women evaluated by 48-h ABPM only once in the first trimester of gestation. Their approach, which we feel is invalid for many reasons [38], utilized a (highly reproducible [34]) first trimester ABPM profile to predict elevated (highly variable and poorly reproducible) clinic BP later in pregnancy. This approach, far from novel, has been used in the past by many other obstetricians [43, 48], as briefly discussed above. When both clinic and ambulatory BP are available, ABPM, but not clinic BP, prevails for diagnosis. This is so because, by comparing clinic and ambulatory BP, one is able to distinguish groups of subjects with normotension, sustained hypertension, isolated clinic (white coat) hypertension, and masked hypertension, characterized by different cardiovascular risk [37, 39, 86]. The inappropriate approach of Vollebregt et al. [85] undoubtedly included women with masked hypertension in their reference population as well as in the comparative group they mistakenly called "normotensive women," making invalid all conclusions drawn from their study. Most important in terms of clinical relevance, the Vollebregt et al. study found perinatal outcome to be more favorable for women with GH than for the ones with normotension, which is just the opposite of what the literature in the field leads anyone to expect.

Previous prospective studies have also documented the ability of the ABPM-derived HBI, but not clinic BP measurements, to differentiate as early as at 20-week gestation women who will develop PE from those who will just develop GH without proteinuria [8, 9]. Accordingly, GH was predicted on the basis of a maximum HBI value exceeding the relatively low specified threshold of 15 mmHg×h, while PE was predicted by the higher HBI threshold of 65 mmHg×h [8].

Clinic versus Ambulatory BP for Diagnosis of Complications in Pregnancy

Another prospective study [8, 9] compared the ABPM profiles and pregnancy outcome between three groups of pregnant women evaluated by 48-h ABPM at the time of recruitment (<16 weeks gestation), and then every 4 weeks thereafter until delivery, namely: (1) "detected" GH, defined as clinic BP ≥140/90 mmHg after 20-week gestation plus maximum HBI consistently above the threshold for diagnosing hypertension in pregnancy provided above (therefore classified as hypertensive by both independent criteria); (2) "undetected" GH (i.e., masked GH), defined as clinic BP <140/90 mmHg *but* HBI above the threshold for diagnosis in each and everyone of the monthly profiles of ABPM obtained after 20-week gestation (therefore considered "normotensive" according to current obstetric guidelines [4, 26], but in actuality considered to be hypertensive by the ABPM-derived HBI criterion); and (3) normotension, defined as clinic BP and maximum HBI both consistently below their respective diagnostic thresholds at all evaluations after 20-week gestation. The demographic and perinatal characteristics of the investigated women are summarized in Table 13.2.

Comparison of the 24-h BP characteristics of "detected" and "undetected" (masked) GH for women sampled during the first trimester of pregnancy revealed

Table 13.2 Demographic and perinatal characteristics of women investigated

Variable	NT	DGH	UGH	p value for comparison of Three groups	DGH vs. UGH
Women, n	234	62	59		
ABPM profiles, n	1404	401	370		
Age, years	30.4±5.5	30.0±4.6	30.8±5.1	0.385	0.726
Weight, kg	63.1±9.7	78.6±17.4	69.6±16.5	<0.001	0.002
Height, cm	161.8±5.5	163.7±7.0	162.3±7.1	0.124	0.194
SBP at first visit, mmHg[a]	119±10	127±10	122±9	<0.001	0.012
DBP at first visit, mmHg[a]	65±7	71±8	68±8	<0.001	0.181
SBP at last visit, mmHg[a]	118±9	142±11	133±7	<0.001	<0.001
DBP at last visit, mmHg[a]	66±7	84±7	79±6	<0.001	<0.001
Gestational age at delivery, weeks	39.4±1.1	38.7±3.4	38.8±3.5	0.044	0.814
Newborn weight, g	3334±447	3088±634	3062±653	<0.001	0.918
Delivery by cesarean section, %	18.4	35.5	40.7	<0.001	0.715
Intrauterine growth retardation, %	5.1	16.1	17.0	<0.001	0.791
Preterm delivery (<37 weeks), %	3.6	9.7	10.2	0.037	0.935
Newborn Apgar score[b] at:					
1 min	8.8±1.0	8.8±0.9	8.7±1.0	0.894	0.682
5 min	9.9±0.4	9.9±0.4	9.8±0.7	0.297	0.334
10 min	10±0.2	10±0.1	9.9±0.2	0.492	0.312

Data from [8, 9]. Values are shown as mean±SD. *NT* normotension, *DGH* "detected" GH, *UGH* "undetected" GH
[a]Values correspond to the average of 3–6 clinic BP measurements obtained by a midwife nurse for each women at the time of their first and last (before delivery) visits to the hospital
[b]The Apgar score is determined by evaluating the newborn with five criteria on a scale from 0 to 2, i.e., appearance, pulse, grimace, activity, and respiration

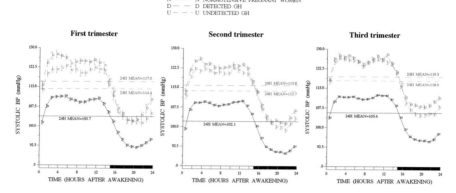

Fig. 13.5 24-h SBP pattern of pregnant women sampled by 48-h ABPM at different stages of pregnancy. Women were divided for comparative purposes into three groups according to the values of clinic BP and maximum HBI at all evaluations after 20-week gestation: (1) normotensives ($N=234$), with both clinic BP and maximum HBI below diagnostic thresholds; (2) "detected" GH ($N=62$), with clinic BP $\geq 140/90$ mmHg plus elevated HBI; "undetected" (masked) GH ($N=59$), with clinic BP $<140/90$ mmHg *but* elevated HBI. Each graph shows hourly means and standard errors of data for each group of women. *Dark shading* along *lower horizontal* axis of graphs denotes the average hours of nighttime sleep across the sample. Updated from [9]

only a small and nonsignificant ($p=0.056$) greater 24-h SBP mean by 2.6 mmHg in "detected" than "undetected" GH (Fig. 13.5, left panel). Differences between groups in the 24-h DBP mean (not shown) only amounted to 0.2 mmHg ($p=0.682$). The hourly means of SBP and DBP did not differ significantly between "detected" and "undetected" GH at any circadian time, as corroborated by t-tests adjusted for multiple testing. In the second trimester, comparisons between the groups of women with "detected" and "undetected" GH failed to reveal any significant differences in the 24-h SBP/DBP means (Fig. 13.5, central panel; $p>0.386$). In the third trimester of pregnancy, differences in the 24-h SBP/DBP means between "detected" and "undetected" GH were even smaller (Fig. 13.5, right panel). Additionally, at all stages of pregnancy, ambulatory BP was highly significantly lower in normotensive pregnant women than in women with either "detected" or "undetected" GH ($p<.001$). Moreover, average newborn weight, gestational age at delivery, plus incidence of preterm delivery, IUGR, and delivery by cesarean section were similar between the two groups of women with "detected" and "undetected" GH (Table 13.2). There were, however, statistically significant differences in all those perinatal outcome variables between these two GH groups and normotensive pregnant women (Table 13.2). Results from this prospective study provide strong evidence to support ABPM as the proper "gold standard," instead of unreliable clinic cuff BP measurements, for the early identification of true hypertension in pregnancy and associated maternal and perinatal complications [8, 9].

Discussion

Although PE has generally received more attention than just hypertension in the absence of any other symptom or complication in pregnancy, the long-term follow-up of women with complicated pregnancies has indicated that GH is associated with highest incidence of subsequent chronic hypertension [87]. Thus, although PE is a more severe obstetric complication, GH may have more important long-term implications. Accordingly, following the common standard applied in most of the cited references in this review, we focused on the identification of BP elevation in pregnancy, whether or not it could be later accompanied by proteinuria. As discussed earlier, clinical studies already substantiate the ability of the HBI to differentiate to some extent, at the end of the first half of pregnancy, women who will develop PE from those who will develop GH [8].

Common to the current definition of all hypertensive complications in pregnancy, independent of how PE might be defined, is the use of the fixed reference threshold of 140/90 mmHg for conventional clinic SBP/DBP measurements obtained at the physician's office [4, 26, 37]. Previous results have consistently documented the poor prognostic value of clinic BP for the early identification of hypertension in pregnancy and prediction of pregnancy outcome [8, 9]. The ideal predictive or diagnostic test should be simple and easy to perform, reproducible, noninvasive, and with high sensitivity and positive predictive value. The tolerance-hyperbaric test described above is noninvasive since it relies on ABPM. Many results summarized in this review are based on ABPM assessed for 48 consecutive hours as opposed to the most common 24 h [40–53]. As a compromise with practicability, monitoring over at least 48 h has been shown to present advantages in the analysis of BP variability, diagnosis of hypertension, and evaluation of patient response to treatment [33]. Moreover, accuracy in the derivation of ABPM characteristics (including mean BP values and HBI) depends markedly on the duration of ABPM [56, 57]. Indeed, sampling requirements for the tolerance-hyperbaric test are not very demanding. While results summarized in this review were obtained with BP series sampled at 20- or 30-min intervals, the HBI can be well-estimated from data sampled at ~2-h intervals with just marginal loss in sensitivity or specificity [57]. Although 15-min sampling for ABPM evaluation in pregnancy has been unjustifiably advocated [40], a longer sampling interval increases compliance and patient acceptability [88]. Additionally, the number of reference subjects needed for estimating stable time-qualified tolerance SBP and DBP intervals is also quite small, as previously documented [58, 89]. Finally, the tolerance-hyperbaric test provides both high sensitivity and positive predictive value as early as in the first trimester of pregnancy [8, 9, 33, 34, 81–84].

Perceived limitations of ABPM stem from the fact that most ambulatory devices, although advanced, are still expensive and most have not been properly validated for specific application in pregnancy. Cost, however, should always be evaluated in relation to potential benefit. Results of the prospective ABPM evaluation studies summarized here indicate the cost–benefit relationship for ABPM is more favorable than clinic BP measurements in pregnancy, simply because ABPM allows proper identification of women at high risk of complications, while clinic BP does not [8, 9, 34]. Tolerability of ABPM has also been discussed as a possible limitation of its use in pregnancy. Although compliance is usually very high [9, 33, 34], reported patient acceptability tends to be lower [88]. Patient acceptability, a potential limitation also discussed when criticizing the utilization of ABPM in general practice [37], is in part related to the ability of the physician to provide useful and convincing information to the patient on the potential advantages of ABPM [39].

Unfortunately, despite the much higher prognostic value of ABPM than clinic BP measurements, the most extended conclusion so far, due to poor results from the diagnostic test when based on 24-h SBP/DBP means ≥130/80 mmHg irrespective of gestational stage, is that ABPM does not provide a proper approach for the early identification of GH or PE, and it should not be used in pregnancy [48]. Thus, from this perspective, it is not surprising that the current obstetric guidelines recommend reliance only upon clinic BP ≥140/90 mmHg after 20-week gestation to establish the diagnosis of GH [4, 26]. However, it must be recognized that these guidelines are obsolete because they have not been updated to acknowledge the consensus recommendations of the European Societies of Hypertension and Cardiology, which specifically state 24-h BP has been shown to be superior to conventional measurements in predicting proteinuria, risk of preterm delivery, infant weight at birth, and in general, outcome of pregnancy [37]. Studies summarized above claiming "poor results" of ABPM are based on the questionable approach to test the ability of the ABPM-derived 24-h mean to predict a diagnosis founded on unreliable clinic BP measurements obtained later in pregnancy. Most important, the significantly lower ambulatory BP of nongravid women as compared to men, the added decrease in ambulatory BP during the second half of gestation in normotensive but not in hypertensive pregnant women, and the 24-h pattern with large amplitude that characterizes BP of healthy and complicated pregnant women at all gestational ages (Fig. 13.3) were not taken into account in studies providing negative results on the use of ABPM in pregnancy. The establishment of proper reference thresholds for the 24-h BP mean derived by taking all those considerations into account has been shown prospectively to markedly increase the sensitivity and specificity of ABPM for the early identification of complications in pregnancy (Fig. 13.4 [78]). Sensitivity and specificity in the early identification of hypertension in pregnancy based on mean BP values can be even further improved by the use of other indexes also derived from ABPM [8, 9, 33, 34]. In particular, the tolerance-hyperbaric test represents a reproducible, noninvasive, and highly sensitive test for the early identification of subsequent hypertension in pregnancy, including PE.

ABPM during gestation, commencing preferably at the time of the first obstetric check-up following positive confirmation of pregnancy, thus provides sensitive endpoints for use in early risk assessment and as a guide for establishing prophylactic or therapeutic intervention [19–23]. Accordingly, ABPM-derived BP measurements have been recently recommended as substitute for the unreliable clinic ones as the "gold standard" for the diagnosis of hypertension in pregnancy and the screening of women at high risk for additional complications, including IUGR and preterm delivery [39].

References

1. Duley L. The global impact of pre-eclampsia and eclampsia. Semin Perinatol. 2009;33:130–7.
2. Roberts CL, Ford JB, Algert CS, et al. Population-based trends in pregnancy hypertension and pre-eclampsia: an international comparative study. BMJ Open. 2011;1, e000101. doi:10.1136/bmjopen-2011-000101.
3. Steegers EA, von Dadelszen P, Duvekot JJ, Pijnenborg R. Pre-eclampsia. Lancet. 2010;376:631–44.
4. Brown MA, Lindheimer MD, de Swiet M, Van Assche A, Moutquin JM. The classification and diagnosis of the hypertensive disorders of pregnancy: statement from The International Society for the Study of Hypertension in Pregnancy (ISSHP). Hypertens Pregnancy. 2001;20:ix–xiv.
5. Hernández-Díaz S, Toh S, Cnattingius S. Risk of pre-eclampsia in first and subsequent pregnancies: prospective cohort study. BMJ. 2009;338:b2255.
6. Roberts CL, Algert CS, Morris JM, Ford JB, Henderson-Smart DJ. Hypertensive disorders in pregnancy: a population-based study. Med J Aust. 2005;182:332–5.
7. Wallis AB, Saftlas AF, Hsia J, Atrash HK. Secular trends in the rates of pre-eclampsia, eclampsia, and gestational hypertension, United States, 1987–2004. Am J Hypertens. 2008;21:521–6.
8. Hermida RC, Ayala DE. Prognostic value of office and ambulatory blood pressure measurements in pregnancy. Hypertension. 2002;40:298–303.
9. Hermida RC, Ayala DE, Iglesias M. Circadian rhythm of blood pressure challengues office values as the "gold standard" in the diagnosis of gestational hypertension. Chronobiol Int. 2003;20:135–56.
10. Roberts CL, Bell JC, Ford JB, Hadfield RM, Algert CS, Morris JM. The accuracy of reporting of the hypertensive disorders of pregnancy in population health data. Hypertens Pregnancy. 2008;27:285–97.
11. Koopmans CM, Bijlenga D, Groen H, et al. Induction of labour versus expectant monitoring for gestational hypertension or mild pre-eclampsia after 36 weeks' gestation (HYPITAT): a multicentre, open-label randomised controlled trial. Lancet. 2009;374:979–88.
12. Dekker GA, Sibai BM. Low-dose aspirin in the prevention of preeclampsia and fetal growth retardation: rationale, mechanisms, and clinical trials. Am J Obstet Gynecol. 1993;168:214–27.
13. Redman CWG, Sargent IL. Pre-eclampsia, the placenta and the maternal systemic inflammatory response—a review. Placenta. 2003;24:s21–7.
14. Sibai BM, Caritis S, Hauth J. What we have learned about preeclampsia. Semin Perinatol. 2003;27:239–46.
15. Walsh SW. Preeclampsia: an imbalance in placental prostacyclin and thromboxane production. Am J Obstet Gynecol. 1985;152:335–40.
16. Duckitt K, Harrington D. Risk factors for pre-eclampsia at antenatal booking: systematic review of controlled studies. BMJ. 2005;330:565.
17. Saftlas AF, Levine RJ, Klebanoff MA, et al. Abortion, changed paternity, and risk of pre-eclampsia in nulliparous women. Am J Epidemiol. 2003;157:1108–14.
18. Skjaerven R, Wilcox AJ, Lie RT. The interval between pregnancies and the risk of pre-eclampsia. N Engl J Med. 2002;346:33–8.
19. Askie LM, Duley L, Henderson-Smart DJ, Stewart LA, Collaborative Group PARIS. Antiplatelet agents for prevention of pre-eclampsia: a meta-analysis of individual patient data. Lancet. 2007;369:1791–8.
20. Ayala DE, Ucieda R, Hermida RC. Chronotherapy with low-dose aspirin for prevention of complications in pregnancy. Chronobiol Int. 2013;30:260–79.
21. Hermida RC, Ayala DE, Iglesias M, et al. Time-dependent effects of low-dose aspirin administration on blood pressure in pregnant women. Hypertension. 1997;30:589–95.

22. Hermida RC, Ayala DE, Fernández JR, et al. Administration time-dependent effects of aspirin in women at differing risk for preeclampsia. Hypertension. 1999;34:1016–23.
23. Hermida RC, Ayala DE, Iglesias M. Administration-time dependent influence of aspirin on blood pressure in pregnant women. Hypertension. 2003;41:651–6.
24. Hofmeyr GJ, Atallah AN, Duley L. Calcium supplementation during pregnancy for preventing hypertensive disorders and related problems. Cochrane Database Syst Rev. 2006;3, CD001059.
25. Cnossen JS, ter Riet G, Mol BW, et al. Are tests for predicting pre-eclampsia good enough to make screening viable? A review of reviews and critical appraisal. Acta Obstet Gynecol Scand. 2009;88:758–65.
26. Lindheimer MD, Taler SJ, Cunningham FG. Hypertension in pregnancy. J Am Soc Hypertens. 2008;2:484–94.
27. Miller RS, Rudra CB, Williams MA. First-trimester mean arterial pressure and risk of pre-eclampsia. Am J Hypertens. 2007;20:573–8.
28. Nijdam ME, Janssen KJ, Moons KG, et al. Prediction model for hypertension in pregnancy in nulliparous women using information obtained at the first antenatal visit. J Hypertens. 2010;28:119–26.
29. Page EW, Christianson R. The impact of mean arterial pressure in the middle trimester upon the outcome of pregnancy. Am J Obstet Gynecol. 1976;125:740–6.
30. Villar MA, Sibai BM. Clinical significance of elevated mean arterial blood pressure in second trimester and threshold increase in systolic or diastolic blood pressure during the third trimester. Am J Obstet Gynecol. 1989;160:419–23.
31. Patterson HR. Sources of error in recording the blood pressure of patients with hypertension in general practice. BMJ. 1984;289:1661–4.
32. Hermida RC, Ayala DE. Diagnosing gestational hypertension and preeclampsia with the 24-hour mean of blood pressure. Hypertension. 1997;30:1531–7.
33. Hermida RC, Ayala DE, Mojón A, et al. Blood pressure excess for the early identification of gestational hypertension and preeclampsia. Hypertension. 1998;31:83–9.
34. Hermida RC, Ayala DE, Fernández JR, Mojón A, Iglesias M. Reproducibility of the tolerance-hyperbaric test for diagnosing hypertension in pregnancy. J Hypertens. 2004;22:565–72.
35. Peek M, Shennan A, Halligan A, Lambert PC, Taylor DJ, De Swiet M. Hypertension in pregnancy: which method of blood pressure measurement is most predictive of outcome? Obstet Gynecol. 1996;88:1030–3.
36. Ayala DE, Hermida RC, Mojón A, Fernández JR, Iglesias M. Circadian blood pressure variability in healthy and complicated pregnancies. Hypertension. 1997;30:603–10.
37. Mancia G, Fagard R, Narkiewicz K, et al. 2013 ESH/ESC Guidelines for the management of arterial hypertension: The Task Force for the management of arterial hypertension of the European Society of Hypertension (ESH) and of the European Society of Cardiology (ESC). J Hypertens. 2013;31:1281–357.
38. Ayala DE, Hermida RC. Ambulatory blood pressure monitoring for the early identificaton of hypertension in pregnancy. Chronobiol Int. 2013;30:233–59.
39. Hermida RC, Smolensky MH, Ayala DE, et al. 2013 ambulatory blood pressure monitoring recommendations for the diagnosis of adult hypertension, assessment of cardiovascular and other hypertension-associated risk, and attainment of therapeutic goals. Joint recommendations from the International Society for Chronobiology (ISC), American Association of Medical Chronobiology and Chronotherapeutics (AAMCC), Spanish Society of Applied Chronobiology, Chronotherapy, and Vascular Risk (SECAC), Spanish Society of Atherosclerosis (SEA), and Romanian Society of Internal Medicine (RSIM). Chronobiol Int. 2013;30:355–410.
40. Shennan A, Halligan A. Ambulatory blood pressure monitoring in pregnancy. Fetal Maternal Med Rev. 1998;10:69–89.
41. Bellomo G, Rondoni F, Pastorelli G, Stangoni G, Narducci P, Angeli G. Twenty four-hour ambulatory blood pressure monitoring in women with pre-eclampsia. J Hum Hypertens. 1995;9:617–21.

42. Bellomo G, Narducci PL, Rondoni F, et al. Prognostic value of 24-hour blood pressure in pregnancy. JAMA. 1999;282:1447–52.
43. Brown MA, Bowyer L, McHugh L, Davis GK, Mangos GJ, Jones M. Twenty-four-hour automated blood pressure monitoring as a predictor of preeclampsia. Am J Obstet Gynecol. 2001;185:618–22.
44. Brown MA, Davis GK, McHugh L. The prevalence and clinical significance of nocturnal hypertension in pregnancy. J Hypertens. 2001;19:1437–44.
45. Churchill D, Perry IJ, Beevers DG. Ambulatory blood pressure in pregnancy and fetal growth. Lancet. 1997;349:7–10.
46. Cugini P, Di Palma L, Battisti P, et al. Describing and interpreting 24-hour blood pressure patterns in physiologic pregnancy. Am J Obstet Gynecol. 1992;166:54–60.
47. Halligan A, O'Brien E, O'Malley K, et al. Twenty-four-hour ambulatory blood pressure measurement in a primigravid population. J Hypertens. 1993;11:869–73.
48. Higgins JR, Walshe JJ, Halligan A, O'Brien E, Conroy R, Darling MRN. Can 24-hour ambulatory blood pressure measurement predict the development of hypertension in primigravidae? Br J Obstet Gynaecol. 1997;104:356–62.
49. Kyle PM, Clark SJ, Buckley D, et al. Second trimester ambulatory blood pressure in nulliparous pregnancy: a useful screening test for pre-eclampsia? Br J Obstet Gynaecol. 1993;100:914–9.
50. Margulies M, Voto LS, Fescina R, Lastra L, Lapidus AM, Schwarcz R. Arterial blood pressure standards during normal pregnancy and their relation with mother-fetus variables. Am J Obstet Gynecol. 1987;156:1105–9.
51. Penny JA, Halligan AWF, Shennan AH, et al. Automated, ambulatory, or conventional blood pressure measurement in pregnancy: which is the better predictor of severe hypertension? Am J Obstet Gynecol. 1998;178:521–6.
52. Tranquilli AL, Giannubilo SR, Dell'Uomo B, Corradetti A. Prediction of gestational hypertension or intrauterine fetal growth restriction by mid-trimester 24-h ambulatory blood pressure monitoring. Int J Gynaecol Obstet. 2004;85:126–31.
53. Waugh J, Perry IJ, Halligan AW, et al. Birth weight and 24-hour ambulatory blood pressure in nonproteinuric hypertensive pregnancy. Am J Obstet Gynecol. 2000;183:633–7.
54. Ayala DE, Hermida RC, Mojón A, et al. Blood pressure variability during gestation in healthy and complicated pregnancies. Hypertension. 1997;30:611–8.
55. Hermida RC, Ayala DE, Iglesias M. Predictable blood pressure variability in healthy and complicated pregnancies. Hypertension. 2001;38:736–41.
56. Hermida RC, Ayala DE, Fontao MJ, Mojón A, Fernández JR. Ambulatory blood pressure monitoring: importance of sampling rate and duration—48 versus 24 hours—on the accurate assessment of cardiovascular risk. Chronobiol Int. 2013;30:55–67.
57. Hermida RC, Ayala DE. Sampling requirements for ambulatory blood pressure monitoring in the diagnosis of hypertension in pregnancy. Hypertension. 2003;42:619–24.
58. Hermida RC, Ayala DE, Mojón A, Fernández JR. Time-qualified reference values for ambulatory blood pressure monitoring in pregnancy. Hypertension. 2001;38:746–52.
59. Hermida RC, Mojón A, Fernández JR, Alonso I, Ayala DE. The tolerance-hyperbaric test: a chronobiologic approach for improved diagnosis of hypertension. Chronobiol Int. 2002;19:1183–211.
60. Fabbian F, Smolensky MH, Tiseo R, Pala M, Manfredini R, Portaluppi F. Dipper and non-dipper blood pressure 24-hour patterns: circadian rhythm-dependent physiologic and pathophysiologic mechanisms. Chronobiol Int. 2013;30:17–30.
61. Hermida RC, Ayala DE, Portaluppi F. Circadian variation of blood pressure: the basis for the chronotherapy of hypertension. Adv Drug Deliv Rev. 2007;59:904–22.
62. Portaluppi F, Tiseo R, Smolensky MH, Hermida RC, Ayala DE, Fabbian F. Circadian rhythms and cardiovascular health. Sleep Med Rev. 2012;16:151–66.
63. Benedetto C, Zonca M, Marozio L, Dolco C, Carandente F, Massobrio M. Blood pressure patterns in normal pregnancy and in pregnancy-induced hypertension, preeclampsia, and chronic hypertension. Obstet Gynecol. 1996;88:503–10.

64. Hermida RC, Ayala DE, Mojón A, et al. Blood pressure patterns in normal pregnancy, gestational hypertension and preeclampsia. Hypertension. 2000;36:149–58.
65. Hermida RC, Ayala DE, Mojón A, et al. Differences in circadian blood pressure variability during gestation between healthy and complicated pregnancies. Am J Hypertens. 2003;16:200–8.
66. Miyamoto S, Shimokawa H, Sumioki H, Touno A, Nakano H. Circadian rhythm of plasma atrial natriuretic peptide, aldosterone, and blood pressure during the third trimester in normal and preeclamptic pregnancy. Am J Obstet Gynecol. 1998;158:393–9.
67. Contard S, Chanudet X, Coisne D, et al. Ambulatory monitoring of blood pressure in normal pregnancy. Am J Hypertens. 1993;6:880–4.
68. Beilin LJ, Deacon J, Michael CA, et al. Circadian rhythms of blood pressure and pressor hormones in normal and hypertensive pregnancy. Clin Exp Pharmacol Physiol. 1982;9:321–6.
69. Redman C, Beilin LJ, Bonnar J. Reversed diurnal blood pressure rhythm in hypertensive pregnancies. Clin Sci Mol Med. 1976;51:687s–9.
70. Ben-Dov IZ, Mekler J, Bursztyn M. Sex differences in ambulatory blood pressure monitoring. Am J Med. 2008;121:509–14.
71. Hermida RC, Ayala DE, Fernández JR, Mojón A, Alonso I, Calvo C. Modeling the circadian variability of ambulatorily monitored blood pressure by multiple-component analysis. Chronobiol Int. 2002;19:461–81.
72. Hermida RC, Ayala DE, Mojón A, Fontao MJ, Chayán L, Fernández JR. Differences between men and women in ambulatory blood pressure thresholds for diagnosis of hypertension based on cardiovascular outcomes. Chronobiol Int. 2013;30:221–32.
73. Vriz O, Lu H, Visentin P, Nicolosi L, Mos L, Palatini P. Gender differences in the relationship between left ventricular size and ambulatory blood pressure in borderline hypertension. The HARVEST study. Eur Heart J. 1997;18:664–70.
74. Wang X, Poole JC, Treiber FA, Harshfield GA, Hanevold CD, Snieder H. Ethnic and gender differences in ambulatory blood pressure trajectories: results from a 15-year longitudinal study in youth and young adults. Circulation. 2006;114:2780–7.
75. Clement DL, De Buyzere ML, De Bacquer DA, et al. Prognostic value of ambulatory blood-pressure recordings in patients with treated hypertension. N Engl J Med. 2003;348:2407–15.
76. Dolan E, Stanton A, Thijs L, et al. Superiority of ambulatory over clinic blood pressure measurement in predicting mortality: the Dublin outcome study. Hypertension. 2005;46:156–61.
77. Hermida RC, Ayala DE, Mojón A, Fernández JR. Decreasing sleep-time blood pressure determined by ambulatory monitoring reduces cardiovascular risk. J Am Coll Cardiol. 2011;58:1165–73.
78. Hermida RC, Ayala DE. Reference thresholds for 24-hour, diurnal, and nocturnal blood pressure mean values in pregnancy. Blood Press Monit. 2005;10:33–41.
79. O'Brien A, Asmar R, Beilin L, et al. European society of hypertension recommendations for conventional, ambulatory and home blood pressure measurement. J Hypertens. 2003;21:821–48.
80. Hermida RC, Mojón A, Fernández JR, Ayala DE. Computer-based medical system for the computation of blood pressure excess in the diagnosis of hypertension. Biomed Instrum Technol. 1996;30:267–83.
81. Benedetto C, Marozio L, Giarola M, Chiarolini L, Maulà V, Massobrio M. Twenty-four hour blood pressure monitoring in early pregnancy: is it predictive of pregnancy-induced hypertension and preeclampsia? Acta Obstet Gynecol Scand. 1998;77:14–21.
82. Carandente F, Angeli A, Massobrio M, et al. Blood pressure and heart rate in pregnancy: comparison between health and pathologic conditions. Prog Clin Biol Res. 1990;341A:575–84.
83. Cornélissen G, Kopher R, Brat P, et al. Chronobiologic ambulatory cardiovascular monitoring during pregnancy in Group Health of Minnesota. In: Proceedings of the 2nd Annual IEEE Symposium on Computer-Based Medical Systems. Minneapolis, MN, June 26–27; 1989;226–237.
84. Shaginian MG. Blood pressure circadian rhythms during development of hypertension in healthy pregnant women. Georgian Med News. 2006;138:84–6.

85. Vollebregt KC, Gisolf J, Guelen I, Boer K, van Montfrans G, Wolf H. Limited accuracy of the hyperbaric index, ambulatory blood pressure and sphygmomanometry measurements in predicting gestational hypertension and preeclampsia. J Hypertens. 2010;28:127–34.
86. Hermida RC, Ayala DE, Mojón A, Fernández JR. Sleep-time blood pressure and the prognostic value of isolated-office and masked hypertension. Am J Hypertens. 2012;25:297–305.
87. Marín R, Gorostidi M, Portal CG, Sánchez M, Sánchez E, Alvarez J. Long-term prognosis of hypertension in pregnancy. Hypertens Pregnancy. 2000;19:199–209.
88. Taylor RS, Freeman L, North RA. Evaluation of ambulatory and self-initiated blood pressure monitors by pregnant and postpartum women. Hypertens Pregnancy. 2001;20:25–33.
89. Hermida RC, Fernández JR. Computation of time-specified tolerance intervals for ambulatorily monitored blood pressure. Biomed Instrum Technol. 1996;30:257–66.

Chapter 14
Ambulatory Blood Pressure in Patients with Chronic Kidney Disease

William S. Asch, Sergio F.F. Santos, and Aldo J. Peixoto

Introduction

Chronic kidney disease (CKD) is a growing global healthcare problem. Recently compiled data from 18 countries worldwide indicate that the prevalence of CKD based on an estimated glomerular filtration rate (eGFR) less than 60 mL/min/1.73 m^2 often exceeds 10 % [1], and it is conceivable that this prevalence will grow further as most of the cases of CKD occur in the setting of diabetes, hypertension, and aging, all conditions of increasing prevalence in modern societies. CKD patients have a significant rate of morbidity and mortality resulting in high utilization of healthcare resources.

Hypertension (HTN) is highly prevalent in CKD, where it is estimated that up to 80 % of patients have elevated blood pressure (BP) by the time they reach advanced stages of kidney disease (glomerular filtration rate <15 mL/min) and is the most important factor in the progression of most chronic renal diseases.

W.S. Asch, M.D., Ph.D.
Section of Nephrology, Yale University School of Medicine, New Haven, CT 06520, USA
e-mail: william.asch@yale.edu

S.F.F. Santos, M.D., Ph.D.
Division of Nephrology, State University of Rio de Janeiro (UERJ),
Rio de Janeiro, RJ 20550-900, Brazil
e-mail: sergioffsantos@globo.com

A.J. Peixoto, M.D. (✉)
Department of Internal Medicine, Section of Nephrology, Yale University School
of Medicine, 330 Cedar Street, New Haven, CT 06520, USA
e-mail: aldo.peixoto@yale.edu

© Springer International Publishing Switzerland 2016
W.B. White (ed.), *Blood Pressure Monitoring in Cardiovascular Medicine
and Therapeutics*, Clinical Hypertension and Vascular Diseases,
DOI 10.1007/978-3-319-22771-9_14

HTN is also highly prevalent in dialysis [2] and kidney transplant [3] patients. Furthermore, cardiovascular diseases are the major cause of death in any stage of renal impairment [4]. Therefore, HTN is a major cardiovascular risk factor during any stage of kidney disease.

Ambulatory blood pressure monitoring (ABPM) is an important tool in hypertension research and clinical practice in view of its better ability to detect target organ damage and to predict prognosis than office blood pressure measurements, which has led some societies to recommend its use as an essential step to the diagnosis of hypertension [5]. Data in patients with kidney disease are still based on comparatively smaller studies, but the literature has grown substantially in the past decade. This chapter will review these relevant findings applicable to patients throughout the spectrum of CKD.

ABPM and Home BP in Chronic Kidney Disease (Stages 1–4, "Pre-Dialysis")

Chronic kidney disease and hypertension commonly coexist. Approximately 80 % of patients reaching stage 5 CKD (glomerular filtration rate <15 mL/min/1.73 m^2) have BP levels above 140/90 mmHg. CKD is currently classified according to the degree of renal function based on estimates of glomerular filtration rate and the presence of albuminuria or structural renal abnormalities. If the eGFR is above 60 mL/min/1.73 m^2, CKD is only diagnosed if there is evidence of albuminuria or other evidence of renal parenchymal disease (e.g., polycystic kidney disease, hematuria, or renal origin). The 2012 KDIGO (Kidney Disease Improving Global Outcomes) guideline stages CKD according to eGFR as follows [6]:

Category (stage) 1—eGFR ≥90 mL/min/1.73 m^2
Category (stage) 2—eGFR 60–89 mL/min/1.73 m^2
Category (stage) 3a—eGFR 45–59 mL/min/1.73 m^2
Category (stage) 3b—eGFR 30–44 mL/min/1.73 m^2
Category (stage) 4—eGFR 15–29 mL/min/1.73 m^2
Category (stage) 5—eGFR <15 mL/min/1.73 m^2 (kidney failure).

The following paragraphs refer to patients with stages 1–4 CKD.

One of the most consistent findings in these patients is the prevalence of abnormal diurnal BP profiles, with blunting of the nocturnal BP dip [7]. In a landmark study, Baumgart et al. showed uniformly blunted circadian BP profiles in patients with various CKD not on dialysis, patients on hemodialysis, and patients with a kidney transplant compared with controls matched for age, sex, office systolic BP, and presence/absence of antihypertensive drug therapy [8]. Average dipping during sleep (SBP%/DBP%) was 7 %/11 % in CKD patients (18 % vs. 24 % in controls), 4 %/8 % in hemodialysis patients (14 % vs. 24 % in controls), and 5 %/9 % in transplantation patients (13 % vs. 18 % in controls) [8]. Since then, many studies have confirmed this trend. One of the most remarkable is the analysis of the African American Study of Kidney Disease (AASK), which included 617 African American

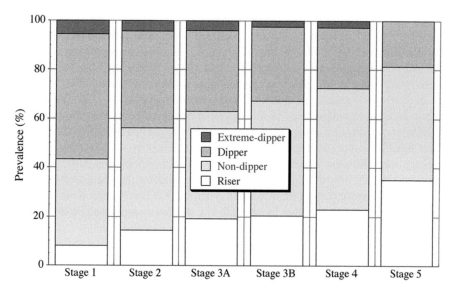

Fig. 14.1 Prevalence of dipping patterns according to stage of chronic kidney disease. Classifications defined in terms of the sleep-time relative SBP decline: ≥20 % (extreme-dipper), 10–20 % (dipper), 0–10 % (non-dipper), <0 % (riser). From Hermida et al. [11], with permission

patients with hypertensive nephrosclerosis with an average iothalamate-measured GFR of 44 mL/min/1.73 m². The investigators observed an 80 % combined prevalence of non-dipping (41 %) or reverse dipping (39 %) in this cohort [9]. Additionally, Mojon et al. demonstrated a 61 % prevalence of non-dipping among 3227 predominantly Caucasian patients from a cohort of less advanced impairment of eGFR (average 59 mL/min/1.73 m²) [10]. The prevalence of non-dipping, and more importantly, reverse dipping, which is associated with the highest risk of cardiovascular events, increases as eGFR falls [11]. Figure 14.1 depicts the proportions of different circadian BP patterns according to the stage of kidney disease.

Evaluation of Adverse Clinical Outcomes in CKD 1–4

Hypertension is a major risk factor for the progression of CKD of any etiology and is a major risk factor for cardiovascular events and death. Because out-of-office BP is a better predictor of target organ damage than office BP and diurnal BP changes may add to this prediction, it was hypothesized that ABPM could be a better predictor of these major adverse events in CKD. This has been evaluated using both overall measures of 24-h BP control and circadian BP patterns.

In a prospective study on the course of events linking BP and albuminuria in type I diabetes, 75 young patients were followed for an average of 63 months and underwent ABPM every two years [12]. There was an increase in nighttime BP in the group who developed microalbuminuria, and this increase in BP preceded the identification of albumin in the urine, raising a possible pathophysiologic link between increase nighttime BP and albuminuria. In a logistic regression model, a 5 mmHg rise in nighttime systolic BP resulted in a 44 % increased risk of development of albuminuria on subsequent examinations. Office BP was unable to detect these differences, and daytime BP was less prominently changed [12]. These findings pointed to the importance of the pattern of nocturnal BP to the progression of renal abnormalities. Likewise, several small studies suggested that the rate of loss of renal function and/or increase in proteinuria was greater in non-dipping than dipping patients with different causes of CKD [13], diabetic nephropathy [14], and IgA nephropathy [15]. However, more recent, larger studies have failed to corroborate the independent importance of non-dipping in predicting CKD progression after adjustments for average BP and other factors [16, 17], as discussed in detail below.

Target-Organ Dysfunction, Morbidity, and Mortality in CKD 1–4

As in essential HTN, ambulatory BP is better than office BP to predict left ventricular mass index in nondiabetic patients with CKD [18]. In hypertensive patients with IgA nephropathy, left ventricular mass was significantly related to nighttime blood pressure and "diurnal index" (% BP decline at night), but there was no relationship with daytime BP [19]. In normotensive patients with autosomal dominant polycystic kidney disease with normal renal function, left ventricular mass was higher as compared to health control subjects. The increase in left ventricular mass index was related to ambulatory BP. The nocturnal decrease in BP was also attenuated in polycystic kidney disease patients, but it was not associated with the increased left ventricular mass [20].

In a cross-sectional analysis of a cohort of 617 African-American patients enrolled in AASK study, ABPM identified patients with more extensive target-organ damage based on nighttime BP levels despite similar clinic and daytime BP [9]. When subjects were divided according to tertiles of nighttime SBP, those in the highest tertile (nighttime SBP >142 mmHg) had significantly lower GFR (41 vs. 44 mL/min/1.73 m^2 compared with lowest tertile), more proteinuria (0.55 vs. 0.17 g/g creatinine), and higher prevalence of LVH on echocardiography (81 % vs. 57 %) [9]. Such differences would not have been captured by clinic or daytime BP, thus making it also unlikely that home BP would have been distinctive. Another cross-sectional study of 232 male patients with CKD has corroborated the stronger association between ABPM with proteinuria than a standardized office BP measurement [21].

There has been progress in identifying the prognostic role of ABPM and home BP monitoring in patients with CKD. Agarwal and Andersen enrolled 217 male patients with CKD due to multiple etiologies, mostly diabetes and hypertension (baseline eGFR 45 mL/min/1.73 m^2), to evaluate the development of ESRD or death according to standardized office BP or home BP [22]. After a median follow-up of

3.5 years, one standard deviation of home systolic BP (21 mmHg) was associated with 84 % increased risk (95 % CI = 1.46–2.32) of death or progression to ESRD after adjustments for demographic factors, office BP, and baseline proteinuria and eGFR [22]. The point estimate of decreased risk for ESRD alone was similar (74 %, 95 % CI = 1.04–2.93). In a companion paper published shortly thereafter, the same authors presented ABPM data for the same cohort showing that one standard deviation increase in 24-h systolic BP (17 mmHg) resulted in a 62 % (95 % CI—1.21–2.18) increase in risk of ESRD or death after adjustment for clinic BP [16]. However, this prognostic advantage did not remain significant after adjustment for other clinical factors (including age, diabetic status, and baseline proteinuria and eGFR). Of the individual components of ABPM, only nighttime systolic BP was a significant predictor of death and ESRD risk after multiple adjustments (hazard ratio 1.79 for ESRD or death, 1.90 for death) [16].

In a multicenter study, Minutolo et al. enlisted 436 patients with CKD of varying etiologies, mostly hypertension, diabetes, and tubulointerstitial diseases (baseline eGFR 43 mL/min/1.73 m^2) [23]. After 4.2 years of follow-up, only ABPM values, not office, were associated with cardiovascular events, progression to ESRD, or death. As noted in Fig. 14.2, there was a progressive increase in the risk of cardio-

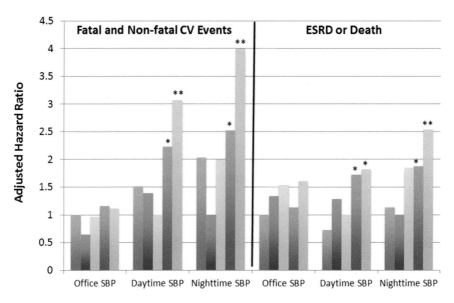

Fig. 14.2 Risk of cardiovascular and renal events in patients with chronic kidney disease according to office or ambulatory BP measurements. *CV* cardiovascular, *ESRD* end-stage renal disease, *SBP* systolic blood pressure. BP categories for each type of measurement (based on quintiles of the distribution): Office SBP (mmHg): <130 (reference), 130–139, 140–149, 150–159, >159. Daytime SBP (mmHg): <118, 118–125, 126–135 (reference), 136–146, >146. Nighttime SBP (mmHg): <106, 106–114 (reference), 115–124, 125–137, >137. Hazard ratios adjusted for age, gender, body mass index, diabetes, cardiovascular disease, hemoglobin, proteinuria, and baseline renal function. *$p < 0.05$, **$p < 0.01$. Data compiled from Minutolo et al. [23]

renal outcomes with increasing levels of baseline daytime and nighttime ambulatory BP, but not office BP. This group has recently published further data on outcomes based on the degree of BP control in the office, on ABPM, both or neither [24]. They considered office BP as being at goal is less than 140/90 mmHg, whereas ABPM was considered at goal if daytime BP was <135/85 mmHg and nighttime BP was <120/70 mmHg. Among the 489 study subjects, 17 % were controlled both at home and office, 22 % were controlled only on ABPM (i.e., a white coat effect), 15 % only in the office (i.e., a masked effect), and 47 % on neither ("uncontrolled"). The group with a "white coat effect" had similar risk of cardiovascular events, dialysis, and death as the referent group (controlled BP in both settings). Conversely, the "masked effect" and uncontrolled groups had 2.3–3.9-fold greater risk of all adverse outcomes than patients with controlled BP on adjusted analyses [24]. The authors also performed several sensitivity analyses using different BP cutoffs that provided relatively similar results.

Finally, the 5-year longitudinal analysis of 617 patients with hypertensive nephrosclerosis enrolled in the AASK study found ABPM to be better than office BP for prediction of loss of renal function and cardiovascular events [17]. Both daytime and nighttime BP remained significant predictors of cardiovascular events despite adjustments for office BP and other covariates. On the other hand, ABPM values were only associated with the composite renal endpoint (doubling of serum creatinine, ESRD or death) in patients with controlled office BP (systolic BP <130 mmHg). The investigators postulated that because they used standardized office BP measurements, this may have decreased the observed differences between ABPM and office BP, and that these differences were only relevant in patients with a possible masked effect (i.e., those with controlled office BP). As previously mentioned, dipping status was not an independent predictor on any outcomes in AASK [17].

In summary, similar to the general population, out-of-office BP measurements, both ABPM and home BP, are better predictors of renal and cardiovascular outcomes in patients with CKD. The studies, however, are not as well-powered as studies in other hypertensive populations, and there are inconsistencies regarding the prognostic value of individual ambulatory BP variables (i.e., daytime vs. nighttime vs. 24-h average vs. dipping status).

ABPM in Hemodialysis and Peritoneal Dialysis

Blood Pressure Profile in Dialysis Patients

Hemodialysis (HD) provides a unique scenario of BP variability making ABPM a potentially valuable diagnostic tool. Fluid gain between HD sessions, represented by the increase in body weight, is removed by ultrafiltration. This reduction in extracellular volume is usually accompanied by a fall in BP [25, 26]. The characteristic intermittence of HD treatments and wide fluctuations of extracellular volume during and between HD sessions produce a unique BP profile in HD patients. In conventional, thrice weekly HD, 44-h interdialytic ABPM shows that both awake and sleep BP increase between HD sessions [27, 28] (Fig. 14.3), and that this is not influenced by HD shift assignment (morning or afternoon) [28]. Although interdialytic fluid retention plays a major role in BP increase [29], several studies failed to find a correlation between interdialytic weight gain and interdialytic BP [28, 30]. Most of the ABPM descriptive studies showed that non-dipping pattern is very common in HD patients; more than two thirds of patients lack the normal diurnal BP rhythm [7]. Limited ABPM data are available in patients receiving more frequent (daily HD) or more prolonged (nocturnal HD) regimens that usually are associated with a better clinic BP control [31].

ABPM has been used to determine reasonable clinic BP references in HD patients, i.e., those BPs taken before (pre-HD BP) and after (post-HD BP) HD sessions that best predict interdialytic BP [32–35]. In a systematic review and meta-analysis which included 18 studies where in-center BP and interdialytic ABPM were available, Agarwal et al. showed that pre-dialysis BP overestimated interdialytic ABPM, while on the other hand post-dialysis underestimated ABPM [33]. Although this meta-analysis raises significant concerns about the use of peri-dialysis BP levels in clinical practice, these are still the only measurements available to most physicians caring for HD patients. Recognizing this, we believe that pre-, post- and intradialytic dialysis BP can be used in a qualitative manner to diagnose interdialytic HTN. Agarwal and Lewis [33] have published clinic BP thresholds that have an accuracy rate of about 80 % to predict a diagnosis of HTN on ABPM ("hypertension" defined as 44-h interdialytic BP >135/85 mmHg). The best sensitivity and specificity are observed using pre-HD BP averages between 140 and 150/80 and 85 mmHg and post-HD BP averages between 130 and 140/70 and 80 mmHg [33]. Data from our group [32] and others [34] indicate that the best estimate of interdialytic BP lies around the average of pre-HD and post-HD BP levels. Indeed, Agarwal et al. [36] validated different indices of peri and intra-dialysis BP measurements and showed that a median of all intradialytic BP measurements including pre and post-dialysis BP was better reproducible and had the best accuracy and precision and the least bias compared to interdialytic ABPM. They also proposed a median intradialytic SBP of ≥140 mmHg (80 % sensitivity and 80 % specificity) and a median intradialytic DBP of ≥80 mmHg (75 % sensitivity and 75 % specificity) as thresholds for diagnosing interdialytic HTN.

Out-of-office BP (ABPM and home BP) is a useful tool to evaluate the efficacy of HTN treatment and to explore the association between BP and interdialytic symptoms. ABPM has been used to monitor dosing periods of antihypertensive drugs and home BP is superior to clinic BP for the titration of antihypertensive therapy in HD patients [37–39]. Moreover, because HD patients often have abnormal intradialytic BP changes, both hypo and hypertension [40], their BP control may be better assessed by interdialytic BP [41]. In an important paper, Battle et al. showed that a substantial portion of HD patients have a delayed BP nadir occurring 4–6 h following HD [41]. Van Buren et al. assessed the interdialytic BP profile of patients with intradialytic HTN (systolic BP increase >10 mmHg from pre- to post-hemodialysis in at least four of six treatments) and compared it with control

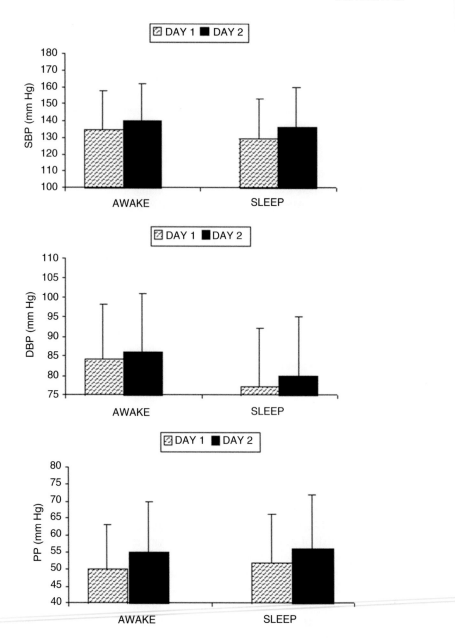

Fig. 14.3 Ambulatory blood pressure values on each interdialytic day during 44-h interdialytic monitoring in hemodialysis patients. *SBP* systolic BP, *DBP* diastolic BP, *PP* pulse pressure, *p<0.05. From: Santos, S.F.F. et al. (2003) Am. J. Nephrol. 23, 96-105, with permission from S. Karger AG, Basel

individuals who had an intradialytic BP fall. Patients with intradialytic HTN had higher mean ambulatory SBP (both daytime and nighttime). Patients with intradialytic HTN had a slight decrease in SBP in the first nocturnal period, while BP increased in the control group. Thereafter, BP increased in both groups [42]. Agarwal and Light used ABPM to evaluate the role of volume overload in intradialytic HTN. They analyzed the intradialytic BP slope at baseline and after probing dry weight [43]. Patients who lost more weight were characterized by an intradialytic rise in BP at baseline. After effective lowering of dry weight, the slope changed to a net BP fall during HD. This observation suggests that lack of BP decline during HD is a sign of covert volume overload.

Decisions about dialysis prescription and timing of antihypertensive drug administration can thereby be made more effectively after understanding the duration of BP control (or even low BP) after each dialysis session. Home BP monitoring is a valuable adjunct in this assessment [44], and we often use it in our practice.

Fluid removal in peritoneal dialysis methods is continuous, and patients do not have large fluctuations in BP related to extracellular volume changes. Therefore, standard methods can be used to assess BP in PD subjects, who are usually seen monthly in the ambulatory setting. ABPM descriptive studies showed a blunted decline in nighttime BP in peritoneal dialysis patients that is very similar to the profile of HD patients [45, 46]. Different PD modalities (conventional ambulatory, cycler assisted) seem to have the same diurnal BP profiles [45, 47]. Differences in BP profile according to peritoneal transport characteristics were explored [48]. While there was substantial difference in the prevalence of HTN and average BP levels (elevated in high and high-average transporters), there were no differences in the diurnal BP profile among groups.

ABPM and Home BP and Target-Organ Dysfunction, Morbidity, and Mortality in Dialysis Patients

The relationship between HTN and outcomes in dialysis patients is complex. While high BP is associated with adverse outcomes, low BP has an even stronger association with mortality, and the optimal levels of BP control are still uncertain for patients on HD or peritoneal dialysis [2]. Despite this uncertainty, HTN remains a central concern in the care of dialysis patients, and ambulatory BP measurements have added substantially to the understanding of the relationships between BP and outcomes in these patients.

Several cross-sectional studies have studied the relationships between office BP, ambulatory BP, and LVH in dialysis patients. Two studies, both in patients undergoing long, slow HD, showed no significant correlation between BP levels, office or ambulatory, and LVH [49, 50]. Others have shown higher correlation coefficients between ambulatory BP and LVH than those linking office BP and LVH in conventional HD patients [26, 27, 51–54], though others have not confirmed this observation [55]. Understanding these differences is not straightforward. Study design, echocardiographic methods, and ABPM techniques were relatively similar among studies. It is possible that the use of a composite of many peri-dialysis readings (or home BP readings for that matter) improves the consistency of the results in such a way that the correlations between LVH and office BPs become indistinguishable from the more consistent and reproducible ABPM values [55, 56]. Furthermore, because dipping is blunted, average casual and ambulatory BPs tend to be more similar, and differences in prediction may be minimized. One last possible factor is that echocardiographic determination of left ventricular mass (LVM) depends on assumptions of cardiac symmetry that are not always present in HD and is dependent on the state of hydration of the patient, which inevitably fluctuates in HD subjects. Echocardiograms underestimate LVM at low LVM values and overestimate it at higher LVM values, a bias that is amplified in patients with higher end-diastolic volumes (a possible indicator of latent volume overload) [57].

Another question that has been addressed by some investigators is whether the circadian BP rhythm matters in the evaluation of LVH in dialysis. Amar et al. did not observe any relationship between dipping status and echocardiographic LVH [58], whereas other investigators have found that the degree of dipping correlates with LVM on univariate, but not multivariate analysis [50], and that nocturnal systolic BP is the strongest predictor of posterior LV wall thickness, though not of other indices of LVH [52]. Wang et al. showed that nocturnal systolic BP load >30 % (% of readings above 125/80 during the night) was the only significant predictor of LVH in a group of peritoneal dialysis patients [47]. In the only available longitudinal study in dialysis, Covic et al. followed echocardiographic and ABPM changes over 12 months and established that patients with a blunted circadian BP rhythm had progressive LV dilatation but no other markers of LV dysfunction on follow-up [59]. Overall, it remains uncertain whether ABPM adds to the evaluation of LVH or if these observations bear any prognostic value to dialysis patients.

Arterial stiffness is a strong predictor of mortality in ESRD [60]. The relationship between ABPM and pulse wave velocity (a marker of arterial stiffness) was studied by Amar et al. in 42 hemodialysis patients [58]. Casual and ambulatory BP had similar correlations with pulse wave velocity. However, non-dipper patients had significantly higher pulse wave velocity than patients with preserved diurnal rhythm (14.1 m/s vs. 11.5 m/s, $p=0.03$). Karpetas et al. [61] performed concomitant 48-h ABPM and pulse wave velocity measurements in a cohort of HD patients. They observed a small increase in pulse wave velocity in the second interdialytic day. Older age and higher ambulatory mean BP were the factors independently associated with higher pulse wave velocity [61]. Agarwal and Light [29] found that arterial stiffness was associated with an overall increase in BP during the interdialytic period, while interdialytic weight gain, which is a predictor of mortality in HD, was associated with interdialytic increase in BP.

ABPM has been evaluated as a predictor of cardiovascular events among dialysis patients [62–65]. In one of the larger studies, Tripepi et al. followed 168 nondiabetic hemodialysis patients who had not sustained a previous cardiovascular event, 49 of whom died during an average follow-up of 38 months. Patients in the highest tertile of the night/day ratio (>1.01, i.e., reverse dippers) had an adjusted hazard ratio of

2.5 for total mortality and 4.3 for cardiovascular mortality [64]. Of relevance, blood pressure (either daytime or nighttime) was not associated with increased mortality risk. In the largest available study to date, Agarwal investigated a prospective cohort of 326 HD patients followed for up to 6 years (median 29 months). Dialysis unit BP (average of 2 weeks), home BP (thrice daily for 1 week), and 44-h ABPM were analyzed as predictors of all-cause mortality. ABPM and home blood pressure were similar predictors of mortality (adjusted hazard ratios for increasing quartiles of ABPM: 2.51, 3.43, 2.62; home BP: 2.15, 1.7, 1.44), and both were better than dialysis unit BP (likelihood ratio test $p=0.009$). Only SBP was predictive of mortality and mortality was lowest when home SBP was between 120 and 130 mmHg and ABPM was between 110 and 120 mmHg [65].

In summary, ABPM and home BP are better predictors of adverse outcomes in dialysis patients as compared to clinic BP.

Technical Issues Specific to Dialysis Patients

Dialysis patients, and more specifically those on hemodialysis, have several features that may make BP measurement and ABPM difficult. These include the presence of arteriovenous grafts or fistulas, which alter blood flow in the extremities, the frequent changes in volume status represented by each dialysis session, and the BP fluctuation in BP throughout the period of 48–72 h separating one dialysis session and the next. Because of these shortcomings, particular concern exists to have devices formally validated in these patients.

In one relevant study, Fagugli et al. monitored 44 patients during the interdialytic period with an ABPM device that is capable of simultaneous oscillometric and auscultatory measurements (A&D Takeda Tm^{2}421) to evaluate the relative accuracy of each technique in hemodialysis patients [66]. The oscillometric component of the device performed better based on several measures: standard deviations of all BP's were lower (18.7 mmHg vs. 20.4 mmHg for systolic, 10.9 mmHg vs. 12.6 mmHg for diastolic, both $p<0.01$); coefficients of variation were also lower (14.6 % vs. 16.1 % for systolic, 14.6 % vs. 17.7 % for diastolic, both $p<0.01$); and percentages of valid BP readings were higher (94 % vs. 72 %, $p=0.001$). The authors concluded that the oscillometric method was preferable in this group of patients. No other study has compared these two methods, but we have validated an oscillometric device in hemodialysis patients (SpaceLabs 90207) with acceptable results [67].

The effects of arteriovenous fistulas or grafts have not been systematically assessed. Nonetheless, in a validation protocol, we demonstrated that an oscillometric device performed equally well in patients with an arteriovenous graft/fistula as in patients with intact arms undergoing hemodialysis via a tunneled venous catheter [67].

Fluctuations in volume status raise issues about the reproducibility of ABPM in hemodialysis patients. To address this question, we evaluated the reproducibility of

ABPM compared with dialysis clinic BP in 21 hemodialysis patients evaluated on average 68 days apart [68]. This study confirmed the wide BP variability in these patients. However, despite this shortcoming, ABPM had lower coefficients of variation and tighter limits of agreement than isolated clinic readings or a composite of readings from the week surrounding the monitoring period. We concluded that ABPM provides more reproducible BP values in hemodialysis patients. When unavailable, a composite of clinic readings are a suitable alternative (investigators have used averages of 1–4 weeks), whereas isolated readings should not be used to make any management decisions [69].

A last but important issue is the need to evaluate the entire interdialytic period and attendant BP fluctuations. This need is compromised by the fact that, in our experience, up to a third of patients are unable to complete a full 2-day monitoring period. As mentioned before, home BP monitoring is a very informative and inexpensive technique, which has the ability to provide comparable information on BP profile and prognosis.

ABPM in Adult Kidney Transplant Recipients

Cardiovascular disease is the leading cause of morbidity and mortality following successful kidney transplantation [70]. Furthermore, cardiovascular disease is a significant cause of death with a functioning allograft [70–74]. Estimates indicate that fatal and nonfatal cardiovascular events are approximately 50-fold more likely in transplant recipients compared with the general population [75]. As poorly controlled hypertension is a well-established risk factor for cardiovascular disease, optimal blood pressure management in the kidney transplant recipient is crucial. Confirming a beneficial effect from management, hypertension control is associated with prolonged allograft survival, even after censoring allograft loss for patient death [76, 77]. As hypertension is a modifiable risk factor, optimal control of blood pressure is essential following kidney transplantation.

Hypertension is present in the majority of kidney transplant recipients [78]. A recent study found only 16 % of recipients to be normotensive without the need for antihypertensive therapy [79]. Consistent with the general population, this study also showed insufficient control of hypertension in 44 %, while 10 % had WCH and 18 % had masked hypertension. Notably, only 16 % of the recipients studied had a normal nocturnal dipping blood pressure pattern. This increased incidence of hypertension is in part a consequence of the immunosuppression regimen. In particular, corticosteroids and the calcineurin inhibitors (cyclosporine more so than tacrolimus) are associated with hypertension [80]. Furthermore, and consistent with native kidney disease, hypertension can be both a cause and a consequence of allograft renal insufficiency.

The RETENAL Study compared assessments of blood pressure control in a cohort of 868 kidney transplant recipients in Spain by ABPM and clinic-based blood pressure measurement [78]. The study found 34 % of participants to have controlled ambulatory blood pressure. Circadian BP patterns showed a high proportion of risers (48 %) in addition to 34 % non-dippers, and only a small proportion (14 %) were dippers [78].

Azancot et al. recently studied the effect of transplantation on hypertension using office BP and ABPM [81]. They hypothesized that the immunosuppressants would lead to a greater degree of hypertension compared to patients with CKD and similar levels of renal insufficiency. The study design required both groups of patients to have moderate impairment in kidney function defined as an eGFR less than 60 mL/min. The office-based blood pressure assessments were comparable between the two groups. Using ABPM, however, a significant difference in both awake and asleep blood pressures was found between the groups, and transplant recipients were less likely to exhibit a normal diurnal blood pressure rhythm (21 % were dippers, compared with 34 % of the patients with CKD) [81]. In summary, nocturnal hypertension and non-dipping, both higher cardiovascular risk blood pressure patterns, were more significant and prevalent in transplant recipients, respectively.

Home Blood Pressure Monitoring (HBPM) has also been investigated following kidney transplantation. Consistent with data from the general population [82], HBPM in kidney transplant recipients more closely correlated with ABPM data than did office-based recordings (72 % concordance vs. 54 %) [83]. Moreover, compared with ABPM reference data, HBPM was both more sensitive and specific at detecting hypertension than office-based BP measurements for the recipients studied.

Limited data are available to compare prognostic accuracy of office and ambulatory BP in renal transplant recipients. As in other groups of patients, ABPM is a better correlate of left ventricular hypertrophy than office BP in renal transplant patients [84, 85]. In a small prospective study of 46 renal transplant recipients undergoing ABPM at 6 and 18 months post-transplantation, ABPM values, but not office BP, were positively correlated with serum creatinine [86]. In a study of 119 transplant recipients, Wadei et al. used ABPM to assess loss of GFR and histological evidence of vascular injury in the allograft 12 months post-transplantation [87]. The analysis focused on circadian BP variability and they did not report on differences in outcomes according to office or average ABPM. As it pertains to circadian variability, they observed that the absence of nocturnal SBP reduction was strongly associated with lower GFR and greater vascular injury in the allograft [87], although this was not observed by another group of investigators using serum creatinine as the outcome variable [88].

The only long-term study evaluating graft failure and cardiovascular events in renal transplant patients included 126 patients followed for 46 months [89]. All patients underwent ABPM at 3 months post-transplantation. In this small study, the presence of a reverse dipper pattern on ABPM was associated with a 3.6-fold increase in risk of loss of allograft or cardiovascular event during follow-up ($p = 0.02$). Neither office BP nor other measures derived from ABPM were associated with the outcomes in question [89].

ABPM in Donor Nephrectomy Candidates

At the present time, there are over 100,000 registrants on the kidney transplant wait-ing list in the United States. This number significantly eclipses the number of deceased donor transplants performed annually, resulting in a significant donor organ shortage. Programs have adapted to this organ shortage through improved utilization of non-standard criteria donor organs, use of organs from deceased donors with cardiac death, and increased efforts to encourage recipients to seek a living donor. Indeed, most programs have a growing experience with allowing donor candidates with well-controlled hypertension to proceed with donor nephrec-tomy. In addition, there has been a significant upward shift in the average age of kidney transplant recipients, and with it an increase in the rate of transplantation from spouse to spouse. As a consequence, more donor candidates in middle and later life are presenting for evaluation. Many will already have a history of hyper-tension or prehypertension. Even more will have an elevated office blood pressure measured during their donor exam, raising concern for undiagnosed hypertension vs. white coat effect.

Multiple studies indicate that donor candidates with hypertension are at risk for worsened BP control following kidney donation [90–92]. Furthermore, one study cor-related the degree of renal function decline associated with kidney donation with the donor's BP prior to the nephrectomy, showing a greater decline in the donors with the higher preoperative BP measurements [92]. Given these findings and concerns, most transplant centers as part of their evaluation will obtain an ABPM study on donor candidates with high blood pressure detected in the office. Ommen et al. reported their experience using ABPM to determine the rates of hypertension, masked hypertension, and white coat hypertension in their single center cohort of potential donors [93]. A diagnosis of WCH was made in 62 % of the donor candidates and masked HTN in 17 %. By screening all of their donor candidates with ABPM, the author's concluded that they had more accurately assessed the medical risk of the donor candidate while at the same time reducing their disqualification rate.

This markedly high incidence of WCH (significantly higher than the expected incidence of WCH for individuals presumed to be in overall good health) in donor nephrectomy candidates has been independently confirmed [94]. Interestingly, the white coat effect was largely absent when donors (who had WCH prior to organ donation) were restudied 6 months postnephrectomy by ABPM [94]. This is consis-tent with the belief that the anxiety associated with consideration of a surgical pro-cedure that one does not require for their own health results in this significantly increased incidence of donor candidates with WCH. To our knowledge, the pres-ence and magnitude of the white coat effect has not been correlated with the strength of the relationship between the donor candidate and their intended recipient.

It is recognized that the absence of nocturnal dipping is associated with increased target organ injury and cardiovascular disease risk in the general population [95]. With studies confirming that the development of end stage renal disease is a rare, albeit increased risk, event in former donors [96, 97], there is continued concern regarding the long-term impact donor nephrectomy has on future cardiovascular disease. Indeed, a group from Norway reported a statistically significant increase in cardiovascular mortality (adjusted hazard ratio 1.40) in their former donors [96].

Prasad et al. studied the impact of donor nephrectomy on BP dipping status 12 months following donation [98]. Fifty one donors were studied; 35 were dippers and 16 were non-dippers predonation. Based on 12-month follow-up data, they reached the conclusion that predonation non-dipping is not associated with adverse consequences. Interestingly, 8 of the predonation dippers studied subsequently became non-dippers, but did so without a statistically significant increase in 24-h blood pressure compared to those who remained dippers. The durability of this change in dipping status, as well as the long-term cardiovascular consequences, remains to be determined.

Mechanistic Considerations on the Blunted Diurnal Rhythm in Renal Disease

As discussed above, non-dipping is the prevailing BP profile in patients with all stages of CKD. The mechanisms responsible for abnormal circadian BP rhythms in CKD patients remain unclear. The key elements appear to be salt-sensitivity (and volume overload), sleep disordered breathing, and sympathetic overactivity [99, 100]. Other possible mechanisms include decreased physical activity [101, 102] and abnormalities in several hormonal and neuroendocrine mediators (catecholamines, renin, aldosterone, insulin, atrial natriuretic peptide, asymmetric dimethylarginine, parathormone), although the strength of these relationships is weak at best [7, 30].

Sodium sensitivity and volume overload appear to be particularly important factors. In patients with essential HTN, a change from a high to a low sodium diet corrects non-dipping in salt-sensitive subjects [103, 104]. In addition, hydrochlorothiazide restores dipping in non-dipper, but not in dipper hypertensive subjects [105]. Thus, it is possible that salt-balance and salt-sensitivity mediate dipping in hypertensive patients without renal disease. However, it is probable that this is not the case in advanced CKD, where multiple studies attempts to correlate interdialytic weight gain with degree of dipping have failed to show any significant correlation [30, 32]. Furthermore, even patients on long-slow hemodialysis, who are characterized by excellent BP control [50, 106] and less marked expansion of extracellular volume than patients on conventional hemodialysis [107], are non-dippers in 50–75 % of cases [108]. Likewise, the transition from standard hemodialysis to short-daily hemodialysis leads to better BP control and decreased extracellular water, but no change in nocturnal dipping [109].

Proteinuria and low GFR seem to interact in the mediation of blunted circadian rhythms. In a study of 336 elderly men, 55 % of whom had CKD (low eGFR or proteinuria) and 45 % did not, patients with low eGFR (<60 mL/min/1.73 m^2) had only 33 % of the circadian variability in systolic BP compared with patients without CKD, while those proteinuria (protein/creatinine ratio >0.22) had only 24 % of the control amplitude [110]. There was further blunting when both low eGFR and proteinuria were present. These results can be interpreted within the context of salt sensitivity and volume excess, as there is growing data on the role of proteinuria mediating sodium avidity through activation of the epithelial sodium channel [111].

Sleep-disordered breathing is a particular problem, especially in advanced CKD, as it is diagnosed in up to 70 % of patients with ESRD [112]. Zoccali et al. showed that HD patients without episodes of nocturnal desaturation had a small decline in sleep BP (by 2.5 %), whereas those with two or more desaturation episodes per hour had a reversal of the BP rhythm (sleep systolic BP increased by 3.9 %) [113]. These observations are relevant because sleep-disordered breathing is associated with left ventricular hypertrophy in dialysis patients [113, 114]. While it is known that intensive dialysis or transplantation can correct the sleep disorder [112, 115], we are not aware of data-linking correction of sleep apnea and normalization of the BP profile in CKD, as has been demonstrated in patients without renal disease. In earlier stages of CKD, this has been assessed in an indirect fashion; one study demonstrated that patients with fragmented sleep patterns due to nocturia have less nocturnal BP decline as compared to the intensity of sleep fragmentation [116].

Chronotherapy in CKD

A possible translation of ABPM to the care of hypertensive patients is the use of chronotherapy, where dosing schedules and/or drug delivery systems are manipulated to mimic the normal circadian BP changes and to minimize the early morning BP rise. In essential hypertension, there is growing evidence of the possible value of shifting medication administration from the morning to night to improve surrogate outcomes [99, 100], and one randomized open-label trial has shown a marked decrease in cardiovascular events [117], though these findings still warrant corroboration.

In CKD patients, non-dipping can be improved or corrected by this chronopharmacologic dosing approach [118–120], although this has not been observed in all studies, as reported among patients with CKD due to hypertensive nephrosclerosis [121]. In some studies, this approach has resulted in potentially relevant results. In a study of 32 non-dipping CKD patients, shifting the administration of one antihypertensive medication from morning to evening resulted in a decrease in the systolic BP night/day ratio from 0.98 to 0.89 ($p < 0.001$) and correction of the non-dipping pattern in most (28 of 32) patients [120]. Moreover, the greater the fall in the night/day ratio induced by the dosing change, the greater the fall in proteinuria during this 8-week study ($r = 0.26$, $p < 0.01$) [120]. Finally, the impact of dose shifting on cardiovascular outcomes was evaluated in 661 patients with early CKD (average eGFR 65 mL/min/1.73 m²) [119]. Patients were randomized to either receiving all medications upon awakening or to receiving at least one drug at bedtime. Bedtime agents

were converting enzyme inhibitors, angiotensin receptor blockers, or calcium channel blockers. After 5.4 years of follow-up, non-dipping frequency was decreased in
the bedtime group (from 65 to 41 %), but not in the awakening group. The primary
endpoint (a composite of death, myocardial infarction, angina pectoris, revascularization, heart failure, arterial occlusion of lower extremities, occlusion of the retinal
artery, and stroke) was decreased by 69 % in the bedtime group (adjusted hazard
ratio 0.31; 95 % CI 0.21–0.46), with significant reductions of most individual
components of the composite. These results were impressive and encouraging; if
corroborated, the practice of bedtime medication dosing may become the standard.

Conclusions

ABPM and home BP allow better understanding of BP behavior, are more reproducible than office BP, and appear to be a better marker of renal and cardiovascular
prognosis in CKD. Further work is necessary to determine which out-of-office measure is most practical in CKD, how often it should be obtained, and for better delin-
eation of reimbursement options remain essential prior to generalization of their
use, in particular in the United States.

References

1. Jha V, Garcia-Garcia G, et al. Chronic kidney disease: global dimension and perspectives.
   Lancet. 2013;382(9888):260–72.
2. Peixoto AJ, Santos SF. Blood pressure management in hemodialysis: what have we learned?
   Curr Opin Nephrol Hypertens. 2010;19(6):561–6.
3. Weir MR, Burgess ED, Cooper JE, et al. Assessment and management of hypertension in
   transplant patients. J Am Soc Nephrol. 2015. doi:10.1681/ASN.2014080834.
4. Gansevoort RT, Correa-Rotter R, Hemmelgarn BR, et al. Chronic kidney disease and cardiovascular risk: epidemiology, mechanisms, and prevention. Lancet. 2013;382(9889):339–52.
5. McManus RJ, Caulfield M, Williams B, National Institute for H, Clinical E. NICE hypertension guideline 2011: evidence based evolution. BMJ. 2012;344:e181.
6. Levin A, Stevens PE. Summary of KDIGO 2012 CKD Guideline: behind the scenes, need for
   guidance, and a framework for moving forward. Kidney Int. 2014;85(1):49–61.
7. Peixoto AJ, White WB. Ambulatory blood pressure monitoring in chronic renal disease:
   technical aspects and clinical relevance. Curr Opin Nephrol Hypertens. 2002;11(5):
   507–16.
8. Baumgart P, Walger P, Gemen S, von Eiff M, Raidt H, Rahn KH. Blood pressure elevation
   during the night in chronic renal failure, hemodialysis and after renal transplantation.
   Nephron. 1991;57(3):293–8.
9. Pogue V, Rahman M, Lipkowitz M, et al. Disparate estimates of hypertension control from
   ambulatory and clinic blood pressure measurements in hypertensive kidney disease.
   Hypertension. 2009;53(1):20–7.
10. Mojon A, Ayala DE, Pineiro L, et al. Comparison of ambulatory blood pressure parameters
    of hypertensive patients with and without chronic kidney disease. Chronobiol Int.
    2013;30(1–2):145–58.

11. Hermida RC, Smolensky MH, Ayala DE, et al. Abnormalities in chronic kidney disease of ambulatory blood pressure 24 h patterning and normalization by bedtime hypertension chronotherapy. Nephrol Dial Transplant. 2014;29(6):1160–7.
12. Lurbe E, Redon J, Kesani A, et al. Increase in nocturnal blood pressure and progression to microalbuminuria in type 1 diabetes. N Engl J Med. 2002;347(11):797–805.
13. Timio M, Venanzi S, Lolli S, et al. "Non-dipper" hypertensive patients and progressive renal insufficiency: a 3-year longitudinal study. Clin Nephrol. 1995;43(6):382–7.
14. Farmer CK, Goldsmith DJ, Quin JD, et al. Progression of diabetic nephropathy—is diurnal blood pressure rhythm as important as absolute blood pressure level? Nephrol Dial Transplant. 1998;13(3):635–9.
15. Csiky B, Kovacs T, Wagner L, Vass T, Nagy J. Ambulatory blood pressure monitoring and progression in patients with IgA nephropathy. Nephrol Dial Transplant. 1999;14(1):86–90.
16. Agarwal R, Andersen MJ. Prognostic importance of ambulatory blood pressure recordings in patients with chronic kidney disease. Kidney Int. 2006;69(7):1175–80.
17. Gabbai FB, Rahman M, Hu B, et al. Relationship between ambulatory BP and clinical outcomes in patients with hypertensive CKD. Clin J Am Soc Nephrol. 2012;7(11):1770–6.
18. Tucker B, Fabbian F, Giles M, Thuraisingham RC, Raine AE, Baker LR. Left ventricular hypertrophy and ambulatory blood pressure monitoring in chronic renal failure. Nephrol Dial Transplant. 1997;12(4):724–8.
19. Szelestei T, Kovacs T, Barta J, Nagy J. Circadian blood pressure changes and cardiac abnormalities in IgA nephropathy. Am J Nephrol. 1999;19(5):546–51.
20. Valero FA, Martinez-Vea A, Bardaji A, et al. Ambulatory blood pressure and left ventricular mass in normotensive patients with autosomal dominant polycystic kidney disease. J Am Soc Nephrol. 1999;10(5):1020–6.
21. Agarwal R, Andersen MJ. Correlates of systolic hypertension in patients with chronic kidney disease. Hypertension. 2005;46(3):514–20.
22. Agarwal R, Andersen MJ. Prognostic importance of clinic and home blood pressure recordings in patients with chronic kidney disease. Kidney Int. 2006;69(2):406–11.
23. Minutolo R, Agarwal R, Borrelli S, et al. Prognostic role of ambulatory blood pressure measurement in patients with nondialysis chronic kidney disease. Arch Intern Med. 2011;171(12):1090–8.
24. Minutolo R, Gabbai FB, Agarwal R, et al. Assessment of achieved clinic and ambulatory blood pressure recordings and outcomes during treatment in hypertensive patients with CKD: a multicenter prospective cohort study. Am J Kidney Dis. 2014;64(5):744–52.
25. Cheigh JS, Milite C, Sullivan JF, Rubin AL, Stenzel KH. Hypertension is not adequately controlled in hemodialysis patients. Am J Kidney Dis. 1992;19(5):453–9.
26. Cannella G, Paoletti E, Ravera G, et al. Inadequate diagnosis and therapy of arterial hypertension as causes of left ventricular hypertrophy in uremic dialysis patients. Kidney Int. 2000;58(1):260–8.
27. Rahman M, Griffin V, Heyka R, Hoit B. Diurnal variation of blood pressure; reproducibility and association with left ventricular hypertrophy in hemodialysis patients. Blood Press Monit. 2005;10(1):25–32.
28. Santos SF, Mendes RB, Santos CA, Dorigo D, Peixoto AJ. Profile of interdialytic blood pressure in hemodialysis patients. Am J Nephrol. 2003;23(2):96–105.
29. Agarwal R, Light RP. Arterial stiffness and interdialytic weight gain influence ambulatory blood pressure patterns in hemodialysis patients. Am J Physiol Renal Physiol. 2008;294(2):F303–8.
30. Peixoto AJ, Sica DA. Ambulatory blood pressure monitoring in end-stage renal disease. Blood Press Monit. 1997;2(6):275–82.
31. Kotanko P, Garg AX, Depner T, et al. Effects of frequent hemodialysis on blood pressure: results from the randomized frequent hemodialysis network trials. Hemodial Int. 2015;2015(5):12255.
32. Mendes RB, Santos SF, Dorigo D, et al. The use of peridialysis blood pressure and intradialytic blood pressure changes in the prediction of interdialytic blood pressure in haemodialysis patients. Blood Press Monit. 2003;8(6):243–8.

33. Agarwal R, Lewis RR. Prediction of hypertension in chronic hemodialysis patients. Kidney Int. 2001;60(5):1982–9.
34. Coomer RW, Schulman G, Breyer JA, Shyr Y. Ambulatory blood pressure monitoring in dialysis patients and estimation of mean interdialytic blood pressure. Am J Kidney Dis. 1997;29(5):678–84.
35. Rodby RA, Vonesh EF, Korbet SM. Blood pressures in hemodialysis and peritoneal dialysis using ambulatory blood pressure monitoring. Am J Kidney Dis. 1994;23(3):401–11.
36. Agarwal R, Metiku T, Tegegne GG, et al. Diagnosing hypertension by intradialytic blood pressure recordings. Clin J Am Soc Nephrol. 2008;3(5):1364–72. doi:10.2215/CJN.01510308. Epub 2008 May 21.
37. Agarwal R. Supervised atenolol therapy in the management of hemodialysis hypertension. Kidney Int. 1999;55(4):1528–35.
38. Agarwal R, Lewis R, Davis JL, Becker B. Lisinopril therapy for hemodialysis hypertension: hemodynamic and endocrine responses. Am J Kidney Dis. 2001;38(6):1245–50.
39. da Silva GV, de Barros S, Abensur H, Ortega KC, Mion Jr D. Home blood pressure monitoring in blood pressure control among haemodialysis patients: an open randomized clinical trial. Nephrol Dial Transplant. 2009;24(12):3805–11.
40. Santos SF, Peixoto AJ, Perazella MA. How should we manage adverse intradialytic blood pressure changes? Adv Chronic Kidney Dis. 2012;19(3):158–65.
41. Batlle DC, von Riotte A, Lang G. Delayed hypotensive response to dialysis in hypertensive patients with end-stage renal disease. Am J Nephrol. 1986;6(1):14–20.
42. Van Buren PN, Kim C, Toto R, Inrig JK. Intradialytic hypertension and the association with interdialytic ambulatory blood pressure. Clin J Am Soc Nephrol. 2011;6(7):1684–91.
43. Agarwal R, Light RP. Intradialytic hypertension is a marker of volume excess. Nephrol Dial Transplant. 2010;25(10):3355–61.
44. Agarwal R. Managing hypertension using home blood pressure monitoring among haemodialysis patients—a call to action. Nephrol Dial Transplant. 2010;25(6):1766–71.
45. Cocchi R, Degli Esposti E, Fabbri A, et al. Prevalence of hypertension in patients on peritoneal dialysis: results of an Italian multicentre study. Nephrol Dial Transplant. 1999;14(6):1536–40.
46. Farmer CK, Goldsmith DJ, Cox J, Dallyn P, Kingswood JC, Sharpstone P. An investigation of the effect of advancing uraemia, renal replacement therapy and renal transplantation on blood pressure diurnal variability. Nephrol Dial Transplant. 1997;12(11):2301–7.
47. Wang MC, Tseng CC, Tsai WC, Huang JJ. Blood pressure and left ventricular hypertrophy in patients on different peritoneal dialysis regimens. Perit Dial Int. 2001;21(1):36–42.
48. Tonbul Z, Altintepe L, Sozlu C, Yeksan M, Yildiz A, Turk S. The association of peritoneal transport properties with 24-hour blood pressure levels in CAPD patients. Perit Dial Int. 2003;23(1):46–52.
49. Covic A, Goldsmith DJ, Georgescu G, Venning MC, Ackrill P. Echocardiographic findings in long-term, long-hour hemodialysis patients. Clin Nephrol. 1996;45(2):104–10.
50. McGregor DO, Buttimore AL, Nicholls MG, Lynn KL. Ambulatory blood pressure monitoring in patients receiving long, slow home haemodialysis. Nephrol Dial Transplant. 1999;14(11):2676–9.
51. Nishikimi T, Minami J, Tamano K, et al. Left ventricular mass relates to average systolic blood pressure, but not loss of circadian blood pressure in stable hemodialysis patients: an ambulatory 48-hour blood pressure study. Hypertens Res. 2001;24(5):507–14.
52. Erturk S, Ertug AE, Ates K, Duman N, Aslan SM, Nergisoglu G, et al. Relationship of ambulatory blood pressure monitoring data to echocardiographic findings in haemodialysis patients. Nephrol Dial Transplant. 1996;11(10):2050–4.
53. Agarwal R, Brim NJ, Mahenthiran J, Andersen MJ, Saha C. Out-of-hemodialysis-unit blood pressure is a superior determinant of left ventricular hypertrophy. Hypertension. 2006;47(1):62–8.
54. Goldsmith DJ, Covic AC, Venning MC, Ackrill P. Ambulatory blood pressure monitoring in renal dialysis and transplant patients. Am J Kidney Dis. 1997;29(4):593–600.

55. Conlon PJ, Walshe JJ, Heinle SK, Minda S, Krucoff M, Schwab SJ. Predialysis systolic blood pressure correlates strongly with mean 24-hour systolic blood pressure and left ventricular mass in stable hemodialysis patients. J Am Soc Nephrol. 1996;7(12):2658–63.
56. Zoccali C, Mallamaci F, Tripepi G, et al. Prediction of left ventricular geometry by clinic, pre-dialysis and 24-h ambulatory BP monitoring in hemodialysis patients: CREED investigators. J Hypertens. 1999;17(12 Pt 1):1751–8.
57. Stewart GA, Foster J, Cowan M, et al. Echocardiography overestimates left ventricular mass in hemodialysis patients relative to magnetic resonance imaging. Kidney Int. 1999;56(6):2248–53.
58. Amar J, Vernier I, Rossignol E, Lenfant V, Conte JJ, Chamontin B. Influence of nycthemeral blood pressure pattern in treated hypertensive patients on hemodialysis. Kidney Int. 1997;51(6):1863–6.
59. Covic A, Goldsmith DJ, Covic M. Reduced blood pressure diurnal variability as a risk factor for progressive left ventricular dilatation in hemodialysis patients. Am J Kidney Dis. 2000;35(4):617–23.
60. Blacher J, Guerin AP, Pannier B, Marchais SJ, Safar ME, London GM. Impact of aortic stiffness on survival in end-stage renal disease. Circulation. 1999;99:2434–9.
61. Karpetas A, Sarafidis PA, Georgianos PI, et al. Ambulatory recording of wave reflections and arterial stiffness during intra- and interdialytic periods in patients treated with dialysis. Clin J Am Soc Nephrol. 2015;10(4):630–8.
62. Amar J, Vernier I, Rossignol E, et al. Nocturnal blood pressure and 24-hour pulse pressure are potent indicators of mortality in hemodialysis patients. Kidney Int. 2000;57(6):2485–91.
63. Liu M, Takahashi H, Morita Y, et al. Non-dipping is a potent predictor of cardiovascular mortality and is associated with autonomic dysfunction in haemodialysis patients. Nephrol Dial Transplant. 2003;18(3):563–9.
64. Tripepi G, Fagugli RM, Dattolo P, et al. Prognostic value of 24-hour ambulatory blood pressure monitoring and of night/day ratio in nondiabetic, cardiovascular events-free hemodialysis patients. Kidney Int. 2005;68(3):1294–302.
65. Agarwal R. Blood pressure and mortality among hemodialysis patients. Hypertension. 2010;55(3):762–8.
66. Fagugli RM, Vecchi L, Valente F, Santirosi P, Laviola MM. Comparison between oscillometric and auscultatory methods of ambulatory blood pressure measurement in hemodialysis patients. Clin Nephrol. 2002;57(4):283–8.
67. Peixoto AJ, Gray TA, Crowley ST. Validation of the SpaceLabs 90207 ambulatory blood pressure device for hemodialysis patients. Blood Press Monit. 1999;4(5):217–21.
68. Peixoto AJ, Santos SF, Mendes RB, Crowley ST, Maldonado R, Orias M, et al. Reproducibility of ambulatory blood pressure monitoring in hemodialysis patients. Am J Kidney Dis. 2000;36(5):983–90.
69. Sankaranarayanan N, Santos SF, Peixoto AJ. Blood pressure measurement in dialysis patients. Adv Chronic Kidney Dis. 2004;11(2):134–42.
70. Ojo AO, Hanson JA, Wolfe RA, Leichtman AB, Agodoa LY, Port FK. Long-term survival in renal transplant recipients with graft function. Kidney Int. 2000;57(1):307–13.
71. Ghods AJ, Ossareh S. Detection and treatment of coronary artery disease in renal transplantation candidates. Transplant Proc. 2002;34(6):2415–7.
72. Ostovan MA, Fazelzadeh A, Mehdizadeh AR, Razmkon A, Malek-Hosseini SA. How to decrease cardiovascular mortality in renal transplant recipients. Transplant Proc. 2006; 38(9):2887–92.
73. Fellström B. Risk factors for and management of post-transplantation cardiovascular disease. BioDrugs. 2001;15(4):261–78.
74. Kasiske BL, Guijarro C, Massy ZA, Wiederkehr MR, Ma JZ. Cardiovascular disease after renal transplantation. J Am Soc Nephrol. 1996;7(1):158–65.
75. Kasiske BL, Chakkera HA, Roel J. Explained and unexplained ischemic heart disease risk after renal transplantation. J Am Soc Nephrol. 2000;11(9):1735–43.
76. Hillebrand U, Suwelack BM, Loley K, et al. Blood pressure, antihypertensive treatment, and graft survival in kidney transplant patients. Transpl Int. 2009;22(11):1073–80.

77. Opelz G, Döhler B, Study CT. Improved long-term outcomes after renal transplantation associated with blood pressure control. Am J Transplant. 2005;5(11):2725–31.
78. Fernandez Fresnedo G, Franco Esteve A, Gómez Huertas E, et al. Ambulatory blood pressure monitoring in kidney transplant patients: RETENAL study. Transplant Proc. 2012; 44(9):2601–2.
79. Czyżewski Ł, Wyzgał J, Kołek A. Evaluation of selected risk factors of cardiovascular diseases among patients after kidney transplantation, with particular focus on the role of 24-hour automatic blood pressure measurement in the diagnosis of hypertension: an introductory report. Ann Transplant. 2014;19:188–98.
80. Miller LW. Cardiovascular toxicities of immunosuppressive agents. Am J Transplant. 2002; 2(9):807–18.
81. Azancot MA, Ramos N, Moreso FJ, et al. Hypertension in chronic kidney disease: the influence of renal transplantation. Transplantation. 2014;98(5):537–42.
82. Masding MG, Jones JR, Bartley E, Sandeman DD. Assessment of blood pressure in patients with Type 2 diabetes: comparison between home blood pressure monitoring, clinic blood pressure measurement and 24-h ambulatory blood pressure monitoring. Diabet Med. 2001;18(6):431–7.
83. Agena F, Prado Eo S, Souza PS, et al. Home blood pressure (BP) monitoring in kidney transplant recipients is more adequate to monitor BP than office BP. Nephrol Dial Transplant. 2011;26(11):3745–9.
84. Covic A, Segall L, Goldsmith DJ. Ambulatory blood pressure monitoring in renal transplantation: should ABPM be routinely performed in renal transplant patients? Transplantation. 2003;76(11):1640–2.
85. Ferreira SR, Moises VA, Tavares A, Pacheco-Silva A. Cardiovascular effects of successful renal transplantation: a 1-year sequential study of left ventricular morphology and function, and 24-hour blood pressure profile. Transplantation. 2002;74(11):1580–7.
86. Jacobi J, Rockstroh J, John S, et al. Prospective analysis of the value of 24-hour ambulatory blood pressure on renal function after kidney transplantation. Transplantation. 2000;70(5):819–27.
87. Wadei HM, Amer H, Taler SJ, et al. Diurnal blood pressure changes one year after kidney transplantation: relationship to allograft function, histology, and resistive index. J Am Soc Nephrol. 2007;18(5):1607–15.
88. Haydar AA, Covic A, Agharazili M, Jayawardene S, Taylor J, Goldsmith DJ. Systolic blood pressure diurnal variation is not a predictor of renal target organ damage in kidney transplant patients. Am J Transplant. 2003;4(2):244–7.
89. Ibernon M, Moreso F, Sarrias X, et al. Reverse dipper pattern of blood pressure at 3 months is associated with inflammation and outcome after renal transplantation. Nephrol Dial Transplant. 2012;27(5):2089–95.
90. Anderson CF, Velosa JA, Frohnert PP, et al. The risks of unilateral nephrectomy: status of kidney donors 10 to 20 years postoperatively. Mayo Clin Proc. 1985;60(6):367–74.
91. Torres VE, Offord KP, Anderson CF, et al. Blood pressure determinants in living-related renal allograft donors and their recipients. Kidney Int. 1987;31(6):1383–90.
92. Talseth T, Fauchald P, Skrede S, et al. Long-term blood pressure and renal function in kidney donors. Kidney Int. 1986;29(5):1072–6.
93. Ommen ES, Schröppel B, Kim JY, et al. Routine use of ambulatory blood pressure monitoring in potential living kidney donors. Clin J Am Soc Nephrol. 2007;2(5):1030–6.
94. DeLoach SS, Meyers KE, Townsend RR. Living donor kidney donation: another form of white coat effect. Am J Nephrol. 2012;35(1):75–9.
95. Routledge FS, McFetridge-Durdle JA, Dean CR, Society CH. Night-time blood pressure patterns and target organ damage: a review. Can J Cardiol. 2007;23(2):132–8.
96. Mjøen G, Hallan S, Hartmann A, et al. Long-term risks for kidney donors. Kidney Int. 2014;86(1):162–7.
97. Muzaale AD, Massie AB, Wang MC, et al. Risk of end-stage renal disease following live kidney donation. JAMA. 2014;311(6):579–86.

98. Prasad GV, Lipszyc D, Huang M, Nash MM, Rapi L. A prospective observational study of changes in renal function and cardiovascular risk following living kidney donation. Transplantation. 2008;86(9):1315–8.
99. Sinha AD, Agarwal R. The complex relationship between CKD and ambulatory blood pressure patterns. Adv Chronic Kidney Dis. 2015;22(2):102–7.
100. Peixoto AJ, White WB. Circadian blood pressure: clinical implications based on the pathophysiology of its variability. Kidney Int. 2007;71(9):855–60.
101. O'Shea JC, Murphy MB. Nocturnal blood pressure dipping: a consequence of diurnal physical activity blipping? Am J Hypertens. 2000;13(6 Pt 1):601–6.
102. Kutner NG, Cardenas DD, Bower JD. Rehabilitation, aging and chronic renal disease. Am J Phys Med Rehabil. 1992;71(2):97–101.
103. Uzu T, Ishikawa K, Fujii T, Nakamura S, Inenaga T, Kimura G. Sodium restriction shifts circadian rhythm of blood pressure from nondipper to dipper in essential hypertension. Circulation. 1997;96(6):1859–62.
104. Higashi Y, Oshima T, Ozono R, et al. Nocturnal decline in blood pressure is attenuated by NaCl loading in salt-sensitive patients with essential hypertension: noninvasive 24-hour ambulatory blood pressure monitoring. Hypertension. 1997;30(2 Pt 1):163–7.
105. Uzu T, Kimura G. Diuretics shift circadian rhythm of blood pressure from nondipper to dipper in essential hypertension. Circulation. 1999;100(15):1635–8.
106. Charra B, Calemard E, Ruffet M, et al. Survival as an index of adequacy of dialysis. Kidney Int. 1992;41(5):1286–91.
107. Katzarski KS, Charra B, Luik AJ, Nisell J, Divino Filho JC, Leypoldt JK, et al. Fluid state and blood pressure control in patients treated with long and short haemodialysis. Nephrol Dial Transplant. 1999;14(2):369–75.
108. Chazot C, Charra B, Laurent G, et al. Interdialysis blood pressure control by long haemodialysis sessions. Nephrol Dial Transplant. 1995;10(6):831–7.
109. Fagugli RM, Reboldi G, Quintaliani G, et al. Short daily hemodialysis: blood pressure control and left ventricular mass reduction in hypertensive hemodialysis patients. Am J Kidney Dis. 2001;38(2):371–6.
110. Agarwal R, Light RP. GFR, proteinuria and circadian blood pressure. Nephrol Dial Transplant. 2009;24(8):2400–6.
111. Peixoto AJ, Orias M, Desir GV. Does kidney disease cause hypertension? Curr Hypertens Rep. 2013;15(2):89–94.
112. Hanly PJ, Pierratos A. Improvement of sleep apnea in patients with chronic renal failure who undergo nocturnal hemodialysis. N Engl J Med. 2001;344(2):102–7.
113. Zoccali C, Benedetto FA, Tripepi G, et al. Nocturnal hypoxemia, night-day arterial pressure changes and left ventricular geometry in dialysis patients. Kidney Int. 1998;53(4):1078–84.
114. Zoccali C, Benedetto FA, Mallamaci F, et al. Left ventricular hypertrophy and nocturnal hypoxemia in hemodialysis patients. J Hypertens. 2001;19(2):287–93.
115. Langevin B, Fouque D, Leger P, Robert D. Sleep apnea syndrome and end-stage renal disease. Cure after renal transplantation. Chest. 1993;103(5):1330–5.
116. Agarwal R, Light RP, Bills JE, Hummel LA. Nocturia, nocturnal activity, and nondipping. Hypertension. 2009;54(3):646–51.
117. Hermida RC, Ayala DE, Mojon A, Fernandez JR. Influence of circadian time of hypertension treatment on cardiovascular risk: results of the MAPEC study. Chronobiol Int. 2010;27(8):1629–51.
118. Portaluppi F, Vergnani L, Manfredini R, degli Uberti EC, Fersini C. Time-dependent effect of isradipine on the nocturnal hypertension in chronic renal failure. Am J Hypertens. 1995;8(7):719–26.
119. Hermida RC, Ayala DE, Mojon A, Fernandez JR. Bedtime dosing of antihypertensive medications reduces cardiovascular risk in CKD. J Am Soc Nephrol. 2011;22(12):2313–21.
120. Minutolo R, Gabbai FB, Borrelli S, et al. Changing the timing of antihypertensive therapy to reduce nocturnal blood pressure in CKD: an 8-week uncontrolled trial. Am J Kidney Dis. 2007;50(6):908–17.
121. Rahman M, Greene T, Phillips RA, et al. A trial of 2 strategies to reduce nocturnal blood pressure in blacks with chronic kidney disease. Hypertension. 2013;61(1):82–8.

Chapter 15
Ambulatory Blood Pressure Monitoring in Coronary Artery Disease and Heart Failure

Fahad Javed and Patrick T. Campbell

Ambulatory blood pressure monitoring (ABPM) is capable of evaluating multiple aspects of blood pressure including 24-h blood pressure, nocturnal blood pressures, dipping patterns, morning surge blood pressures, postprandial hypotension, and BP variability. ABPM has been shown to be highly effective for the diagnosis and management of hypertension. ABPM and specifically nocturnal blood pressure has demonstrated superior predictive and prognostic value for target organ dysfunction and cardiovascular events. While there is an abundance of data on ABPM in hypertension, stroke, diabetes, and chronic kidney disease, there is relatively little data on ABPM in coronary artery disease (CAD) or heart failure (HF).

In this chapter, we summarize much of the available data, discuss the diagnostic and therapeutic benefits offered by ABPM, and will suggest future avenues for research.

Hypertension in Heart Failure

Hypertension (HTN) has long been recognized as one of the most prevalent modifiable risk factors for the development of both heart failure with preserved ejection fraction (HFpEF) and heart failure with reduced ejection fraction (HFrEF). In the

F. Javed, M.D.
Ochsner Heart and Vascular Institute, 1514 Jefferson Highway,
New Orleans, LA 70121, USA

P.T. Campbell, M.D. (✉)
Heart Failure and Transplant Cardiology, Transplant Institute Baptist Health,
9500 Kanis Road, Little Rock, AR 72205, USA
e-mail: patcamp23@hotmail.com

© Springer International Publishing Switzerland 2016
W.B. White (ed.), *Blood Pressure Monitoring in Cardiovascular Medicine and Therapeutics*, Clinical Hypertension and Vascular Diseases,
DOI 10.1007/978-3-319-22771-9_15

Framingham Heart Study, the presence of elevated blood pressure (BP) was associated with twice the risk of developing HF compared with normotension [1].

The prevalence of hypertension in the U.S. is approximately 30 % of people over the age of 18 and current statistics demonstrate that less than 50 % are achieving adequate control. This is a staggering 95 million Americans at risk for the development of heart failure from hypertension. Patients with hypertension are considered to be Stage A heart failure by current guidelines, at risk for heart failure without structural disease or symptoms, and aggressive management of risk factors is recommended by the current guidelines [2]. Patients with evidence of structural heart disease, including Left Ventricular Hypertrophy (LVH), Left Atrial Enlargement (LAE), reduced systolic function, diastolic dysfunction, valvular disease, and coronary artery disease (CAD), even without symptoms, are classified as being Stage B heart failure and require additional therapies beyond BP control; however, anti-hypertensive therapies remain an integral component of their management. For patients with Stage C Heart Failure (structural heart disease and current or history of HF symptoms), maximally titrated guideline-directed therapy is the mainstay of treatment [2]. In those who have progressed to refractory heart failure (Stage D), specialized therapies are required and the benefit of ABPM may be limited as patients are often on inotropic support or have mechanical circulatory support.

Hypertensive heart disease is associated with both HFrEF and HFpEF. The exact mechanisms and triggers that precipitate the progression from LVH to heart failure remain poorly understood. Hypertension can result in either concentric LVH (increased wall thickness) or eccentric LVH (dilation of the LV cavity). Traditional teachings hold that LVH progresses from concentric LVH to dilated LV cavity and subsequent reduced LV function; however, more recent data suggests that while patients can progress down the classical pathway to HF, the majority of patients develop either concentric LVH or eccentric LVH with little crossover [3]. The reasons for the dichotomy remain unclear, but are likely related to a multitude of simultaneously interacting factors including: patient characteristics, concomitant disease processes, variable neurohormonal milieu, variability of pressure and volume load, and currently unrecognized genetic factors. Concentric LVH is associated with higher systolic blood pressures (SBP), peripheral vascular resistance (PVR), and elevated renin levels, while eccentric LVH may be more related to volume loads [4, 5]. Concentric LVH and HFpEF have been correlated with abnormal changes in the extracellular matrix driven by mineralocorticoid receptor activation and increased collagen deposition from dysregulation of matrix metaloproteinases [3]. In patients with eccentric LVH and HFrEF, an initial insult to the myocardium (infection, MI, toxin, hypertension) results in a decline in LV function. This decline activates the sympathetic nervous system (SNS) and the renin-angiotensin-aldosterone system (RAAS) that cause salt and water retention, vasoconstriction, increased afterload, and increased contractility of healthy myocardium. The compensatory mechanisms ultimately lead to deleterious LV remodeling with LVH, LV chamber dilation, and myocardial fibrosis. The remodeling results in reduced efficiency and further decline in LVH function [6] (Fig. 15.1).

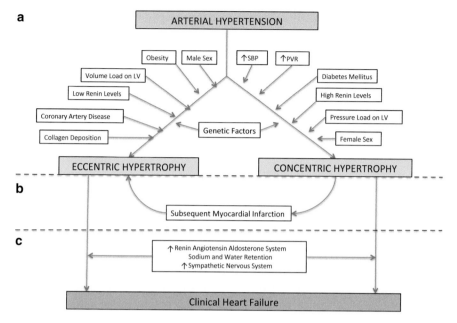

Fig. 15.1 Pathophysiology of hypertension and heart failure. Schematic of the progression from hypertension to LVH to the clinical syndrome of heart failure. (**a**) The exact mechanisms that determine LV geometry are unclear; however, there are a variety of factors that may play a role in the progression to eccentric or concentric hypertrophy. (**b**) While the transition from concentric to eccentric hypertrophy can occur, most commonly the transition requires an interceding ischemic event. C: The subsequent maladaptive neurohormonal responses result in progression from LVH to overt heart failure symptoms. *SBP* systolic blood pressure, *PVR* peripheral vascular resistance, *LV* left ventricle, *RAAS* renin angiotensin aldosterone system, *SNS* sympathetic nervous system, *LVH* left ventricular hypertrophy

Arterial hypertension is the most common risk factor present prior to the development of heart failure. In the Framingham Heart Study, the vast majority (90 %) of patients diagnosed with heart failure had antecedent hypertension [6]. The same risk was seen in patients with asymptomatic LV dysfunction with 65 % of patients having a prior history of hypertension [7]. In the original Framingham cohort, the presence of hypertension doubled the risk of developing clinical heart failure.

The silver-lining to these bleak statistics comes from data demonstrating that the treatment and control of hypertension reduces the risk of developing heart failure by 50 % [8, 9], reduce the incidence of LVH by EKG, and slows the progression from Stage A / B to Stage C heart failure [10, 11]. In the SHEP Trial [10], the treatment of HTN resulted in a 50 % reduction in the incidence of HF with even greater benefit (80 % reduction) seen in patients with a history of myocardial infarction (MI). While this benefit has been seen most dramatically in the elderly, modification of risk is of the utmost importance to reduce the incidence of heart failure in the entire population. The benefit of BP control is seen irrespective of the anti-hypertensive strategy used, with the exception of alpha-blockers. The treatment of HTN with diuretics, angiotensin-converting enzyme [ACE] inhibitors, angiotensin II receptor blockers [ARBs], diuretics, Calcium Chanel Blockers [CCBs], β-blockers all reduce the incidence of heart failure. However, current data demonstrates that ACEIs and ARBs are most effective at improving the detrimental LV remodeling and improving outcomes in patients with reduced LV function [12], followed by beta-blockers to a lesser extent.

The Basics of ABPM in Heart Failure

The application of ABPM to congestive heart failure has been limited to date, with much of the data having been gathered prior to the current era of guideline-directed medical therapy (GDMT). The data that has been published has focused mainly on describing the 24-h, nocturnal blood pressure and blood pressure variability in heart failure; there is almost no data regarding the management and outcomes of patients treated by ABPM. There remains little basic data comparing the variation in BP readings between office, ambulatory and home blood pressure monitoring in heart failure, or the prevalence of white coat hypertension and masked hypertension. These basic analyses are required to aid in the application of ABPM to heart failure. Guidelines for ABPM have established lower definitions for hypertension and treatment goals compared to office and home blood pressure measurements. To date, there has been no similar studies to define appropriate blood pressure levels in heart failure by ABPM. Some limited data has described the prognostic benefits of ABPM in evaluating heart failure patients. The studies are small and limited in scope. The potential advantages of ABPM compared to traditional office blood pressure monitoring in congestive heart failure include: identification of White Coat Hypertension, Masked hypertension, nocturnal hypertension, describing dipping profiles, evaluation of possible orthostatic hypotension, monitoring of heart failure medication effectiveness, and titration of GDMT. Some small studies have suggested that ABPM, specifically nocturnal blood pressures, may be superior to office blood pressure measurements in predicting hospitalization for heart failure; large scale studies are needed to confirm these findings [13].

As with many chronic diseases, early identification and prevention are keys to reducing the incidence and decreasing the negative impact of the disease on society. The use of ABPM to assess patients at risk for heart failure may identify individuals that could potentially benefit from intensified therapy and life-style modifications to reduce their risk. ABPM correlates more strongly with LVH than office BP measurements [14] and has been inversely related to diastolic dysfunction [15]. LV afterload pressures, which can be detected during ambulatory blood pressure readings, may play a significant role in the development of LV dysfunction. 24-h ambulatory blood pressures have been strongly correlated to early left ventricular filling parameters [16], which can identify patients that may benefit from tighter blood pressure control and afterload reduction. In fact, the reduction in average BP recorded by ABPM has been shown to correlate with regression of LVH [17], demonstrating that early intervention may decrease the risk for developing heart failure. However, the limitation of much of this data is that long-term evaluation of heart failure outcomes has not been studied. While data has shown that ABPM may help identify patients with greater risk and that treatment has decreased surrogate markers (structural abnormalities) that may be precursors to heart failure, there are no studies that have shown a direct correlation between treatment and outcomes based on ABPM. While the use of GDMT has demonstrated significant benefit in the progression of heart failure and development of heart failure in patients at risk, the application of ABPM may provide further insight into therapeutic strategies and targets in the future.

One of the earliest signs of progression of heart failure is hypotension and the inability to tolerate GDMT. The need to withdraw or reduce heart failure medications portends poor prognosis in patients. In several small clinical trials, patients with higher blood pressure [18] had better outcomes and patients with NYHA Class IV heart failure with higher mean 24-h, awake and sleeping blood pressures had better prognosis compared to those with lower blood pressures [19]. Furthermore many heart failure symptoms, fatigue, dizziness, lightheadedness, and decreased exercise tolerance, can also be symptoms of hypotension. The presence of persistent or prolonged periods of hypotension, which may result from heart failure therapies, may predispose patients to increased risk of target organ dysfunction. The combination of low cardiac output and significant hypotension may increase the risk of renal dysfunction, pre-syncope, syncope, and altered mental status. The application of ABPM could possibly aid in determining optimal dosing and timing of GDMT to reduce potential side-effects and maintain optimal therapies. Currently, there remains a paucity of large randomized data, demonstrating the potential benefits of utilizing ABPM to optimize treatment in heart failure.

Circadian Variation in Heart Failure

The importance of circadian variations in blood pressure was first described almost four decades ago and the literature supporting prognostic impact of ABPM in cardiovascular disease continues to grow. In healthy subjects, BP is highest in the early morning hours and declines to its lowest levels at night. Normal circadian rhythms are dictated by various mechanisms including the sympathetic nervous system, postural position, baroreflexes, physical activity, tobacco use, sodium intake, alcohol use, and neurohormones. Over the ensuing decades, the superiority of circadian blood pressures, specifically nocturnal BPs, has been repeatedly demonstrated for cardiovascular outcomes in many disease states including hypertension, diabetes, stroke, and kidney disease.

The two most influential circadian patterns for cardiovascular disease are early morning surge BP and the nocturnal dipping profile. As with the majority of ABPM

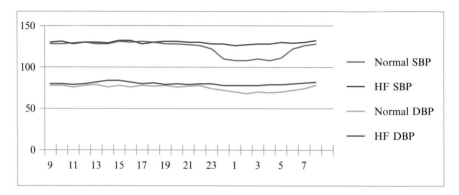

Fig. 15.2 24-h Blood pressure curve in normal controls compared to heart Failure. An illustration of the blunted circadian variation in both systolic and diastolic blood pressure in patients with Heart Failure compared to normotensive controls. *SBP* systolic blood pressure, *DBP* diastolic blood pressure, *HF* heart failure

data, there is a relative paucity of information regarding the risk and benefits of ambulatory circadian variation in heart failure, and much of the data that exists were obtained prior to the current era of GDMT. Current guidelines do not discuss the potential role of circadian variation in heart failure management [20].

Early studies that assessed the circadian variation in heart failure have demonstrated a correlation between circadian BP and left ventricular dysfunction; however, the risk or outcomes attributed to ambulatory readings were not assessed [21]. The current literature suggests that heart failure patients have depressed circadian variation compared to normal controls (Fig. 15.2). In heart failure up-regulated neurohormones, increased sympathetic activity, salt and water retention, and impaired baroreceptors may impact the normal circadian rhythm. Heart failure pharmacologic therapies that modulate the neurohormonal milieu, such as beta-blockers and ACEI, may also play a role in the altered circadian rhythms. The findings regarding average 24-h blood pressure in heart failure patients have been conflicted, which impacts the assessment of ambulatory circadian variation. Several small studies have demonstrated different average daytime blood pressures ranging from 108/72 mmHg [19] to 131/77 mmHg [22]. The data obtained by Borne et al. [21] demonstrated even lower ambulatory daytime and nocturnal blood pressures in NYHA Class III-IV patients. These conflicting data highlight the need for large studies to assess the circadian blood pressure patterns in the heart failure population, especially in the current era of GDMT. The effects of neurohormonal activity, LV function, gender, etiology of cardiomyopathy, functional class, and medication need to be better understood to appropriately apply ABPM data in heart failure. While much is still poorly understood, some data exists as a starting point, demonstrating that neurohormonal activity was indirectly related to circadian variations while ventricular function was directly associated with greater variability [22]. Furthermore, the severity of HF has been linked to decreased circadian variation, as heart failure progresses the degree of circadian variation in BP also declines.

Dipping Profile in Heart Failure

In healthy controls, the normal circadian pattern is one of nocturnal dipping or a decline in BP from ambulatory daytime BPs. Typically, this decline is approximately 20 % compared with awake readings; however, the general consensus is that a decline or a "dip" of <10 % from day to night BP readings is considered abnormal and is associated with poor CV outcomes [20]. Current literature classifies patients based on their nocturnal dipping profile: (1) Dippers, a normal decline in BP from day to night, (2) Non-Dippers, a 0–10 % decline in nocturnal BP, (3) Extreme dippers, those with >20 % decline in BP, and (4) Risers, an increase in nighttime BP from daytime readings. Dippers and extreme dippers have the lowest cardiovascular risk, while non-dippers and risers have the highest, incrementally.

While these definitions have been applied to heart failure patients, there is no consensus on what constitutes a normal dipping profile in heart failure. In a large cohort of NYHA Class II–III heart failure patients, the majority had an abnormal dipping profile using the standard definitions. In the same cohort, the presence of an abnormal dipping profile was an independent predictor HF outcomes. Non-dippers and risers had a 1.6 and 2.7 times increased risk of death or hospitalization compared to dippers, respectively [13]. Interestingly, in this cohort the majority of patients were on GDMT, which included metoprolol as a beta-blocker. If up-regulation of the sympathetic nervous system indeed plays a role in the altered circadian rhythm in heart failure, the use of alpha-adrenergic blockade along with beta-blockade (such as carvedilol) may help to normalize the dipping profile in these patients. There is, however, no data demonstrating benefit in restoration of a normal dipping pattern in HF. In fact, there is some data that suggests a normal dipping profile may be detrimental in heart failure. Canesin MF et al. [19] studied the effect of dipping profile on survival in 38 NYHA Class IV HF patients. Patients who had ≤6 mmHg decline in mean nighttime BP or nocturnal systolic BP had better prognosis at 6 months. More importantly, patients with a sleep SBP <105 mmHg were almost eight times more likely to die. While these findings cannot be extrapolated to patients with less severe heart failure (NYHA Class I–III), they do raise considerable questions regarding the normal dipping profile in HF patients. Large-scale assessment of dipping profiles in HF patients with varying severity is required. Establishing values to define dippers and non-dippers in HF is essential; it is possible that a dip of <10 % is beneficial in HF. Establishing these definitions are important in ultimately determining if pharmacotherapy can be used to normalize the dipping profile and improve outcome. Chronotherapy may play a significant role in the future of heart failure management. The administration of ACEI at bedtime has been shown to normalize dipping profiles in refractory hypertensives, and while it has become widely accepted to dose ACEI twice daily in heart failure therapy, adjusting the dosing between morning and evening doses may provide further benefit in the dipping profile in this population.

Morning Surge BP and Heart Failure

After a normal decline in blood pressure during the quiescence of sleep, a physiologic increase in BP upon wakening should occur. The physiologic increase in neurohormones, cortisol, and heart rate are likely triggers for the increase in BP. An increase in cardiovascular events, including stroke and MI, has been associated with this rise in morning blood pressure. Morning surge BP is an exaggerated rise in morning blood pressures to levels significantly higher than mean daytime values and may add incremental risk beyond the normal morning rise. There is limited recommendation on the application of morning surge BP in clinical practice.

The prevalence and degree of morning surge BP is undefined in heart failure. The use of GDMT that inhibit the SNS and regulate neurohormonal activity may blunt the morning rise; however, the altered baroreceptor reflex and chronic adrenergic up-regulation may result in significantly higher morning BP elevations.

In a sub-study of the PRAISE trial [23], the authors evaluated the timing of sudden cardiac death (SCD) in NYHA Class III–IV patients. The analysis of the data revealed a non-uniform distribution of SCD with a peak occurring in the evening not in the early morning. The evening peak was seen only in those with an ischemic etiology. The data suggests that the chronically elevated neurohormones resulted in a more uniform distribution. The study did not assess for heart failure admissions or cardiovascular mortality. The presence of an early morning surge may suggest suboptimal neurohormonal blockade and the spike in catecholamines may result in more rapid progression of heart failure.

Studies evaluating the impact of early morning BP surge on heart failure outcomes and long-term progression of the disease process may provide important clinical information and offer a potential target for future therapies. Chronotherapy aimed at reducing the morning surge may prove beneficial in the management of chronic heart failure.

White Coat Hypertension and White Coat Effect

White coat hypertension (WCH) is the presence of elevated BPs during contact with medical professionals, with otherwise normotensive BPs on ABPM in patients not currently on anti-hypertensive therapies. While it remains controversial, the general consensus is that white coat hypertension places patients at increased cardiovascular risk compared to the general population. Given that the majority of heart failure patients, including Stage A HF, are likely to be on some anti-hypertensive therapy, establishing guidelines for WCH in heart failure may be limited. However, in the rare patient with risk factors not actively on therapy, the presence of WHC may prompt closer monitoring of blood pressure and reemphasis on the importance of life-style modifications for preventing progression of the disease. Current data do not support treating WCH with pharmacologic therapies.

White coat effect (WCE) is the presence of higher BPs during clinic visits with lower, although still elevated, BPs on ambulatory readings in patients on therapy. Current consensus is that WCE >20 mmHg systolic and >10 mmHg diastolic are clinically relevant [20]. To the authors knowledge, there is no evidence demonstrating the presence of WCE in heart failure patients, nor demonstrating any increased risk from its presence. The lack of evidence highlights the gaps in knowledge regarding ABPM and HF. The importance of identifying patients with WCE would be to prevent unnecessary titration of medications, which may place patients at increased risk for adverse events. Patients identified to have WCE may require closer monitoring of BPs with more frequent home BP monitoring or repeat ABPM. In the treatment of Stage C heart failure, current guidelines recommend titrating GDMT to maximum tolerated doses, which should be performed regardless of the presence or absence of WCE. Therefore, defining WCE may be of limited benefit in these patients.

Masked Hypertension

Masked hypertension (MH) is traditionally defined as having normal office blood pressure (<140/90 mmHg) in the presence of elevated daytime ambulatory BPs (>135/85 mmHg) [20]. While current hypertension guidelines have recommended values for the diagnosis of MH in the general population, there are no data specifically in heart failure patients. Patients with heart failure, diabetes, LVH, obesity, and other comorbid conditions are more likely to have MH; the exact prevalence of MH in the heart failure population requires defining.

This definition is traditionally applied to those not currently receiving therapy, as HTN clearly cannot be defined as "masked" if indeed it is being treated. However, in the heart failure population using the term "masked" hypertension, or some derivation thereof, may play an important role. If patients with Stage A or B heart failure only have blood pressure readings in the office, the presence of elevated ambulatory BPs may result in undertreatment of an important risk factor for the progression of the disease. The use of ambulatory monitoring may identify those patients who would benefit from intensified pharmacologic and life-style therapies. In patients with Stage C HF, the guidelines clearly recommend forced titration of GDMT to maximum tolerable doses [2]; however, clinicians may not be comfortable pushing the doses of many of the medications if office BP readings are controlled. Elevated daytime ambulatory BPs in the presence of controlled office readings would reassure the clinician that continued dose titration will be tolerated and repeated ABPM could demonstrate appropriate response to the therapies. Without data demonstrating the presence of "masked" hypertension or the benefit of treatment on heart failure outcomes, recommendations cannot be made. Future investigations should establish the prevalence of MH, the incremental risk associated with MH, and determine if normalization of ABPM readings in the presence of lower office BPs would confer benefit.

Ambulatory Hypotension

ABPM can provide important information regarding the presence of daytime ambulatory hypotension. While short/intermittent episodes of hypotension or orthostatic changes may not be captured during ambulatory monitoring, the identification of patients with prolonged periods of hypotension is possible. Heart failure is common in the elderly who are at risk for hypotension due to baroreceptor and autonomic dysfunction. The symptoms of hypotension, lightheadedness or presyncope from decreased cerebral perfusion and decreased exercise tolerance, may also be symptoms of worsening heart failure. Identification of patients with ambulatory hypotension could aid in the titration of GDMT and prevent target organ dysfunction.

Postprandial hypotension is the decline in systolic blood pressure within 90 min of ingesting a meal. The current literature does not specify a clear clinical definition of Postprandial hypotension, yet in certain populations it is more common than orthostatic hypotension. It has been associated with syncope, falls and cardiovascular events. Postprandial hypotension is common in the elderly, with one study demonstrating it in nearly 70 % of a geriatric population [24]; its prevalence in the heart failure population in unclear. In healthy subjects, cardiac output can increase by as much as 20 % after a meal; in patients with impaired ventricular function and reduced cardiac reserve, cardiac output may not be able to increase sufficiently. Typically, in heart failure this manifests as early satiety and decreased appetite; however, it may also result in postprandial hypotension. The prevalence and effect of postprandial hypotension should be evaluated in the heart failure population. Recommendations such as smaller more frequent meals may reduce the incidence and decrease the risk of adverse events.

GDMT may precipitate prolonged periods of hypotension which may not be recognized in the clinic depending on timing of the medications. Many patients take all of their medications in the morning and the onset of action of multiple anti-hypertensive medications may result in periods of hypotension. If discovered during ambulatory monitoring, the clinician could adjust the timing of medications to avoid unnecessary periods of low blood pressure while maintaining appropriate GDMT. Volume depletion from diuretic therapies could also increase the risk of ambulatory hypotension, which could prompt adjustment of the timing or dose of diuretic therapies. Little data exist regarding ambulatory hypotension in the heart failure population and studies should focus on defining the prevalence and risk associated with daytime hypotension.

Hypertension and Ischemic Heart Disease

Ischemic Heart Disease: Morbidity and Mortality

Ischemic heart disease (IHD) remains one of the most common chronic fatal illnesses with death rates of nearly 530,000 per year in United States of America [25]. According to National Hospital Ambulatory Medical care Survey, about 11,883,000 people visited a physician's office for ischemic heart disease in the US 2001. IHD is an all-too-common initial step on a pathway that leads to various detrimental cardiovascular outcomes that negatively impact both the longevity and quality of life. IHD, or coronary artery disease (CAD), is a condition which results from atherosclerosis and resultant plaque build-up in the coronary arteries. This plaque narrows the arteries with time and reduces coronary blood flow which presents as chest pain, resulting from myocardial ischemia. Eventually, an area of plaque can rupture causing thrombosis formation which itself can block local coronary blood flow or can dislodge to distant coronary artery resulting in embolic obstruction, with resultant myocardial infarction.

Risk Factors of IHD

There are several modifiable and some non-modifiable risk factors that predispose to the development of ischemic heart disease. Important risk factors include, but are not limited to, age, serum cholesterol, hypertension, tobacco use, sedentary lifestyle, diabetes mellitus, stress, obesity, family history, left ventricular hypertrophy, and various genetic factors [26–29]. These predisposing factors are advantageous in identifying people who are at increased risk of ischemic heart disease and who should be targeted for specific life-style and pharmacologic interventions aimed at prevention and treatment to reduce the incidence of IHD. The non-modifiable risk factors are age, gender, and family history of IHD. Among many, one of the most well-documented and important modifiable risk factors is arterial hypertension [30]. There are several epidemiological studies that have documented the strong correlation between hypertension and ischemic heart disease [31–33].

Impact of Hypertension

Hypertension is one of the most common causes of premature death worldwide and the problem continues to grow; in 2025, an estimated 1.56 billion adults will be living with hypertension [34]. The trend towards increasing obesity, sedentary lifestyles, and an aging population contribute to the increased incidence of arterial hypertension. The overall prevalence of hypertension is similar in women and men based on recent NHANES data, though the prevalence varies by age [35]. Over 65 million Americans age 20 or older have hypertension, which translates into one in every three adults [36]. The prevalence of hypertension also varies with ethnicity and is several fold higher in the African American population [37]. In recently published US population data, the prevalence of hypertension after age 60 years is 60 % in Caucasians and 70 % in African Americans. According to the Framingham study on risk stratification, hypertension was the most significant risk factor leading to 40 % of coronary events in men and 68 % in women [38]. The relationship between hypertension and risk of cardiovascular events is continuous, consistent, and independent of other risk factors [46]. The higher the blood pressure, the greater the chance of ischemic heart disease, heart failure, and stroke. High blood pressure was a primary or contributing cause of death for more than 360,000 Americans in 2013—which is nearly 1000 deaths each day [36]. Of greater concern is the overall poor awareness and control of hypertension; recent data from a large multinational study consisting of 142,042 participants demonstrated that 46.5 % of the participants with hypertension were aware of the diagnosis, but only 32.5 % of those were being treated [39]. In U.S. only, about half (52 %) of people with high blood pressure have their condition under control [40]. These findings suggest substantial room for improvement in hypertension diagnosis and treatment. Hypertension, often referred to as the "silent killer," results in progressive and unrecognized vascular damage increasing the risk of cardiovascular morbidity and mortality. Consistent and regular monitoring of blood pressure in patients with risk factors for CV disease allows for early identification of patients who may benefit from lifestyle modification and pharmacologic therapy that may prevent the development of chronic morbidity and mortality.

Correlation of IHD with Systolic and Diastolic Blood Pressures

Population-based observational data has consistently demonstrated a strong correlation between increased systolic blood pressure (SBP) and diastolic blood pressure (DBP) with ischemic heart disease [41, 42]. Data from the Framingham Heart Study [43] supported by more recent data [44, 45] indicates that SBP increases continuously across all age groups, whereas DBP increases until age 60 years and then begins to decrease steadily. We know that coronary arteries are perfused predominantly during diastole and significant variations in DBP affect coronary circulation directly. During systole, the contracting LV myocardium compresses intramyocardial vessels and obstructs its own blood flow. There is sufficient data demonstrating a J-curve relationship between IHD and mortality when DBP was either too high or too low [46]. This simply extrapolates to an increased mortality from myocardial infarctions in patient on either side of range of optimum DBP [47]. As the prevalence of hypertension increases with age, adequate control of both SBP and pulse pressure rather than DBP in the elderly has become the dominant public health imperative. A large study including 902 patients with moderate to severe HTN reported the nadir of the J-Curve in DBP to be 85–90 mmHg, while no such J-curve relationship has been found between SBP and IHD; the risk of IHD increases steeply with increasing SBP [47]. In the Chicago Heart Association Detection Project in Industry, men 18 to 39 years of age at baseline with a BP of 130–139/85–89 mmHg or with stage 1 hypertension (SBP 140–159/ 90=99 mmHg) accounted for nearly 60 % of all excess IHD, overall cardiovascular disease, or all-cause mortality [33]. Effective control of both systolic and diastolic blood pressure with the use of life-style modification and antihypertensive therapies has resulted in major reductions in cardiovascular morbidity and mortality over the past 50 years [48].

Randomized trials have shown that lowering BP results in rapid reductions in cardiovascular risks [49]. As an illustration, a 10-mmHg–lower usual SBP (or a 5-mmHg–lower usual DBP) would predict a 50–60 % lower risk of fatal stroke and an approximately 40–50 % lower risk of death due to ischemic heart disease or other vascular causes at middle age [50].

Pathophysiology of IHD: Role of Hypertension

Pathophysiology relating to the development of ischemic heart disease in hypertension involves increased myocardial oxygen demand and decreased coronary blood flow. When SBP is elevated, there is an increase in both LV output impedance and intra-myocardial wall tension, which increases LV pressure load and cardiac work—leading to LV hypertrophy (Fig. 15.3). Arterial hypertension exerts strain on the

Fig. 15.3 The pathophysiology of hypertension induced ischemic heart disease

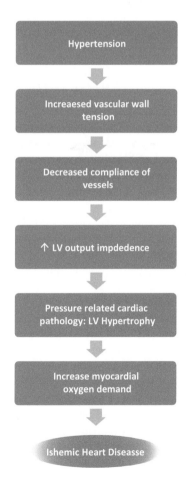

arterial wall leading to fragmentation, thinning, and fracture of elastin fibers, as well as increased collagen deposition in arteries, which results in decreased compliance of these vessels and overtime development of atherosclerosis [51, 52]. Atherosclerosis leads to diminished coronary blood flow or, at least, a diminished coronary flow reserve. In addition to these structural abnormalities, endothelial dysfunction, which develops over time as a consequence of both aging and hypertension, contributes functionally to increased rigidity of arterial wall [53]. Many of the mechanisms of the initiation and maintenance of hypertension are also those that mediate damage to target organs, including the coronary vessels and the myocardium. These mechanisms include increased sympathetic nervous system and renin-angiotensin-aldosterone system (RAAS) activity; deficiencies in release and/or activity of vasodilators, for example, nitric oxide, prostacyclin, and the natriuretic peptides; structural and functional abnormalities in conductance and resistance arteries, particularly endothelial dysfunction; and increased expression of growth factors and inflammatory cytokines in the arterial tree [54]. All of these factors either increase myocardial demand or decrease oxygen supply to myocardium, leading to chronic stable angina at one end of the spectrum and acute myocardial infarction at the other end depending on the time lapse for which myocardium is deprived of oxygen.

Role of ABPM in IHD

The identification and management of hypertension is of prime importance for both primary as well as the secondary prevention of IHD. As such, the accurate measurement of blood pressure is of paramount importance for determination of overall 24-h control, efficacy of therapies, and the identification of those at increased risk of IHD [55–57]. Various errors in measurement of office blood pressure have been reported including errors due to manometer, cuff size, observer's error, or even errors due to the patient [55]. Studies that have compared office, self-measured, and ambulatory blood pressures have documented substantial, but nonsystematic, differences between these measurements [55]. Over the last 50 years, it has become increasingly recognized that isolated clinic blood pressure measurements may not be adequately representative of the daily blood pressure load away from the medical environment [56]. Ambulatory blood pressure monitoring (ABPM) has evolved as one of the most reliable noninvasive assessment of a person's average blood pressure (BP) in modern era [57]. Because ABPM provides large numbers of measurements, researchers have sought to analyze data beyond just the average of BP values during 24 h or even over more restricted periods such as the day, night, or morning. Discrepancies between office and out-of-office blood pressure have resulted in the description of four clinically important blood pressure profiles: normotension, sustained hypertension, white coat hypertension, and masked hypertension.

There is growing evidence to suggest that target-organ-damage is more closely associated with 24-h ABPM than with office blood pressure, especially in the

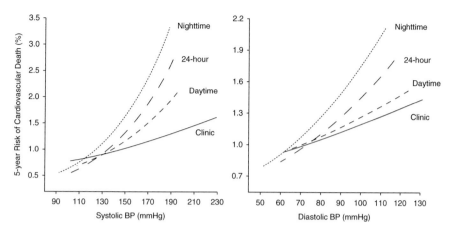

Fig. 15.4 Risk of cardiovascular mortality: comparison of clinic and ambulatory blood pressure. Adjusted 5-year risk of cardiovascular death in the study cohort of 5292 patients for CBPM and ABPM. Using multiple Cox regression, the relative risk was calculated with adjustment for baseline characteristics including gender, age, presence of diabetes mellitus, history of cardiovascular events, and smoking status. The 5-year risks are expressed as number of deaths per 100 subjects *From Dolan E. et al. Superiority of Ambulatory Over Clinic Blood Pressure Measurements in Predicting Mortality. The Dublin Outcome Study. Hypertension. 2005;46:156–161*

prediction of IHD [58–60] (Fig. 15.4). Various studies have pointed out that not only mean ambulatory blood pressure levels but also degree of blood pressure variability, or circadian variations, may have an independent and significant relationship with IHD [61]. Multiple components of the ABPM have been shown to be involved in the complex interplay of IHD, including BP increases induced by stress at work [62], rate of BP rise during early morning [63, 64], Daytime BP variations [65], Night time BP fall (dipping) [66, 67], or no change (non-dipping) [68].

Circadian BP Variations in Sustained Hypertension and IHD

ABPM has shown that the circadian BP is variable and not uniform in patients with hypertension. Blood pressure values tend to peak during the daytime hours and then fall to a nadir after midnight. BP normally decreases ("dips") during sleep, and people whose BP dips ≤10 % from their daytime baseline BP have been referred to as "nondippers." Nighttime blood pressure (BP) dipping can further be quantified as the ratio of mean nighttime (sleep) BP to mean daytime (awake) BP. During last decade, four dipping categories have been described, based on the night–day blood pressure ratio from 24-h ambulatory blood pressure recordings: extreme dippers (night–day blood pressure ratio < or=0.8), dippers (0.8 < ratio < or=0.9), nondippers (0.9 < ratio < or=1.0), and reverse dippers (ratio > 1.0).

Early Morning BP Surge and IHD

In the early morning hours with awakening and resuming activities, blood pressure rises sharply, with daytime levels being reached within a relatively short period. The circadian pattern of numerous cardiovascular events (myocardial infarction, sudden cardiac death, stroke) reveals a peak in the early hours of the morning, which may well be explained by early morning higher BP. This circadian rhythm BP peaking in the morning has also been shown to trigger so-called silent myocardial ischemia, which occurs in more than 20 % of patients with arterial hypertension and can only be regularly detected by ABPM [69].

Nocturnal Dipping and IHD

It has been observed that degree of nocturnal dipping, which also contributes to the magnitude of overall 24-h blood pressure variability, is inversely related to severity of end organ damage of hypertension especially IHD. In patients with hypertension, non-dipping is associated with target organ damage and higher cardiovascular events independent of the overall BP [70]. Non-dipping may be a risk factor for cardiovascular disease even when the 24-h BP average is not elevated. In a small study of men with angiographically proven coronary artery disease, 72 % exhibited a non-dipping BP pattern compared with 46 % of matched controls without known coronary artery disease [71]. Another study showed that levels of von Willebrand factor, D-dimer, fibrinogen, and P-selectin were significantly higher among patients with documented coronary artery disease who were non-dippers [72]. This clearly extrapolates that high ABP or non-dipping pattern of circadian BP per se is an important pathophysiologic factor that may influence cardiovascular risk by altering hemostasis or endothelial function [56] as discussed earlier in Fig. 15.1. Furthermore, non-dippers experience a greater "BP load" over 24 h than dippers with the same daytime BP and, hence, may be more likely to develop target organ damage in the form of IHD.

White Coat Hypertension and IHD

White coat hypertension is a phenomenon in which patients exhibit elevated blood pressure in a clinical setting. It is believed that this is due to the anxiety and stress some people experience during a clinic visit [73]. The diagnosis of white coat hypertension (also called isolated clinic or office hypertension) is applied to patients with office readings that average more than 140/90 mmHg and reliable out-of-office readings that average less than 140/90 mmHg. The effect of isolated white coat hypertension on cardiovascular risk has been controversial. White coat hypertension is found to be associated with more advanced cardiovascular target organ damage as compared to people who are normotensive [74], but certain studies have denied this association [75]. The effect of isolated white coat hypertension on cardiovascular risk still needs further investigation to determine the necessity of treating it with anti-hypertensives. Therefore, patients with white coat hypertension should be identified to prevent unnecessary medication implementation. One of the most important indications for ABPM is to exclude white coat hypertension [76] as the use of ABPM has added a new source of information about out-of-office blood pressure to end the debate and conflicting ideas which revolve around whether or not it would be feasible to treat white coat hypertension [77].

Masked Hypertension and IHD

Over the last decade, masked hypertension (MH) has gained interest in its relation to increase risk of ischemic heart disease. According to international guidelines, MH is defined as elevated daytime ambulatory BP (at least 135 or at least 85 mmHg) in the face of normal office BP (less than 140 and less than 90 mmHg) [78]. It is believed that clinical blood pressure of the patient with masked hypertension would underestimate the risk of cardiovascular disease [79]. Studies have reported that associations between MH and cardiovascular diseases are as strong as those found for sustained hypertension [80]. MH has also been hypothesized to be a transient status which progresses to sustained (and detectable) hypertension when a sufficient time lapse has occurred [80]. A recent study showed that out of all the patients seen in hypertensive clinic, about one third of those had masked hypertension, and over a 5-year follow-up period, their relative risk of cardiovascular events was 2.28 as compared with the patients whose blood pressure was adequately controlled [81]. ABPM provides a useful tool to identify patients with MH whose office BP measurement systematically fail to identify them and who should be treated as hypertensive to avoid progression to develop IHD [82].

Role of ABPM in Anti-Hypertensive Drug Therapy

IHD can be prevented or reversed when aggressive targets are achieved for major cardiovascular disease risk factors [31]. The distinction between primary and secondary prevention is arbitrary, because the major therapeutic objective in any individual is to delay or reverse the underlying atherosclerotic disease process of which hypertension is a major contributor. Furthermore, existing therapies are the same for both primary or secondary cardiac protection. The effectiveness of any therapy is judged by the degree of reduction in the surrogate BP and the ability of the chosen regimen to reduce ischemic events [83].

As mentioned above, several studies have persistently shown an association between nocturnal BP decline (non-dipper BP pattern) and escalating incidence of fatal and nonfatal CVD events. These findings documenting the risk of CVD events are influenced not only by ambulatory BP elevation, but also by blunted nocturnal BP decline, even within the normotensive range, thereby supporting ABPM as a necessity for appropriate and opportune assessment of CVD risk in the general population. However, myocardial ischemic events are less frequent during the night than they are during the day; nevertheless studies suggest that there is increased frequency of cardiovascular ischemic events in hypertensive patients with nocturnal blood pressure variation [84]. And these were especially true for non-dippers, probably because persistently raised BP during the night favored myocardial ischemia by increasing oxygen demand.

Keeping in mind these variations, it may be beneficial to implement chronotherapy as a method of adjusting treatment accordingly based on blood pressure variability and dipping-profile. Though currently little data supports improved outcomes by utilizing chronotherapy based on dipping profile, it remains possible that non-dippers may benefit from a subtly different dosing regimen compared to extreme-dippers and that adjusting the timing of medications could reduce the risk of CV events. In one study that assessed BP control between a once-daily evening dose in comparison with a single morning dose, ingestion of angiotensin receptor blockers and angiotensin-converting enzyme inhibitors results in greater therapeutic effect on asleep BP, without impacting overall 24-h control, independently of the terminal half-life of each individual medication [85]. Thus, the impact of hypertension treatment-time on sleep-time BP regulation might be clinically relevant. The previously reported results of the randomized part of the MAPEC study indicate that treatment with one medication at bedtime was significantly associated with greater asleep BP reduction and significantly lower CVD risk than treatment with all hypertension medications upon awakening [86].

ABPM: A Useful Tool for Both Primary and Secondary Prevention of IHD

In nutshell, ABPM is extremely beneficial in enabling the clinician to monitor multiple aspects of the blood pressure profile, including 24-h average BP, circadian variation, early morning surge and dipping profile, and in patients with hypertension and aids assessing the risk of IHD and even ACS. Furthermore, ambulatory blood pressure monitoring allows the clinician to assess the response to anti-hypertensive medication and possibly suggesting a benefit of chronotherapy such as switching to an evening dose of ACEI to improve dipping profile or adding an additional agent that will prevent early morning surge of BP. Lack of adequate BP control is a major clinical issue which predicts a high risk of future cardiovascular events; therefore, ABPM is a helpful tool in keeping record and analyzing the changes in blood pressure throughout 24-h and adjusting the doses of anti-hypertensive agents accordingly, thereby enabling more effective control of arterial hypertension.

References

1. Lloyd-Jones DM, Larson MG, Leip EP, et al. Lifetime risk for developing congestive heart failure—The Framingham Heart study. Circulation. 2002;106:3068–72.
2. Yancy CW, Jessup M, Bozkurt B, et al. ACCF/AHA guideline for the management of heart failure. J Am Coll Cardiol. 2013;62(16):e147–239.
3. Drazner MH. The progression of hypertensive heart disease. Circulation. 2011;123:327–34.
4. Ganau A, Devereux RB, Roman MJ, et al. Patterns of left ventricular hypertrophy ad geometric remodeling in essential hypertension. J Am Coll Cardiol. 1992;19:1550–8.
5. Davila DF, Donis JH, Oderman R, Gonzalez M, Landaeta A. Patterns of left ventricular hypertrophy in essential hypertension: should echocardiography guide the pharmacological treatment? Int J Cardiol. 2008;124:134–8.
6. Goldberg LR, Jessup M. Stage B Heart Failure Management of asymptomatic left ventricular systolic dysfunction. Circulation. 2006;113:2851–60.
7. Wang TJ, Levy D, Benjamin EJ, Vasan RS. The epidemiology of "asymptomatic" left ventricular systolic dysfunction: implications for screening. Ann Intern Med. 2003;138:907–16.
8. Sciarretta S, Palano F, Tocci G, Baldini R, Volpe M. Antihypertensive treatment and development of heart failure in hypertension: a Bayesian network meta-analysis of studies in patients with hypertension and high cardiovascular risk. Arch Intern Med. 2011;171(5):384–94.
9. Baker DW. Prevention of heart failure. J Card Fail. 2002;8:333–46.
10. Kostis JB, Davis BR, Cutler J, et al. Prevention of heart failure by antihypertensive drug treatment in older persons with isolated systolic hypertension. SHEP Cooperative Research Group. JAMA. 1997;278(3):212–6.
11. Yusuf S, Sleight P, Pogue J, et al. Effects of an angiotensin-converting-enzyme inhibitor, Ramipril, on cardiovascular events in high risk patients: the heart outcomes prevention evaluation study investigators. N Engl J Med. 2000;342:145–53.
12. The SOLVD Investigators. Effect of enalapril on mortality and the development of heart failure in asymptomatic patients with reduced left ventricular ejection fractions. N Engl J Med. 1992;327:685–91.
13. Shin J, Kline S, Moore M, et al. Association of diurnal blood pressure pattern with risk for hospitalization or death in men with heart failure. J Card Fail. 2007;13(8):656–62.
14. Verdecchia P, Porcellati C, Schilliaci G, et al. Ambulatory Blood Pressure. An independent predictor of prognosis in essential hypertension. Hypertension. 1994;24(6):793–801.
15. White WB, Dey HM, Schulman P. Assessment of the daily blood pressure load as a determinant of cardiac function in patients with mild-moderate hypertension. Am Heart J. 1989;118(4):782–95.
16. Verdecchia P, Schillaci G, Guerrieri M, et al. Prevalence and determinants of left ventricular diastolic filling abnormalities in an unselected hypertensive population. Eur Heart J. 1990;11(8):679–91.
17. Mancia G, Zanchetti A, Agabiti-Rosei E, et al. Ambulatory blood pressure is superior to clinic blood pressure in predicting treatment induced regression of left ventricular hypertrophy. SAMPLE Study on Ambulatory Monitoring of Blood Pressure and Lisinopril Evaluation. Circulation. 1997;95(6):1464–70.
18. Mosterd A, Cost B, Hoes AW, et al. The prognosis of heart failure in the general population. The Rotterdam Study. Eur Heart J. 2001;15:1318–27.
19. Canesin MF, Giorgi D, Oliveira Jr MT, et al. Ambulatory blood pressure monitoring of patients with heart failure. A new prognostic marker. Arq Bras Cardiol. 2002;78(1):83–9.
20. O'Brien E, Parati G, Sterigou G, Asmar R, Beilin L, Bilo G, et al. European society of hypertension position paper on ambulatory blood pressure monitoring. J Hypertens. 2013;31:1731–68.
21. Borne P, van de Abramowicz M, Degre S, et al. Effects of chronic congestive heart failure on 24-hour blood pressure and heart rate patterns: a hemodynamic approach. Am Heart J. 1992;123:998–1004.

22. Giles TD, Roffidal L, Quiroz A, Sander G, Trenznewsky O. Circadian variation in blood pressure and heart rate in nonhypertensive congestive heart failure. J Cardiovasc Pharmacol. 1996;28(6):733–40.
23. Carson PA, O'Connor CM, Miller AB, et al. Circadian rhythm and sudden death in heart failure results from prospective randomized amlodipine survival trial. J Am Coll Cardiol. 2000;36:541–6.
24. Vloet LC, Pel-Littel RE, Jansen PA, Jansen RWMM. High prevalence of postprandial and orthostatic hypotension among geriatric patients admitted to Dutch hospitals. J Gerontol A Biol Sci Med Sci. 2005;60A:1271–7.
25. Wei R, Curtin LR, Arias E, Anderson RN. U.S. decennial life tables for 1999–2001: methodology of the United States Life Tables. Natl Vital Stat Rep. 2008;57(4):1–9.
26. Gordon T, Kannel WB. Multiple risk functions for predicting coronary heart disease: the concept, accuracy, and application. Am Heart J. 1982;103:1031–9.
27. Kannel WB, McGee DL. Diabetes and glucose tolerance as risk factors for cardiovascular disease: the Framingham Study. Diabetes Care. 1979;2:120–6.
28. Expert Panel on Detection, Evaluation, and Treatment of High Blood Cholesterol in Adults. Summary of the second report of the National Cholesterol Education Program (NCEP) expert panel on detection, evaluation, and treatment of high blood cholesterol in adults (Adult Treatment Panel II). JAMA. 1993;269:3015–23.
29. Anderson KM, Wilson PWF, Odell PM, Kannel WB. An updated coronary risk profile: a statement for health professionals. Circulation. 1991;83:356–62.
30. Yusuf S. Preventing vascular events due to elevated blood pressure. Circulation. 2006;113:2166–8.
31. Chobanian AV, Bakris GI, Black HR, Joint National Committee on Prevention, Detection, Evaluation, and Treatment of High Blood Pressure, National Heart, Lung, and Blood Institute, National High Blood Pressure Education Program Coordinating Committee, et al. Seventh report of the Joint National Committee on Prevention, detection, evaluation, and treatment of high blood pressure. Hypertension. 2003;42:1206–52.
32. Vasan RS, Beiser A, Seshadri S, et al. Residual lifetime risk for developing hypertension in middle-aged women and men: the Framingham Heart Study. JAMA. 2002;287:1003–10.
33. Miura K, Daviglus ML, Dyer AR, et al. Relationship of blood pressure to 25-year mortality due to coronary heart disease, cardiovascular diseases, and all causes in young adult men: the Chicago Heart Association Detection Project in Industry. Arch Intern Med. 2001;161:1501–8.
34. WHO Regional Office for South East Asia. Hypertension fact sheet. http://www.searo.who.int/linkfiles/non_communicable_diseases_hypertension-fs.pdf. Accessed 21 Mar 2012.
35. Mozaffarian D, Benjamin EJ, Go AS, et al. Heart disease and stroke statistics—2015 update: a report from the American Heart Association. Circulation. 2015;131(4):e29–322. doi:10.1161/CIR.0000000000000152. Epub 2014 Dec 17.
36. Nwankwo T, Yoon SS, Burt V, Gu Q. Hypertension among adults in the US: National Health and Nutrition Examination Survey, 2011-2012. NCHS Data Brief, No. 133. Hyattsville, MD: National Center for Health Statistics/Centers for Disease Control and Prevention/US Dept of Health and Human Services; 2013.
37. Javed F, Aziz EF, Sabharwal MS, et al. Association of BMI and cardiovascular risk stratification in the elderly African-American females. Obesity (Silver Spring). 2011;19(6):1182–6. doi:10.1038/oby.2010.307.
38. Franklin SS, Larson MG, Khan SA, et al. Does the relation of blood pressure to coronary heart disease risk change with aging? The Framingham Heart Study. Circulation. 2001;103:1245–9.
39. Chow CK, Teo KK, Rangarajan S, PURE (Prospective Urban Rural Epidemiology) Study investigators, et al. Prevalence, awareness, treatment, and control of hypertension in rural and urban communities in high-, middle-, and low-income countries. (Prospective Urban Rural Epidemiology) Study investigators. JAMA. 2013;310(9):959–68. doi:10.1001/jama.2013.184182.

40. Farley TA, Dalal MA, Mostashari F, Frieden TR. Deaths preventable in the U.S. by improvements in the use of clinical preventive services. Am J Prev Med. 2010;38(6):600–9.
41. Joint National Committee on the Detection, Evaluation, and Treatment of High Blood Pressure. The sixth report of the Joint National Committee on prevention, detection, evaluation, and treatment of high blood pressure. Arch Intern Med. 1997;157:2413–46.
42. Stamler J, Neaton JD, Wentworth DN. Blood pressure (systolic and diastolic) and risk of fatal coronary heart disease. Hypertension. 1989;13(suppl I):I-2–12.
43. Franklin SS, Gustin IV W, Wong ND, et al. Hemodynamic patterns of age-related changes in blood pressure: the Framingham Heart Study. Circulation. 1997;96:308–15.
44. Tate RB, Manfreda J, Krahn AD, Cuddy TE. Tracking of blood pressure over a 40-year period in the University of Manitoba Follow-up Study, 1948–1988. Am J Epidemiol. 1995;142: 946–54.
45. Lee ML, Rosner BA, Vokonas PS, Weiss ST. Longitudinal analysis of adult male blood pressure: the Normative Aging Study, 1963–1992. J Epidemiol Biostat. 1996;1:79–87.
46. Farnett L, Mulrow CD, Linn WD, Lucey CR, Tuley MR. The J-curve phenomenon and the treatment of hypertension. Is there a point beyond which pressure reduction is dangerous? JAMA. 1991;265:489–95.
47. Cruickshank JM, Thorp JM, Zacharias FJ. Benefits and potential harm of lowering high blood pressure. Lancet. 1987;1:581–4.
48. Rosendorff C, Black HR, Cannon CP, et al. Treatment of hypertension in the prevention and management of ischemic heart disease: a scientific statement from the American Heart Association Council for High Blood Pressure Research and the Councils on Clinical Cardiology and Epidemiology and Prevention. Circulation. 2007;115(21):2761–88. Epub 2007 May 14.
49. Neal B, MacMahon S, Chapman N, Blood Pressure Lowering Treatment Trialists' Collaboration. Effects of ACE inhibitors, calcium antagonists, and other blood-pressure-lowering drugs: results of prospectively designed overviews of randomized trials. Lancet. 2000;356:1955–64.
50. Lewington S, Clarke R, Qizilbash N, Peto R, Collins R, Prospective Studies Collaboration. Age-specific relevance of usual blood pressure tovascular mortality: a meta-analysis of individual data for one million adults in 61 prospective studies [published correction appears in Lancet. 2002;361:1060]. Lancet. 2002;360:1903–13.
51. Chobanian AV. Vascular effects of systemic hypertension. Am J Cardiol. 1992;69:3E–7.
52. Chobanian AV, Lichtenstein AH, Nilakhe V, Haudenschild CC, Drago R, Nickerson C. Influence of hypertension on aortic atherosclerosis in the Watanabe rabbit. Hypertension. 1989;14:203–9.
53. Todd ME. Hypertensive structural changes in blood vessels: do endothelial cells hold the key? Can J Physiol Pharmacol. 1992;70:536–51.
54. Opari S, Zaman MA, Calhoun DA. Pathogenesis of hypertension. Ann Intern Med. 2003;139:761–76.
55. James PA, Oparil S, Carter BL, et al. Evidence-Based Guideline for the Management of High Blood Pressure in Adults: report from the Panel Members Appointed to the Eighth Joint National Committee (JNC 8). JAMA. 2014;311(5):507–20.
56. Ayman D, Goldshine AD. Blood pressure determinations by patients with essential hypertension, I: the difference between clinic and home readings before treatment. Am J Med Sci. 1940;200:465–74.
57. Pickering TG, Shimbo D, Haas D. Ambulatory blood pressure monitoring. N Engl J Med. 2006;354:2368–74. PubMed: 16738273.
58. Perloff D, Sokolow M, Cowan R. The prognostic value of ambulatory blood pressures. JAMA. 1983;249(20):2792–8. doi:10.1001/jama.1983.03330440030027.
59. Hansen TW, Jeppesen J, Rasmussen S, Ibsen H, Torp-Pedersen C. Ambulatory blood pressure and mortality: a population based study. Hypertension. 2005;45:499–504.
60. Clement DL, De Buyzere ML, De Bacquer DA, et al. Prognostic value of ambulatory blood-pressure recordings in patients with treated hypertension. N Engl J Med. 2003;348:2407–15.

61. Mancia G, Parati G, Albini F, Villani A. Circadian blood pressure variations and their impact on disease. J Cardiovasc Pharmacol. 1988;12 suppl 7:S11–7.
62. Devereaux R, Pickering TG, Harshfield GA, et al. Left ventricular hypertrophy in patients with hypertension: importance of blood pressure response to regularly recurring stress. Circulation. 1983;68:470–6.
63. Khoury AF, Sunderajan P, Kaplan NM. The early morning rise in blood pressure is related mainly to ambulation. Am J Hypertens. 1992;5:339–44.
64. Rocco MB, Nadel EG, Selvyn AP. Circardian rhythms and coronary artery disease. Am J Cardiol. 1987;59:13C–7.
65. Verdecchia P, Gatteschi C, Benemi G, Bodrini F, Guerreri M, Porcellati C. Circadian blood pressure changes and left ventricular hypertrophy in essential hypertension. Circulation. 1990;81:528–36.
66. Verdecchia P, Schillaci G, Gatteschi C, et al. Blunted nocturnal fall in blood pressure in hypertensive women in future cardiovascular morbid events. Circulation. 1993;88:986–92.
67. Viera AJ, Lin FC, Hinderliter AL, et al. Nighttime blood pressure dipping in young adults and coronary artery calcium 10-15 years later: the coronary artery risk development in young adults study. Am J Hypertens. 2015;28(1):42–9.
68. O'Brien E, Sheridan J, O'Malley K. Dippers and non-dippers. Lancet. 1988;2:397.
69. Uen S, Un I, Fimmers R, Vetter H, Mengden T. Myocardial ischemia during everyday life in patients with arterial hypertension: prevalence, risk factors, triggering mechanism and circadian variability. Blood Press Monit. 2006;11(4):173–82.
70. Ohkubo T, Hozawa A, Yamaguchi J, et al. Prognostic significance of the nocturnal decline in blood pressure in individuals with and without high 24-h blood pressure: the Ohasama Study. J Hypertens. 2002;20:2183–9.
71. Mousa T, El-Sayed MA, Motawea AK, Salama MA, Elhendy A. Association of blunted nighttime blood pressure dipping with coronary artery stenosis in men. Am J Hypertens. 2004;17:977–80.
72. Lee KW, Blann AD, Lip GY. High pulse pressure and nondipping circardian blood pressure in patients with coronary artery disease: relationship to thrombogenesis and endothelial damage/dysfunction. Am J Hypertens. 2005;18:104–15.
73. Jhalani J, Goyal T, Clemow L, et al. Anxiety and outcome expectations predict the white-coat effect. Blood Press Monit. 2005;10(6):317–9.
74. Glen S, Elliott H, Curzio J, Lees K, Reid J. White-coat hypertension as a cause of cardiovascular dysfunction. Lancet. 1996;348(9028):654–7.
75. Pierdomenico SD, Cuccurullo F. Prognostic value of white-coat and masked hypertension diagnosed by ambulatory monitoring in initially untreated subjects: an updated meta analysis. Am J Hypertens. 2011;24(1):52–8.
76. O'Brien E, Asmar R, Beilin L, et al. European Society of Hypertension recommendations for conventional, ambulatory and home blood pressure measurement. J Hypertens. 2003; 21(5):821–48.
77. Pickering T. Blood pressure measurement and detection of hypertension. Lancet. 1994;344(8914):31–5.
78. O'Brien E, Asmar R, Beilin L, et al. Practice guidelines of the European Society of Hypertension for clinic, ambulatory and self blood pressure measurement. J Hypertens. 2005; 23(4):697–701.
79. Fagard RH, Cornelissen VA. Incidence of cardiovascular events in white-coat, masked and sustained hypertension versus true normotension: a meta-analysis. J Hypertens. 2007; 25(11):2193–8.
80. Mancia G, Bombelli M, Facchetti R, et al. Long-term risk of sustained hypertension in white-coat or masked hypertension. Hypertension. 2009;54(2):226–32.
81. Pierdomenico SD, Lapenna D, Bucci A, et al. Cardiovascular outcome in treated hypertensive patients with responder, masked, false resistant, and true resistant hypertension. Am J Hypertens. 2005;18:1422–8.

82. Verberk WJ, Thien T, de Leeuw PW. Masked hypertension, a review of the literature. Blood Press Monit. 2007;12(4):267–73.
83. Sytkowski PA, Kannel WB, D'Agostino RB. Changes in risk factors and the decline in mortality from cardiovascular disease: the Framingham Heart Study. N Engl J Med. 1990; 322:1635–41.
84. Pierdomenico SD, Bucci A, Costantini F, Lapenna D, Cuccurullo F, Mezzetti A. Circadian blood pressure changes and myocardial ischemia in hypertensive patients with coronary artery disease. J Am Coll Cardiol. 1998;31:1627–34.
85. Smolensky MH, Hermida RC, Ayala DE, Tiseo R, Portaluppi F. Administration-time-dependent effect of blood pressure-lowering medications: basis for the chronotherapy of hypertension. Blood Press Monit. 2010;15:173–80.
86. Hermida RC, Ayala DE, Mojón A, Fernández JR. Influence of circadian time of hypertension treatment on cardiovascular risk: results of the MAPEC study. Chronobiol Int. 2010; 27:1629–51.

Chapter 16
Ambulatory Blood Pressure Monitoring in Special Populations: Masked Hypertension

Anthony J. Viera

Introduction

The pairing of the average of blood pressure (BP) measurements derived from out-of-office BP monitoring with office BP measurements yields four possible diagnostic categories (Table 16.1). White coat hypertension refers to elevated office measurements with non-elevated out-of-office measurements and is familiar to most clinicians. The opposite phenomenon, "masked hypertension," is more recently described, and the best strategy for detecting and addressing it has not been established. This chapter will review the definition, prevalence, and outcomes associated with masked hypertension as well as possible diagnostic strategies.

Definition

The term "masked hypertension" refers to elevated average ambulatory BP coinciding with a non-elevated office BP [1]. The definition originally applied to people with the described BP measurements who were not taking antihypertensive therapy. However, patients on antihypertensive therapy may also exhibit the same BP measurement pattern. The term "masked uncontrolled hypertension" is now suggested to describe patients on BP-lowering treatment who exhibit non-elevated office but elevated ambulatory BP [2].

For either group (masked hypertension and masked uncontrolled hypertension), non-elevated office BP is typically defined as <140/90 mmHg, usually by an average

A.J. Viera, M.D. (✉)
Department of Family Medicine and Hypertension Research Program, University of North Carolina at Chapel Hill, Chapel Hill, NC, USA
e-mail: anthony_viera@med.unc.edu

© Springer International Publishing Switzerland 2016   323
W.B. White (ed.), *Blood Pressure Monitoring in Cardiovascular Medicine and Therapeutics*, Clinical Hypertension and Vascular Diseases,
DOI 10.1007/978-3-319-22771-9_16

Table 16.1 Four diagnostic categories pairing office with Out-of-Office BP

		Office BP average	
		Not elevated above threshold	*Elevated above threshold*
Out-of-office BP average	*Not elevated above threshold*	Sustained ("true") normotension	White coat hypertension
	Elevated above threshold	Masked hypertension	Sustained hypertension

Note that classification is based on either systolic, diastolic, or both

of repeated measurements [3]. The threshold for defining elevated ambulatory BP varies somewhat in the literature [4, 5], but the most widely used threshold has been a mean awake ambulatory BP $\geq 135/85$ mmHg [6, 7]. If the 24-h BP average is used, the threshold is typically an average of $\geq 130/80$ mmHg [3].

The nighttime BP average has also been incorporated into the definition of masked hypertension. According to the European Society of Hypertension, elevated nighttime BP is defined as $\geq 120/70$ mmHg [2]. Thus, individuals with non-elevated office BP with elevated mean awake ambulatory BP and/or elevated mean 24-h ambulatory BP, and/or elevated mean nighttime ambulatory BP are said to exhibit masked hypertension.

Prevalence of Masked Hypertension

Masked hypertension is present in approximately 10 % of the general adult population [4, 6, 8, 9]. Among the general adult population of those with non-elevated office BP, it is present in approximately 15–30 % [10]. The first cross-sectional study of masked hypertension in the general population was conducted in Ohasama, a small community in Japan [11]. Among 969 adults (some under treatment for hypertension), 13 % of those with normal office BPs had masked hypertension detected by ambulatory BP monitoring (ABPM). A second study conducted in Italy examined 3200 adults and found a 9 % prevalence of masked hypertension by ABPM (Sega et al. [12]). A third study ($N = 1400$) conducted in Spain used home BP monitoring for the out-of-office BP measurements and also found a 9 % prevalence of masked hypertension [13]. Other studies have examined the prevalence in certain subpopulations. In a worksite study of 267 men, 14 % had masked hypertension by ABPM [14]. In a study of 319 healthy adult volunteers with normal office BP, 23 % had masked hypertension detected by ABPM [15]. Among 578 Swedish men 70-years of age, 14 % had masked hypertension [8]. In national and international databases, the prevalence of masked hypertension among people with normal office BP ranges from 9 to 54.5 % [16]. The variability in prevalence estimates is due to the heterogeneous definition of masked hypertension as well as differences in the sample characteristics across studies.

Among certain clinical subgroups, masked hypertension may be even more common. Diabetics have a higher prevalence of masked hypertension [17–19]. In the International Database of Ambulatory Blood Pressure in Relation to Cardiovascular Outcomes (IDACO), among the 7826 participants not taking BP-lowering medications, the prevalence of masked hypertension (clinic BP < 140/90 mmHg and daytime ambulatory BP average ≥135/85 mmHg) was higher in the clinic normotensive participants with diabetes (29 %) than in those without diabetes (19 %) [17].

Masked hypertension also appears more common among patients with chronic kidney disease (CKD). One Spanish study of 5693 hypertensive patients with CKD showed that the proportion of individuals with masked hypertension was 7 % among all the patients and 32 % among patients with clinic normotension [20]. In a cross-sectional study of 617 treated hypertensive African Americans with CKD, the prevalence of masked uncontrolled hypertension was 70 % among individuals with controlled clinic BP [21].

Obstructive sleep apnea (OSA) may also be associated with masked hypertension. In one study of 133 newly diagnosed OSA patients taking no medications, 30 % exhibited masked hypertension using mean 24-h ambulatory pressures [22]. In another study of 61 otherwise healthy men with normal clinic BP, obstructive sleep apnea was associated with masked hypertension even using mean awake ambulatory BP, suggesting that OSA adversely affects ambulatory BP beyond the sleep period [23].

Target Organ Damage and Outcomes

Several studies have examined target organ damage and outcomes associated with masked hypertension, finding that the risk associated with masked hypertension approaches that of sustained hypertension. In a study published in 1999, left ventricular mass index (LVMI) and carotid plaque were measured among people with masked hypertension and compared to those with true normotension and those with sustained hypertension [24]. The LVMI was 73 g/m^2 in the true normotensives, 86 g/m^2 in the masked hypertensives, and 90 g/m^2 in the sustained hypertensives. Carotid plaque was present in 15 % of true normotensives and in 28 % of both the masked and sustained hypertensives. In another study, LVMI in people with masked hypertension was 91 g/m^2 compared to 79 g/m^2 in true normotensives and 94 g/m^2 in people with sustained hypertension [12]. The association with carotid atherosclerosis was also confirmed in a 2007 study [25]. Thus, masked hypertension is associated with target organ damage on an order of magnitude approaching that associated with sustained hypertension.

More importantly, there is also evidence of increased cardiovascular disease (CVD) events (stroke, myocardial infarction, cardiovascular mortality) occurring in people with masked hypertension. A meta-analysis of seven studies including a total of 11,502 subjects followed over a mean of 8 years showed a twofold higher incidence of CVD events (HR 2.00; 95 % CI 1.58–2.52) in people with masked

Table 16.2 Target organ damage and cardiovascular events [12, 24, 26]

	True normotension	Masked hypertension	Sustained hypertension
Left ventricular mass index (g/m^2)	73–79	86–91	90–94
Carotid plaque (%)	15	28	28
Cardiovascular events hazard ratio (95 % CI)	1.0	2.00 (1.58–2.52)	2.28 (1.87–2.78)

hypertension compared to those with true normotension [26]. This risk approaches the risk conferred by sustained hypertension (HR 2.28; 95 % CI 1.87–2.78). Table 16.2 summarizes the target organ damage associations and cardiovascular event rates in true normotension, masked hypertension, and sustained hypertension.

In another analysis, individual-level data from the IDACO was used to examine differences in CVD risk among 7030 people comparing white coat hypertension, masked hypertension, and sustained hypertension. At a median follow-up of 9.5 years (64,958 person years), compared to people with sustained normotension, the adjusted hazard ratios for CVD events were 1.22 (95 % CI 0.96–1.53) for those with white coat hypertension, 1.62 (95 % CI 1.35–1.96) for those with masked hypertension, and 1.80 (95 % CI 1.59–2.03) for those with sustained hypertension [27]. Notably, the hazard ratios between masked hypertension and sustained hypertension were not significantly different ($p = 0.14$).

Diagnosis of Masked Hypertension

Missing from the current literature is any evidence that identification and treatment of masked hypertension reduces CVD events or mortality. In order to conduct such studies, a practical approach to detecting masked hypertension is needed. At the very least, identification of people with masked hypertension may allow earlier, more aggressive lifestyle modifications and closer monitoring for progression to overt (sustained) hypertension. However, there is limited evidence on how best to identify people with masked hypertension. One approach would be to perform ABPM on all adults, perhaps over a certain age, with non-elevated office BP. Given the relatively new recommendations that ABPM ought to be performed in adults before diagnosing hypertension (in order to exclude white coat hypertension) [28, 29], an approach that also uses ABPM among people with "normal" office BP would in effect mean everyone would be getting ABPM. Such an approach is not practical.

An alternative detection strategy would be to target ABPM to people who are at high risk for having masked hypertension. While some factors associated with masked hypertension have been observed, they are not consistent, and no validated risk assessment tool has yet been developed. The most reliable risk factor may simply be the office BP level. Recent evidence suggests that the BP cutoff that may have the most reasonable tradeoff between sensitivity and specificity is approximately 126 mmHg systolic [30]. Similarly, other studies have shown that office BP in the upper prehypertensive range predicts masked hypertension [31]. Another study examined the diagnostic overlap between masked hypertension and prehypertension (systolic BP 120–139 mmHg or diastolic BP 80–89 mmHg) [7]. Among 813 participants not on antihypertensive medications, 769 participants had non-elevated clinic BP. The overall prevalence of masked hypertension in the participants with non-elevated clinic BP was 15 % using a cutoff of 135/85 mmHg for mean awake ambulatory BP. The prevalence of masked hypertension was only 4 % in participants with office BP <120/80 mmHg. In the subgroup of participants with prehypertension, the prevalence of masked hypertension increased to 34 % and reached 52 % in the upper prehypertensive range (systolic BP 130–139 mmHg or diastolic BP 80–89 mmHg). Other studies have shown a similarly high prevalence of masked hypertension among patients with borderline prehypertensive office BP levels [32, 33].

Thus, one diagnostic approach may be to assess individuals for masked hypertension if their office BP is in the prehypertensive range (Fig. 16.1). If office BP is <120/80 mmHg, there may be no need to do ABPM since the likelihood of masked hypertension, especially of any clinical significance, is low. Another potential approach would be to perform targeted testing among subgroups who exhibit a higher prevalence of masked hypertension, including those with diabetes, OSA, and possibly CKD.

Another potential strategy for detecting masked hypertension would be to use home BP monitoring (HBPM). Like ABPM, measurements from HBPM correlate better with CVD prognosis. HBPM has also been used in a number of studies to define masked hypertension [34–37] However, it is not clear that HBPM and ABPM are interchangeable for identifying masked hypertension. In one study, the congruence of the diagnosis of masked hypertension comparing awake ABPM to HBPM among 420 adults 30 years and older was 72 % ($k=0.36$) [33]. In the PAMELA study, home BP was elevated (defined as $\geq 135/83$ mmHg) in only half of the patients diagnosed with masked hypertension by mean 24-h ambulatory BP (defined as $\geq 125/79$ mmHg), again suggesting limited agreement between ABPM and HBPM in diagnosing masked hypertension [4]. Finally, HBPM may not be an ideal methodology for identifying masked hypertension due to its inability to determine nighttime (sleep) BP [4].

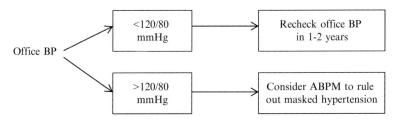

Fig. 16.1 A possible strategy for detecting masked hypertension

Conclusions

Masked hypertension is associated with an increased risk of cardiovascular target organ damage, CVD events, and mortality compared to sustained normotension. It appears that 15–30 % of adults have masked hypertension, yet the condition goes undetected because the office BP is "normal." The paradigm for detecting hypertension may need to be changed. Already, enough evidence has accumulated such that guideline groups recommend ABPM to confirm hypertension in patients with elevated office BP [28, 29]. The evidence is growing such that in time, it may also be commonplace to use ABPM—at least for some groups—to ensure that masked hypertension is not present.

References

1. Pickering TG, Davidson K, Gerin W, Schwartz JE. Masked hypertension. Hypertension. 2002;40(6):795–6.
2. O'Brien E, Parati G, Stergiou G, et al. European society of hypertension position paper on ambulatory blood pressure monitoring. J Hypertens. 2013;31(9):1731–68.
3. O'Brien E, Asmar R, Beilin L, et al. Practice guidelines of the European Society of Hypertension for clinic, ambulatory and self blood pressure measurement. J Hypertens. 2005;23(4):697.
4. Mancia G, Facchetti R, Bombelli M, Grassi G, Sega R. Long-term risk of mortality associated with selective and combined elevation in office, home, and ambulatory blood pressure. Hypertension. 2006;47:846–53.
5. Hansen TW, Jeppesen J, Rasmussen S, Ibsen H, Torp-Pedersen C. Ambulatory blood pressure monitoring and risk of cardiovascular disease: a population based study. Am J Hypertens. 2006;19(3):243–50.
6. Ohkubo T, Kikuya M, Metoki H, et al. Prognosis of "masked" hypertension and "white-coat" hypertension detected by 24-h ambulatory blood pressure monitoring 10-year follow-up from the Ohasama study. J Am Coll Cardiol. 2005;46(3):508–15.
7. Shimbo D, Newman JD, Schwartz JE. Masked hypertension and prehypertension: diagnostic overlap and interrelationships with left ventricular mass: the Masked Hypertension Study. Am J Hypertens. 2012;25(6):664–71.
8. Bjorklund K, Lind L, Zethelius B, Andren B, Lithell H. Isolated ambulatory hypertension predicts cardiovascular morbidity in elderly men. Circulation. 2003;107(9):1297–302.
9. Hanninen M-RA, Niiranen TJ, Puukka PJ, Johansson J, Jula AM. Prognostic significance of masked and white-coat hypertension in the general population: the Finn-Home Study. J Hypertens. 2012;30:705–12.
10. Peacock J, Diaz KM, Viera AJ, Schwartz JE, Shimbo D. Unmasking masked hypertension: prevalence, clinical implications, diagnosis, correlates and future directions. J Hum Hypertens. 2014;28(9):521–8.
11. Imai Y, Tsuji I, Nagai K, et al. Ambulatory blood pressure monitoring in evaluating the prevalence of hypertension in adults in Ohasama, a rural Japanese community. Hypertens Res. 1996;19(3):207–12.
12. Sega R, Trocino G, Lanzarotti A, et al. Alterations of cardiac structure in patients with isolated office, ambulatory, or home hypertension: Data from the general population (Pressione Arteriose Monitorate E Loro Associazioni [PAMELA] Study). Circulation. 2001;104(12): 1385–92.

13. Márquez Contreras E, Casado Martínez JJ, Pardo Alvarez J, Vázquez I, Guevara B, Rodríguez J. Prevalence of white-coat hypertension and masked hypertension in the general population, through home blood pressure measurement. Aten Primaria. 2006;38(7):392–8.
14. Belkić KL, Schnall PL, Landsbergis PA, et al. Hypertension at the workplace—an occult disease? The need for work site surveillance. Adv Psychosom Med. 2001;22:116–38.
15. Selenta C, Hogan BE, Linden W. How often do office blood pressure measurements fail to identify true hypertension? An exploration of white-coat normotension. Arch Fam Med. 2000;9:533–40.
16. Gorostidi M, Vinyoles E, Banegas JR, de la Sierra A. Prevalence of white-coat and masked hypertension in national and international registries. Hypertens Res. 2015;38(1):1–7.
17. Franklin SS, Thijs L, Li Y, et al. Masked hypertension in diabetes mellitus: treatment implications for clinical practice. Hypertension. 2013;61(5):964–71.
18. Leitao CB, Canani LH, Silveiro SP, Gross JL. Ambulatory blood pressure monitoring and type 2 diabetes mellitus. Arq Bras Cardiol. 2007;89:315–21; 347–54.
19. Ben-Dov IZ, Ben-Ishay D, Mekler J, Ben-Arie L, Bursztyn M. Increased prevalence of masked blood pressure elevations in treated diabetic subjects. Arch Intern Med. 2007;167:2139–42.
20. Gorostidi M, Sarafidis PA, de la Sierra A. et al; Spanish ABPM Registry Investigators. Differences between office and 24-hour blood pressure control in hypertensive patients with CKD: A 5,693-patient cross-sectional analysis from Spain. Am J Kidney Dis. 2013;62(2):285–94.
21. Pogue V, Rahman M, Lipkowitz M, et al. Disparate estimates of hypertension control from ambulatory and clinic blood pressure measurements in hypertensive kidney disease. Hypertension. 2009;53:20–7.
22. Baguet JP, Levy P, Barone-Rochette G, et al. Masked hypertension in obstructive sleep apnea syndrome. J Hypertens. 2008;26(5):885–92.
23. Drager LF, Diegues-Silva L, Diniz PM, et al. Obstructive sleep apnea, masked hypertension, and arterial stiffness in men. Am J Hypertens. 2010;23(3):249–54.
24. Liu JE, Roman MJ, Pini R, Schwartz JE, Pickering TG, Devereux RB. Cardiac and arterial target organ damage in adults with elevated ambulatory and normal office blood pressure. Ann Intern Med. 1999;131(8):564–72.
25. Matsui Y, Eguchi K, Ishikawa J, Hoshide S, Shimada K, Kario K. Subclinical arterial damage in untreated masked hypertensive subjects detected by home blood pressure measurement. Am J Hypertens. 2007;20:385–91.
26. Fagard RH, Cornelissen VA. Incidence of cardiovascular events in white-coat, masked and sustained hypertension versus true normotension: a meta-analysis. J Hypertens. 2007;25(11):2193–8.
27. Hansen TW, Kikuya M, Thijs L, et al. Prognostic superiority of daytime ambulatory over conventional blood pressure in four populations: a meta-analysis of 7,030 individuals. J Hypertens. 2007;25(8):1554–64.
28. National Clinical Guideline Centre (UK). Hypertension: The Clinical Management of Primary Hypertension in Adults: Update of Clinical Guidelines 18 and 34. London: Royal College of Physicians; 2011.
29. Piper MA, Evans CV, Burda BU, Margolis KL, O'Connor E, Whitlock EP. Diagnostic and predictive accuracy of blood pressure screening methods with consideration of rescreening intervals: a systematic review for the US Preventive services task force. Ann Intern Med. 2015;162(3):192–204.
30. Viera AJ, Lin FC, Tuttle LA, et al. Levels of office blood pressure and their operating characteristics for detecting masked hypertension based on ambulatory blood pressure monitoring. Am J Hypertens. 2015;28(1):42–9.
31. Hanninen M-RA, Niiranen TJ, Puukka PJ, Mattila AK, Jula AM. Determinants of masked hypertension in the general population: the Finn-Home study. J Hypertens. 2011;29:1880–8.
32. Viera AJ, Hinderliter AL, Kshirsagar AV, Fine J, Dominik R. Reproducibility of masked hypertension in adults with untreated borderline office blood pressure: comparison of ambulatory and home monitoring. Am J Hypertens. 2010;23(11):1190–7.

33. Viera AJ, Lin FC, Tuttle LA, Olsson E, Stankevitz K, Girdler SS, Klein JL, Hinderliter AL. Reproducibility of masked hypertension among adults 30 years or older. Blood Press Monit. 2014;19(4):208–15.
34. Bobrie G, Chatellier G, Genes N, et al. Cardiovascular prognosis of "masked hypertension" detected by blood pressure self-measurement in elderly treated hypertensive patients. JAMA. 2004;291:1342–9.
35. Zhuo S, Wen W, Li-Yuan M, Shu-Yu W, Yi-Xin W. Home blood pressure measurement in prehypertension and untreated hypertension: comparison with ambulatory blood pressure monitoring and office blood pressure. Blood Press Monit. 2009;14:245–50.
36. Stergiou GS, Argyraki KK, Moyssakis I, et al. Home blood pressure is as reliable as ambulatory blood pressure in predicting target-organ damage in hypertension. Am J Hypertens. 2007;20:616–21.
37. Matsui Y, Eguchi K, Ishikawa J, Hoshide S, Shimada K, Kario K. Subclinical arterial damage in untreated masked hypertensive subjects detected by home blood pressure measurement. Am J Hypertens. 2007;20(4):385–91.

Chapter 17
White Coat Hypertension

Lawrence R. Krakoff

Introduction

Arterial pressure varies, from heart beat to heart beat, from minute to minute, hour to hour, and day to day. This fundamental property of systolic and diastolic pressure has been recognized since the work of Harvey who first measured blood pressure in equine arteries [1]. During the nineteenth century, astute physicians (Bright, Mahomet) observed high pressures in patients with chronic kidney disease and then in a fraction of the population without kidney disease, but destined to die of stroke or heart disease. (They assessed pressure by feeling the pulse or use of primitive devices for semi-quantitative measurements [2].

Development of the Riva-Rocci device and use of the stethoscope to hear Korotkof sounds markedly expanded approximation of the arterial pressure in the clinic leading to the more general recognition that higher arterial pressure, i.e., hypertension, was highly prevalent in the population at large and clearly associated with cardiovascular and renal diseases. These studies were based on measurement in the clinic. While variation in arterial pressure from visit to visit may have been recognized, its significance for clinical diagnosis implied the need for measurement not only in the clinic but in "real life" where 99 % of any patient's life is spent, at home, work, or other locations and activities.

Ayman and Goldshine made the initial observation that clinic or office blood pressures were often much higher than pressures measured at home. Their patients were trained to take their own pressure using the stethoscope and mercury manometer [3]. There was no effective treatment at that time. These authors suggested that

L.R. Krakoff, M.D. (✉)
Icahn School of Medicine at Mount Sinai,
One Gustave L Levy Place, Box 1030, New York, NY 10029-6574, USA
e-mail: Lawrence.krakoff@mountsinai.org

© Springer International Publishing Switzerland 2016
W.B. White (ed.), *Blood Pressure Monitoring in Cardiovascular Medicine and Therapeutics*, Clinical Hypertension and Vascular Diseases,
DOI 10.1007/978-3-319-22771-9_17

those with lower home pressures might be less at risk to develop target organ pathology or die prematurely compared with those with high pressures in both environments. Ayman and Goldshine's report, published in 1940, had little apparent impact at the time, most likely due to the world's attention to the onset of World War II and, in the United States, the extraordinary Presidential election (Roosevelt versus Wilkie) with Roosevelt seeking an unprecedented third term.

The development of a portable recording device (Remmler) for measuring blood pressure throughout the day was a major step forward for evaluating blood pressure during ordinary activities, but required manual inflation of the cuff [4]. Perlow and Sokolow used the Remmler to collect daytime ambulatory blood pressures for nearly 1000 participants with clinic hypertension and followed this cohort for many years to characterize patterns of subsequent cardiovascular disease. Those with ambulatory pressures greater than clinic pressures in this prospective cohort study had a higher incidence of cardiovascular events, compared with those whose ambulatory pressures were lower than their clinic pressure [5]. Since then, several large prospective surveys have amply confirmed the importance of ambulatory blood pressure monitoring for superior prognostic accuracy in predicting cardiovascular disease in [6–8].

The presence of a physician can increase blood pressure and intra-arterial blood pressure in the clinic or a medical intensive care unit [9, 10]. Pickering and colleagues studied a large number of hypertensive patients and compared clinic and 24-h ambulatory pressures. They found that many of their participants with clinic hypertension had much lower pressures during the day and night at work or home as revealed by ambulatory blood pressure monitoring. They coined the "White Coat Hypertension" as a useful diagnosis for those with high clinic pressures and normal out-of-office pressures [11]. From 1988 until the present time, recognition of White Coat Hypertension has grown progressively with more than 1000 publications in English listed in PubMed. "White Coat Hypertension" (WCH) is now widely recognized as a distinct diagnostic entity (ICD 9 code 796.2) that is highly useful for assessment of patients initially thought to be hypertensive on the basis of screening programs or limited clinic assessment. The "White Coat Effect" in treated patients describes those with pressures above goal in the clinic, but below the goal for treatment when out-of-the- office.

Does WCH indicate that future cardiovascular risk is the same as that of those with normal clinic pressures? When WCH is present, is anti-hypertensive drug therapy warranted or can it be withheld and for how long? For treated patients, when a White Coat Effect (WCE) is present, which pressure is best related to prognosis; should treatment be based on the clinic pressure or the out-office-pressure? Few of these questions have been put to rest, despite the progress that has been made in diagnosis and treatment of hypertension since initial recognition of White Coat Hypertension, 30 years ago. This review will summarize current knowledge of White Coat Hypertension and the White Coat Effect. Our goal is to enhance awareness and usefulness of these diagnoses for better management of hypertension.

Defining White Coat Hypertension and the White Coat Effect

Table 17.1 summarizes the definition of these terms as reflected in recent guidelines and reports from consensus groups. Alternate terms have sometimes been used. "Isolated office hypertension" and "Isolated ambulatory hypertension" convey the same meaning as WCH or Masked Hypertension, respectively.

Most hypertensive patients have slightly higher office pressures compared to either daytime ABPM or HBPM explaining the differences between threshold pressures in Table 17.2. Occasionally, these differences are large with office systolic pressures higher by >20 mmHg than out-of-office daytime pressures. Normal participants and many hypertensive patients have 10–20 % lower nighttime pressures (dipper pattern) that account for the lower threshold pressures for 24 h ABPM compared to either daytime ABPM or Home pressures.

For those patients >60 years of age, some recent guidelines, for clinic pressures, have accepted systolic pressures of 145–150 mmHg as thresholds for both diagnosis and on-treatment goal pressure [12, 13]. It is not yet established whether or not there should be changes in current thresholds for arterial pressure when measured out-of-the office by ABPM or HBPM.

Table 17.1 Arterial pressure categories based on relation between Clinic and Out-of-Office measurement for *untreated* patients [16, 17]

Classification	Normal	White coat hypertension[a]	Sustained hypertension
Location			
Clinic Pressures	Normal	High	High
	<140/90 mmHg	≥140/90 mmHg	≥140/90 mmHg
Daytime ABPM or Home BP	Normal	Normal	High
	<135/85 mmHg	<135/85 mmHg	≥135/85 mmHg
24 h ABPM	<130/80 mmHg	<130/80 mmHg	≥130/80

[a]Alternate-isolated office hypertension

Table 17.2 Arterial pressure categories based on relation between Clinic and Out-of-Office measurement for *treated* patients [17, 18]

Classification	Normal-controlled	White coat effect	Sustained hypertension[a]
Location			
Clinic pressures	Normal	High	High
	<140/90 mmHg	≥140/90 mmHg	≥140/90 mmHg
Daytime ABPM or Home BP	Normal	Normal[b]	High[c]
	<135/85 mmHg	<135/85 mmHg	≥135/85 mmHg
24 h ABPM	<130/80 mmHg	<130/80 mmHg	≥130/80

[a]Alternate-Isolated office hypertension
[b]Pseudo-resistant hypertension, if taking multiple medications at usual therapeutic doses
[c]Resistant hypertension if patients are prescribed with three or more drugs at usual therapeutic doses [19]

Definitions for WCH or WCE are currently based only on the level or blood pressure observed in clinic and out-of-the office. The degree of difference is not included. Thus, a 55-year-old patient with an office pressure of 160/100 mmHg and a home pressure average of 138/84 is still considered to be hypertensive despite the substantially lower pressure outside the office. The presence or absence of the normal nocturnal dip in blood pressure is, likewise, not presently considered in the criteria for WCH or WCE despite its significance for prognosis [14, 15].

Causes of WCH or WCE

Anxiety in anticipation of or during the clinic visit has been linked to WCH or the WCE during treatment, especially when the doctor measures the pressure. While some patients have a generalized anxiety syndrome or panic disorder, a sudden increase in pressure in the office may be, in part, a conditioned reflex [20]. Older patients may be more likely to have anxiety-related White Coat response, but in those with dementia the response is less prominent [21].

WCH/WCE Methods

Clinic Pressures Measured by Providers (Assistants, Nurses, Physicians Using Auscultation)

The diagnosis of White Coat Hypertension or the White Coat effect for treated patients depends on comparing the clinic pressures and out-of-office pressures. For a valid comparison, pressures measured in both settings should be accurate, but representative of each setting. Only one or two pressures are taken at a usual clinic visit by varying personnel (medical assistant, nurse, or physician) on either arm and in the sitting position. The limitations for clinic pressure have been amply documented [22] and include inaccurate devices, incorrect cuff size, lack of training and observer bias if auscultation is used rather than a device [23]. Since the virtual disappearance of mercury column sphygmomanometers due to concern about contamination, many clinics now use either an aneroid sphygmomanometer with auscultation or a device that inflates the cuff has a sensor in the cuff and displays pressure. In general, pressures measured by the physician are higher than those measured by trained nurses, resulting in a greater likelihood of WCH or WCE when out-of-office measurements are obtained for comparison [22].

Use of Devices in the Clinic/Office

Measuring more blood pressures with an accurate device at the clinic visit can reduce the chance of a false positive diagnosis of WCH or WCE. Bias is eliminated. Several approaches have been explored. Patients referred to the Mayo Clinic have been evaluated by a 6-h recording using the SpaceLabs ambulatory blood pressure monitor. There was excellent correlation with measurements made by trained nurses for systolic pressure. Diastolic pressures were about 7 mmHg higher for 6 h average compared to nurse measurements. Results were not compared with either out-of-office measurement by ABPM or HBPM [24].

Extensive studies have been reported for use of the BpTru device for clinic pressures. The BpTru consists of a cuff with pressure detector by oscillometry, inflation pump, and recording software that uses a programmed sequence of pressure measurements, then calculates the average pressures. The first measurement is discarded. Average pressures are then calculated from the following five measurements, usually taken at 1–2 min intervals [25]. In a series of 400 patients evaluated by both daytime ABPM and in clinic by BpTru, average systolic and diastolic pressures were very similar and highly correlated: systolic pressure $r=0.640$ and diastolic pressure $r=0.693$ for comparison between daytime ABPM and BpTru using 1 min intervals. However, the absolute differences for individuals were often >5 mmHg for systolic or diastolic pressure and nearly 20 % had differences of >10 mmHg. The widely available Omron device has been compared to the BpTru for clinic assessment. Both devices give very similar systolic and diastolic pressure measurements when taken at 1-min intervals. When taken at 2-min intervals, systolic pressures were similar, but the average diastolic pressures were higher for the BpTru device [26].

Out-of-Office ABPM or HBPM

The generally accepted "gold standard" for measuring out-of-office pressure is non-invasive 24-h ambulatory blood pressure monitoring. Several accurate and well-validated devices for this purpose are now available. Protocols for use of ABPM have been described in guidelines and recommend measurements every 15–20 min during the day and every 30 min during the night. Use of ABPM requires well-trained staff, patient education to minimize errors (i.e., exercise), and computers for programing the monitors, collecting stored results and preparing reports. In general, patients go to a practice or station for placement of monitors and return the devices after a day of monitoring. This results in some degree of inconvenience in requiring two visits per ABPM determination. The costs for resources and personnel to maintain and ABPM program are small, by Western standards, but steep for developing nations. At present, US Medicare and other insurance providers pay for ambulatory blood pressure monitoring when the diagnosis of WCH is suspected.

Home blood pressure monitoring (HBPM) is most accurate and reliable when automated devices are used (i.e., Omron et al.). There is very good correlation between HBPM and daytime ABPM. Devices must be checked for accuracy. Patients need to be trained for use of the devices, recording of results (if devices don't have memory), and transmission of results as data sheets or by telemetry (an increasing trend). Feedback and counseling can be done by phone or e-mail (security necessary) so that there is less need for clinic visits. An average of 10–20 home measurements is needed for comparison with clinic pressures to determine presence or absence of WCH/WCE [27]. Most insurance providers don't support purchase of HBPM devices. Prices are in the range of $70–100 for devices with automatic inflation and memory for storing results. Devices are widely available in pharmacies and medical supply stores. Combining HBPM with transmission of results directly to the provider by telemetry is now available in some programs. One advantage for HBPM with telemetry for treated patients is that patients can evaluate the effect of treatment and even participate in drug titration during follow-up care, reducing unnecessary medication that might be prescribed if only office pressures were available [28–31].

WCH/WCE Epidemiology

WCH occurs in about 30 % of untreated patients suspected of being hypertensive on the basis of office/clinic measurements. Those most likely to have WCH are women, younger patients with recent onset of office hypertension [32], and older patients with varying systolic pressure [33]. The WCE in treated hypertensive patients may occur less often; recent meta-analyses suggest prevalence rates of 15–20 % [34–36].

WCH and WCE in African-American Hypertensives

African-Americans have not been extensively studied for prevalence of WCH or WCE. However, in those with chronic kidney disease, the AASK trial found that 33 % of those treated had WCE based on comparison of daytime ambulatory pressure with clinic pressure. However, only 23 % had WCE when nighttime pressures were considered the basis for controlling hypertension [37]. A study of young (average age 30) White and African-American participants found that sustained hypertension, WCH, and Masked hypertension all occurred in <5 % of either group without significant differences between the groups [38]. However, average nighttime systolic and diastolic pressures were significantly higher in African-Americans compared to Whites and nighttime dipping in pressure was significantly less for African-Americans. There is a pressing need for more studies of ABPM and HBPM to assess WCH and WCE in African-American and other less well-studied adult populations.

WCH and WCE in Diabetes

Presence of WCH is associated with greater risk of pre-diabetes and adult (type-2) diabetes compared to normal participants in prospective observational studies [39].

WCH in Pregnancy

Pregnant women who are hypertensive based on office measurements may have either pregnancy-induced hypertension or hypertension that was present prior to pregnancy (chronic hypertension). Either condition requires close monitoring of blood pressure by office and either ABPM or HBPM for optimal management [40]. Detection of WCH by ABPM early in pregnancy of women initially considered to have chronic hypertension may help to select those who might not need anti-hypertensive medication during pregnancy. Those with WCH in early pregnancy have fewer complications during their pregnancies than those with sustained hypertension [41, 42]. However, it is recommended that ABPM in early pregnancy is not accurate enough to predict either pregnancy-induced hypertension or incidence of pre-eclampsia, so that HBPM is required for close follow-up. HBPM combined with telemetry is a very promising strategy for monitoring blood pressure during pregnancy and detecting WCH, but also for early detection of true hypertension [43].

WCH/WCE in Chronic Renal Disease

Hypertension occurs often in chronic renal disease (CRD), irrespective of the specific cause of the nephropathy. Uncontrolled or resistant hypertension contributes to disease progression resulting in the need for renal replacement therapy or cardiovascular pathology. Nearly all patients with CRD are treated for hypertension. The prevalence of WCE in CRD is in the range of 20–30 % and conveys a better prognosis when compared to sustained hypertension [44].

Progression to Sustained Hypertension

WCH may persist without progression to sustained hypertension for many years [45]. However, in prospective surveys, baseline presence of WCH is associated with a nearly twofold increased incidence of sustained hypertension during an 8–10 year follow-up, compared to those with normal pressure [46–48]. Annual re-evaluation for those with WCH by HBPM is an effective strategy to detect the transition to sustained hypertension [47].

Progression to sustained hypertension from WCE while on anti-hypertensive drug treatment has not been well-studied, but might be due to reduced adherence to medication [49] or to genuine resistance to current treatment [50].

WCH/WCE Prognosis for CVD and Mortality

Perloff reported, in 1983, that out-of-office daytime blood pressures were superior to office pressures for predicting cardiovascular outcomes in hypertensive patients [5]. In 1994, Verdecchia et al. published results of a prospective survey using 24-h

ABPM comparing normals to those with WCH (19 %) and two groups with
sustained hypertension. Those with sustained hypertension had either a normal fall
in pressure at night during sleep (Dipper pattern) or a lack of nocturnal (Non-
dippers). During the 7.5 year follow-up period, incidence of CVD in WCH was
almost identical to that of the normals [6]. Since then a number of individual surveys
and several meta-analyses have supported the conclusion that WCH, at baseline, is
associated with less future CVD and mortality compared to sustained hypertension
[18, 34, 35]. It is less certain whether or not WCH confers a greater risk for CVD
than normal blood pressure. Figure 17.1 displays hazard ratios and p values for risk
ratios for pooled results from two recent meta-analyses [34, 35]. Hazard ratios for
WCH tend to be slightly higher than for normal blood pressure, but statistical
significance is not always met.

Not all those classified as WCH are the same, with respect to all available
pressures. In subgroup analyses, a large cohort with "true WCH" (normal home and
24- h ABPM pressures) were compared to "partial WCH" (normal 24-h ABPM, and

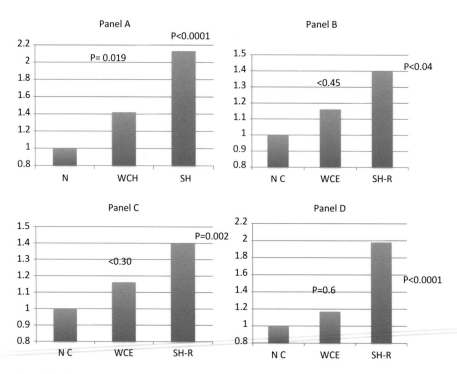

Fig. 17.1 Hazard ratios for cardiovascular events during follow-up from two recent meta-analyses
are shown. (**a, b**) Data from Stergiou et al. [35] show hazard ratios for WCH or WCE versus N
(normal) or sustained hypertension. (**c, d**) show hazard ratios from Franklin et al. [34] for WCH or
WCE. *P* values for comparison of WCH or WCE with normal states are shown. (**a, c**) *N* untreated,
normal pressure, *WCH* white coat hypertension, *S* sustained hypertension. (**b, d**) *NC* normal, controlled on treatment, *WCE* white coat effect on treatment, *SH-R* sustained resistant hypertension on
treatment

high home pressures). Those with "true" WCH had hazard ratios for CVD and mortality similar to normals, whereas hazard ratios for "partial WCH" were significantly above that of the normal group but lower than for sustained hypertension [48]. The results are best explained by differences in pressures; all available pressures tend to be higher in "partial WCH" compared to "true WCH." The prognosis is then best related to average out-of-office pressures rather than the less precise label, "WCH" [8].

WCE in Treated Patients

In treated patients, prognosis for mortality and morbidity in those with normal pressures (well-controlled) is similar to those with normal out-of-office pressures and far better than for sustained-treated hypertension [7, 18, 34, 35]. However, the risk of future CVD or mortality for those with normal pressure on treatment remains significantly above that for those with normal pressure without need for drug treatment.

Treatment of WCH or WCE in Treated Patients

It is reasonable to recommend life-style improvement, for those with WCH and to evaluate these patients for other cardiovascular risk factors. Other risk factors may be found in a substantial fraction of those with WCH, especially older patients [51]. A study of placebo administration during a clinical trial reported that women with a large WCE at entry had a significant fall in office pressure on follow-up without a change in ABPM, whereas men had a much smaller fall in office pressure [52]. It is uncertain whether anti-hypertensive medications reduce cardiovascular risk in WCH, but some have advocated drug treatment despite lack of trial evidence [53]. Patients with WCH or WCE on treatment and prominent anxiety or panic symptoms might benefit from strategies to reduce symptoms, some form of behavior modification with appropriate anti-anxiety medication.

WCH and Cost-Effectiveness

Testing for WCH or the WCE (during treatment) has costs, but these are relatively low compared to cost of diagnostic tests and medication for control of hypertension. Economic forecasts indicate that use of 24-h ABPM for detection of WCH is cost-effective [54]. This strategy may be valuable even when ABPM is repeated annually for those with WCH to evaluate these patients for transition to sustained hypertension [55]. Home Blood pressure monitoring may be even more effective and cost-effective both for initial diagnosis and annual follow-up for transition to sustained hypertension [56].

Conclusions–Recommendations

Office blood pressure measurement may be misleading. WCH or isolated office hypertension should be detected to avoid overdiagnosis of hypertension as a false positive classification. Ambulatory blood pressure monitoring has become the standard of care for detection of WCH. British and US guidelines for management of hypertension now recognize this conclusion [57, 58]. Future risk for cardiovascular disease in those with WCH is minimally above that of those with normal pressure. It is not known whether or not drug treatment alters the prognosis of WCH or intensification of drug treatment alters prognosis for WCE with normal pressures. However, WCH is more likely to progress to sustained hypertension, so that annual re-evaluation is needed using either ambulatory blood pressure monitoring or home blood pressure monitoring.

References

1. Frank RGJ. Harvey and the Oxford physiologists. Berkeley: University of California Press; 1980.
2. Pickering G. Systemic arterial hypertension. In: Fishman AP, Richards DW, editors. Circulation of the blood: men and ideas. New York: Oxford University Press; 1964. p. 487–541.
3. Ayman D, Goldshine AD. Blood pressure determinations by patients with essential hypertension: the difference between clinic and home readings before treatment. Am J Med Sci. 1940;200:465–70.
4. Perloff D, Sokolow M. The representative blood pressure: usefulness of office, basal, home, and ambulatory readings. Cardiovasc Med. 1978;3:655–68.
5. Perloff D, Sokolow M, Cowan R. The prognostic value of ambulatory blood pressures. JAMA. 1983;249:2792–8.
6. Verdecchia P, Porcellati C, Schillaci G, et al. Ambulatory blood pressure: an independent predictor of prognosis in essential hypertension. Hypertension. 1994;24:793–801.
7. Clement D, De Buyzere M, De Bacqer DA, et al. Prognostic value of ambulatory blood-pressure recordings in patients with treated hypertension. N Engl J Med. 2003;348:2407–15.
8. Dolan E, Stanton A, Thijs L, et al. Superiority of ambulatory over clinic blood pressure measurement in predicting mortality: the Dublin outcome study. Hypertension. 2005;46(1):156–61.
9. Mancia G, Bertinieri G, Grassi G, et al. Effects of blood pressure measurement by the doctor on patient's blood pressure and heart rate. Lancet. 1983;2:695–8.
10. Simons RJ, Baily RG, Zelis R, Zwillich CW. The physiologic and psychologic effects of the bedside presentation. N Engl J Med. 1989;321:1273–5.
11. Pickering TG, James GD, Boddie C, Harshfield GA, Blank S, Laragh JH. How common is white coat hypertension? JAMA. 1988;259:225–8.
12. Aronow WS, Fleg JL, Pepine CJ, et al. ACCF/AHA 2011 expert consensus document on hypertension in the elderly: a report of the American College of Cardiology Foundation Task Force on Clinical Expert Consensus Documents. Circulation. 2011;123(21):2434–506.
13. James PA, Oparil S, Carter BL, et al. 2014 evidence-based guideline for the management of high blood pressure in adults: report from the Panel Members Appointed to the Eighth Joint National Committee (JNC 8). JAMA. 2013;311:507–20.
14. Fagard RH, Celis H, Thijs L, et al. Daytime and nighttime blood pressure as predictors of death and cause-specific cardiovascular events in hypertension. Hypertension. 2008;51(1):55–61.

15. Verdecchia P, Schillaci G, Borgioni C, et al. Adverse prognostic value of a blunted circadian rhythm of heart rate in essential hypertension. J Hypertens. 1998;16(9):1335–43.
16. Parati G, Pickering TG. Home blood-pressure monitoring: US and European consensus. Lancet. 2009;373(9667):876–8.
17. Kikuya M, Hansen TW, Thijs L, et al. Diagnostic thresholds for ambulatory blood pressure monitoring based on 10-year cardiovascular risk. Circulation. 2007;115:2145–52.
18. Franklin SS, Thijs L, Hansen TW, O'Brien E, Staessen JA. White-coat hypertension: new insights from recent studies. Hypertension. 2013;62(6):982–7.
19. Achelrod D, Wenzel U, Frey S. Systematic review and meta-analysis of the prevalence of resistant hypertension in treated hypertensive populations. Am J Hypertens. 2014.
20. Ogedegbe G, Pickering TG, Clemow L, et al. The misdiagnosis of hypertension: the role of patient anxiety. Arch Intern Med. 2008;168(22):2459–65.
21. Mario B, Massimiliano M, Chiara M, Alessandro S, Antonella C, Gianfranco F. White-coat effect among older patients with suspected cognitive impairment: prevalence and clinical implications. Int J Geriatr Psychiatry. 2008;24(5):509–17.
22. Graves JW, Sheps SG. Does evidence-based medicine suggest that physicians should not be measuring blood pressure in the hypertensive patient? Am J Hypertens. 2004;17(4):354–60.
23. Bruce NG, Shaper AG, Walker M, Wannamethee G. Observer bias in blood pressure studies. J Hypertens. 1988;6:375–80.
24. Graves JW, Nash CA, Grill DE, Bailey KR, Sheps SG. Limited (6-h) ambulatory blood pressure monitoring is a valid replacement for the office blood pressure by trained nurse clinician in the diagnosis of hypertension. Blood Press Monit. 2005;10(4):169–74.
25. Myers MG, Valdivieso M, Kiss A. Optimum frequency of office blood pressure measurement using an automated sphygmomanometer. Blood Press Monit. 2008;13(6):333–8.
26. Myers MG, Valdivieso M, Kiss A, Tobe SW. Comparison of two automated sphygmomanometers for use in the office setting. Blood Press Monit. 2009;14(1):45–7.
27. Niiranen TJ, Johannsson JK, Reunanen A, Jula A. Optimal schedule for home blood pressure measurement based on prognostic data: the Finn-Home Study. Hypertension. 2011;57:1081–6.
28. Margolis KL, Asche SE, Bergdall AR, et al. Effect of home blood pressure telemonitoring and pharmacist management on blood pressure control: a cluster randomized clinical trial. JAMA. 2013;310(1):46–56.
29. Neumann CL, Menne J, Rieken EM, et al. Blood pressure telemonitoring is useful to achieve blood pressure control in inadequately treated patients with arterial hypertension. J Hum Hypertens. 2011.
30. McManus RJ, Mant J, Bray EP, et al. Telemonitoring and self-management in the control of hypertension (TASMINH2): a randomised controlled trial. Lancet. 2010;376(9736):163–72.
31. Parati G, Omboni S, Albini F, et al. Home blood pressure telemonitoring improves hypertension control in general practice. The TeleBPCare study. J Hypertens. 2009;27(1):198–203.
32. Khattar RS, Senior R, Lahiri A. Cardiovascular outcome in white-coat versus sustained mild hypertension: a 10 year follow-up. Circulation. 1998;98:1892–7.
33. Ruddy MC, Bialy GB, Malka ES, Lacy CR, Kostis JB. The relationship of plasma renin activity to clinic and ambulatory blood pressure in elderly people with isolated systolic hypertension. J Hypertens. 1988;6:S412–5.
34. Franklin SS, Thijs L, Hansen TW, et al. Significance of white-coat hypertension in older persons with isolated systolic hypertension: a meta-analysis using the International Database on Ambulatory Blood Pressure Monitoring in Relation to Cardiovascular Outcomes population. Hypertension. 2012;59(3):564–71.
35. Stergiou GS, Asayama K, Thijs L, et al. Prognosis of white-coat and masked hypertension: International Database of Home blood pressure in relation to cardiovascular outcome. Hypertension. 2014;63(4):675–82.
36. Ben-Dov IZ, Kark JD, Mekler J, Shaked E, Bursztyn M. The white coat phenomenon is benign in referred treated patients: a 14-year ambulatory blood pressure mortality study. J Hypertens. 2008;26(4):699–705.

37. Pogue V, Rahman M, Lipkowitz M, et al. Disparate estimates of hypertension control from ambulatory and clinic blood pressure measurements in hypertensive kidney disease. Hypertension. 2009;53(1):20–7.
38. Muntner P, Lewis CE, Diaz KM, et al. Racial differences in abnormal ambulatory blood pressure monitoring measures: results from the Coronary Artery Risk Development in Young Adults (CARDIA) study. Am J Hypertens. 2014.
39. Mancia G, Bombelli M, Facchetti R, et al. Increased long-term risk of new-onset diabetes mellitus in white-coat and masked hypertension. J Hypertens. 2009;27(8):1672–8.
40. Brown MA, McHugh L, Mangos G, Davis G. Automated self-initiated blood pressure or 24-hour ambulatory blood pressure monitoring in pregnancy? BJOG. 2004;111(1):38–41.
41. Brown MA, Mangos G, Davis G, Homer C. The natural history of white coat hypertension during pregnancy. BJOG. 2005;112(5):601–6.
42. Brown MA. Is there a role for ambulatory blood pressure monitoring in pregnancy? Clin Exp Pharmacol Physiol. 2014;41(1):16–21.
43. Denolle T, Weber JL, Calvez C, et al. Diagnosis of white coat hypertension in pregnant women with teletransmitted home blood pressure. Hypertens Pregnancy. 2008;27(3):305–13.
44. Agarwal R. Home and ambulatory blood pressure monitoring in chronic kidney disease. Curr Opin Nephrol Hypertens. 2009;18(6):507–12.
45. Martin K, Phillips RA, Krakoff LR. Persistant white coat hypertension. Am J Hypertens. 1994;7:368–70.
46. Mancia G, Bombelli M, Facchetti R, et al. Long-term risk of sustained hypertension in white-coat or masked hypertension. Hypertension. 2009;54(2):226–32.
47. Ugajin T, Hozawa A, Ohkubo T, et al. White-coat hypertension as a risk factor for the development of home hypertension: the Ohasama study. Arch Intern Med. 2005;165(13):1541–6.
48. Mancia G, Bombelli M, Brambilla G, et al. Long-term prognostic value of white coat hypertension: an insight from diagnostic use of both ambulatory and home blood pressure measurements. Hypertension. 2013;62(1):168–74.
49. Kronish IM, Ye S. Adherence to cardiovascular medications: lessons learned and future directions. Prog Cardiovasc Dis. 2013;55(6):590–600.
50. Redon J, Campos C, Rodicio JL, Pascual JM, Ruilope LM. Prognostic value of ambulatory blood pressure monitoring in refractory hypertension: a prospective study. Hypertension. 2001;31:712–8.
51. Pierdomenico SD, Cuccurullo F. Ambulatory blood pressure monitoring in type 2 diabetes and metabolic syndrome: a review. Blood Press Monit. 2010;15(1):1–7.
52. Loeb EN, Diamond JA, Krakoff LR, Phillips RA. Sex difference in response of blood pressure to calcium antagonism in the treatment of moderate-to-severe hypertension. Blood Press Monit. 1999;4:209–12.
53. Moser M. White-coat hypertension- to treat or not to treat: a clinical dilemma. Arch Intern Med. 2001;161:2655–6.
54. Lovibond K, Jowett S, Barton P, et al. Cost-effectiveness of options for the diagnosis of high blood pressure in primary care: a modelling study. Lancet. 2011;378:1219–30.
55. Krakoff LR. Cost-effectiveness of ambulatory blood pressure: a reanalysis. Hypertension. 2006;47(1):29–34.
56. Mallick S, Kanthety R, Rahman M. Home blood pressure monitoring in clinical practice: a review. Am J Med. 2009;122(9):803–10.
57. Ritchie LD, Campbell NC, Murchie P. New NICE guidelines for hypertension. Br Med J. 2011;343:d5644.
58. Piper MA, Evans CV, Burda BU, Margolis KL, O'Connor E, Whitlock EP. Diagnostic and predictive accuracy of blood pressure screening methods with consideration of rescreening intervals: an updated systematic review for the U.S. Preventive Services Task Force. Ann Intern Med. 2015;162(3):192–204.

Chapter 18
Gender and Circadian Rhythms in Cardiovascular Function

Björn Lemmer

Introduction

Progress has been made in studying gender-specific differences in the symptoms and treatment of cardiovascular diseases. There is also increasing evidence that mechanisms of regulation of cardiovascular functions are sex-dependent both in animal and in man. However, the data published are still not sufficient to draw final conclusions on whether drug treatment should consider gender-dependency and whether pre- and postmenopausal women should be treated differently.

Clinical Observations

Hypertension, myocardial infarction, and stroke are well-known risk factors influencing the life span of an individual. Ambulatory blood pressure measurements greatly helped not only to better understand mechanisms of blood pressure (BP) and heart rate (HR) regulation, but also gave more insight into the way of antihypertensive treatment. The dipping or non-dipping BP profile greatly determines the choice and the circadian timing of a drug and its application in order not only to reduce elevated BP, but also to normalize a pathological BP profile (see [1–5]). However, there are no data convincingly demonstrating that the 24-h BP pattern is different between male and female persons, in contrast to rats (see below). Conversely, there is overwhelming evidence that BP increases and severity of cardiovascular disease

B. Lemmer, M.D. (✉)
Faculty of Medicine Mannheim, Institute of Experimental & Clinical Pharmacology & Toxicology, Ruprecht-Karls University of Heidelberg,
Maybachstr,14, Mannheim 68169, Germany
e-mail: bjoern.lemmer@medma.uni-heidelberg.de

© Springer International Publishing Switzerland 2016
W.B. White (ed.), *Blood Pressure Monitoring in Cardiovascular Medicine and Therapeutics*, Clinical Hypertension and Vascular Diseases,
DOI 10.1007/978-3-319-22771-9_18

343

are higher in women after menopause than in age-matched men [6–8]. After menopause, women catch up with the higher cardiovascular risk observed in men indicating the important role of sex hormones on vascular functions. The Framingham study has shown that cardiovascular risk factors are increased after menopause when compared to premenopausal women [6].

Importantly however, hormone replacement therapy does not reduce BP in most cases of postmenopausal women [9]. On one hand, this indicates that other factors than the loss of estrogens are involved in higher BP development [9]. On the other hand, an important chronobiological point which has not been challenged by a clinical study to the best of my knowledge: Estrogens are administered to postmenopausal women as *slow release* (e.g., *retard*) formulations, which is not the physiological way these hormones are secreted in premenopausal women; all sex hormones are secreted in a rhythmic fashion, both in a circadian and monthly pattern. It is well-known that the physiological function of a hormone/transmitter can be abolished when these compounds are applied in zero order kinetics and not in their rhythmic pattern. Hence, it would be worthwhile to address such an issue in a clinical study.

It is now well-documented that the vasodilator nitric oxide (NO) plays an important role in regulating the vascular bed. Nitric oxide production occurs in a circadian phase-dependent fashion with peak values in the early afternoon. In healthy men, NO marker molecules such as urinary nitrate and cGMP secretion increase in the morning concomitantly with the morning increase in BP and show peak values in the early afternoon, indicating that NO may buffer the BP increase [10]. In patients with peripheral arterial occlusive disease and in hypertensive patients, these rhythms are abolished and this disturbed rhythmic NO production may contribute to the BP increases [10].

We recently studied in 10 healthy male and female subjects at an age of 21–23 years simultaneously the 24-h BP and HR profiles by ambulatory BP monitoring (ABPM) together with circadian pattern in plasma catecholamines and the nitrate/nitrite (NOx) excretion in urine [11]. The subjects exhibited a normal 24-h profile and there was no gender-dependent differences in the normal BP and HR data [11] (Fig. 18.1).

Concerning the plasma norepinephrine concentrations, however, there was a clear sex-dependent difference, the early morning rise in norepinephrine was significantly steeper in males than in females though both groups were normotensive (Fig. 18.2). In males, this observation could be an early sign of a genetically set greater early morning drive in sympathetic tone, which is often found in white coat hypertensive patients [12].

The sex-dependent difference was even greater for the NOx concentration determined in 6-h portions in the urine over 24 h in male and female subjects (Fig. 18.3). In both groups, NOx concentration displayed a 24-h rhythm with a peak value in the activity phase, similar to the rhythm in nitrate and cGMP secretion described by Bode-Boger et al. [10].

These data clearly demonstrate that at an early age and under normotensive conditions, the important co-regulator of the vascular bed, NO, displays sex-dependent variations with higher values in female subjects, possibly allowing

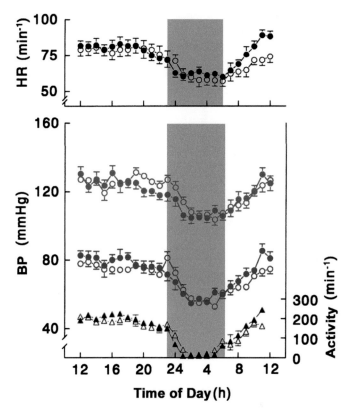

Fig. 18.1 24-h patterns in heart rate (HR) and systolic and diastolic BP (upper/lower BP curve) in ten male (*closed*) and ten female (*open*) healthy volunteers of an age of 21–23 years, motility was registered to control sleep activity. Data from [11] with permission

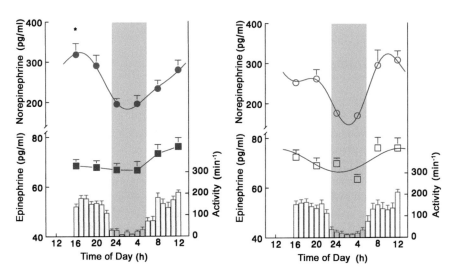

Fig. 18.2 24-h values in plasma norepinephrine and epinephrine concentrations and motility in healthy young (21–23 years) subjects. Figure from [11] with permission

Fig. 18.3 Amount of NOx (nitrate/nitrite) in 6-h portions of urine in 10 female (*filled*) and 11 male (*open*) healthy volunteers. Note: NOx is significantly higher in females than males ($p < 0.05$). Figure from [11] with permission

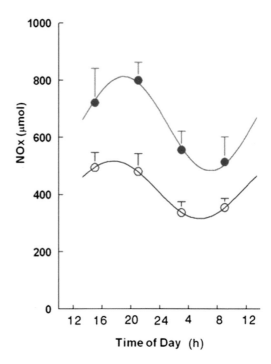

a better buffering capacity for BP changes for females than for males. This observation could contribute to the increasing data that show that the setting of the cardiovascular system is different between males and females. Though the therapeutic consequences are not clear at the moment, future clinical research must concentrate on cardiovascular factors associated with gender in more detail than has been the case in the past.

Data from Animal Experiments

Basic research in the cardiovascular system of experimental animals has been greatly improved by the availability of telemetric blood pressure monitoring devices. They are regarded as the gold standard today allowing in vivo experimentation in freely moving unrestrained animals [13–16], which is not the case for the tail-cuff method [17, 18]. Radiotelemetry also allows a closer look on the rhythmic organization of the cardiovascular system. These clinical experiments in small animals mainly used males. Thus, the data on cardiovascular effects and mechanisms in female rats are sparce. By 1993, we could demonstrate specific circadian rhythms in BP and HR in four different strains of rats, both normotensive and hypertensive [15]. In this study, there was evidence that in a transgenic rat strain (TGR), a dissociation occurred between BP and HR; whereas HR peaked in the activity phase of the animals at night, BP showed peak values in the resting phase during daytime [15], exhibiting a BP pattern known as non-dippers in humans. Thus, this rat strain displayed an internal desychronization concerning BP and HR.

Maris et al. studied by radiotelemerty BP and HR in normotensive Wistar-Kyoto (WKY) and spontaneous hypertensive (SHR) rats [19]. In both strains and in males and females, they show significant daily variations, HR was higher in female WKY than in all other groups, and male SHR had higher systolic BP than the females [19]. Very similar to these findings, we describe that under control conditions of 12:12 h of light and darkness, the HR was higher in pro-estrous females than in age-mached male SHRs, whereas BP was inversely higher in males than in females [20] (Fig. 18.4). Urinary NO excretion was about threefold higher in female than in male SHR with peak value in the dark span [20]. Additionally, eNOS expression in the aortae of females was significantly higher than in males (relative expression 42.9 ± 7.3 vs. 25.2 ± 1.0, $p < 0.05$), indicating that elevated NOx excretion in females in comparison to males is linked to higher eNOS expression [20]. The beta-receptor blocking drug metoprolol was also more effective in decreasing HR and BP in females than in males. These animal data greatly support the notion that sex-dependent variations have to be taken into account as they contribute to the regulation and drug effectiveness within the cardiovascular system, both in animal and in humans.

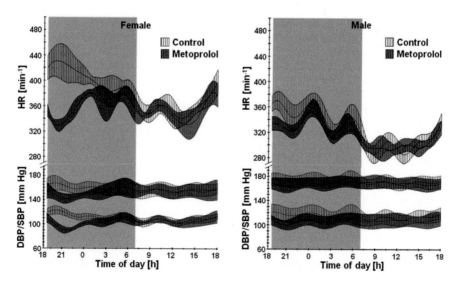

Fig. 18.4 Heart rate, systolic and diastolic BP after intraperitoneal application of 30 mg/kg MET at 19.00 h to female ($n = 7$) and male SHR ($n = 13$). Shown are mean values ± 95 % confidence intervals. The dark period is highlighted. Data from [20] with permission

Conclusion

There is increasing evidence that cardiovascular factors are associated with sex and sex-related modifications within circadian systems. Unfortunately, both in clinical studies and in basic research, mainly male subjects and animals have been studied in the past. In light of recent data that women and female animals use different mechanisms of regulation in the cardiovascular system and may differ in drug sensitivity and drug effectiveness [6, 21–23], future research should focus more on females in clinical research.

References

1. White WB. Utilizing ambulatory blood pressure recordings to evaluate antihypertensive drug therapy. Am J Cardiol. 1992;69(13):E8–12.
2. White WB, LaRocca GM. Chronopharmacology of cardiovascular therapy. Blood Press Monit. 2002;7(4):199–207.
3. Smolensky MH, Hermida RC, Ayala DE, Tiseo R, Portaluppi F. Administration-time-dependent effects of blood pressure-lowering medications: basis for the chronotherapy of hypertension. Blood Press Monit. 2010;15(4):173–80.
4. Lemmer B. Chronobiology and chronopharmacology of hypertension: importance of timing of dosing. In: White WB, editor. Blood pressure monitoring in cardiovascular medicine and therapeutics. 2nd ed. Totowa, NY: Humana Press; 2007. p. 410–35.
5. Portaluppi F, Lemmer B. Chronobiology and chronotherapy of ischemic heart disease. Adv Drug Deliv Rev. 2007;59(9-10):952–65.
6. Kannel WB, Hjortland MC, McNamara PM, Gordon T. Menopause and risk of cardiovascular disease: the Framingham study. Ann Intern Med. 1976;85(4):447–52.
7. Dubey RK, Oparil S, Imthurn B, Jackson EK. Sex hormones and hypertension. Cardiovasc Res. 2002;53(3):688–708.
8. Safar ME, Smulyan H. Hypertension in women. Am J Hypertens. 2004;17(1):82–7.
9. Reckelhoff JF. Gender differences in the regulation of blood pressure. Hypertension. 2001;37(5):1199–208.
10. Bode-Boger SM, Boger RH, Kielstein JT, Loffler M, Schaffer J, Frolich JC. Role of endogenous nitric oxide in circadian blood pressure regulation in healthy humans and in patients with hypertension or atherosclerosis. J Invest Med. 2000;48(2):125–32.
11. Lemmer B. The importance of biological rhythms in drug treatment of hypertension and sex-dependent modifications. Chron Physiol Ther. 2012;2:9–18.
12. Middeke M, Lemmer B. Office hypertension: abnormal blood pressure regulation and increased sympathetic activity compared with normotension. Blood Press Monit. 1996; 1:403–7.
13. Brockway BP, Mills PA, Azar SH. A new method for continuous chronic measurement and recording of blood pressure, heart rate and activity in the rat via radio-telemetry. Clin Exp Hypertens A. 1991;13(5):885–95.
14. Lemmer B, Mattes A. Evaluation of the dose-response relationship and circadian phase-dependency of antihypertensive drugs in normotensive and hypertensive rats by use of telemetry. Baltic Meeting on Pharmacology; Vilnius, Litauen, Abstr pp. 57–58; 1992.
15. Lemmer B, Mattes A, Bohm M, Ganten D. Circadian blood pressure variation in transgenic hypertensive rats. Hypertension. 1993;22(1):97–101.

16. van den Buuse M. Circadian rhythms of blood pressure, heart rate, and locomotor activity in spontaneously hypertensive rats as measured with radio-telemetry. Physiol Behav. 1994;55(4):783–7.
17. Abu-Taha I, Lemmer B. Superiority of radiotelemetry over the tail-cuff method in evaluating control and drug-induced values in cardiovascular functions in rats. Naunyn-Schmiedeberg's Arch Pharmacol. 2007;375 Suppl 1:R313.
18. Grundt A, Grundt C, Gorbey S, Thomas MA, Lemmer B. Strain-dependent differences of restraint stress-induced hypertension in WKY and SHR. Physiol Behav. 2009;97(3–4):341–6.
19. Maris ME, Melchert RB, Joseph J, Kennedy RH. Gender differences in blood pressure and heart rate in spontaneously hypertensive and Wistar-Kyoto rats. Clin Exp Pharmacol Physiol. 2005;32(1–2):35–9.
20. Grundt C, Meier K, Lemmer B. Gender dependency of circadian blood pressure and heart rate profiles in spontaneously hypertensive rats: effects of beta-blockers. Chronobiol Int. 2006;23(4):813–29.
21. Mendelsohn ME, Karas RH. Molecular and cellular basis of cardiovascular gender differences. Science. 2005;308(5728):1583–7.
22. Hermida RC, Ayala DE, Mojon A, Fontao MJ, Chayan L, Fernandez JR. Differences between men and women in ambulatory blood pressure thresholds for diagnosis of hypertension based on cardiovascular outcomes. Chronobiol Int. 2013;30(1–2):221–32.
23. Meyer MR, Haas E, Barton M. Gender differences of cardiovascular disease: new perspectives for estrogen receptor signaling. Hypertension. 2006;47(6):1019–26.

Part IV
Applications of Out-of-Office Blood Pressure Monitoring

Chapter 19
Home (Self) Monitoring of Blood Pressure in Clinical Trials

George S. Stergiou and Angeliki Ntineri

Introduction

Although the conventional measurement of blood pressure by the doctor in the office remains the cornerstone for the diagnosis and management of hypertension worldwide, it is recognized that this method can be misleading and evaluation of blood pressure out of the office using 24-h ambulatory or self-home monitoring by patients is often necessary for optimal decision making. The limitations of conventional office blood pressure measurement have a strong impact on the precision of hypertension clinical trials, which can be considerably improved by the application of out-of-office blood pressure monitoring. This chapter presents the features of self-home blood pressure monitoring (HBPM) that are important for the design of clinical trials and how they can be applied in hypertension research (Table 19.1).

Advantages of Self-Home Blood Pressure Monitoring

HBPM has the unique advantage of providing multiple readings obtained over several days, weeks, or months, in the individual's usual environment. On the contrary, office or clinic blood pressure measurement provides only few readings taken in an artificial and potentially stressful setting. Twenty-four hour ambulatory blood pressure monitoring (ABPM) also provides multiple measurements away from the office, yet these are crowded during a single day and cannot be frequently repeated. Because of these features, HBPM, as well as ABPM, are

G.S. Stergiou, M.D. (✉) • A. Ntineri, M.D.
Third University Department of Medicine, Hypertension Center STRIDE-7, Sotiria Hospital,
152 Mesogion Avenue, Athens 11527, Greece
e-mail: gstergi@med.uoa.gr

© Springer International Publishing Switzerland 2016
W.B. White (ed.), *Blood Pressure Monitoring in Cardiovascular Medicine
and Therapeutics*, Clinical Hypertension and Vascular Diseases,
DOI 10.1007/978-3-319-22771-9_19

Table 19.1 Advantages of home blood pressure compared to office and ambulatory blood pressure in clinical trial design

	HBP	OBP	ABP
Reproducibility, study power, and sample size	+++	+	+++
Exclusion of white coat hypertension	+++	−	+++
Observer bias elimination	+++ (automated devices or tele-monitoring)	+	+++
Placebo effect elimination	+++	−	+++
Assessment of magnitude of BP changes	+++	+	+++
Assessment of duration of antihypertensive drug action	++	+	+++
Time-course of BP lowering effect (days)	++	+	−
Assessment of homogeneity of antihypertensive drug action (smoothness index)	−	−	+++
Assessment of morning hypertension	+++	+	+++
Assessment of nocturnal hypertension—detection of non-dippers	++ (devices which monitor asleep BP)	−	+++
Identification of masked uncontrolled hypertension	+++	−	+++
Diagnosis of true resistant hypertension	++	+	+++
Assessment of short-term variability	−	−	++
Assessment of mid-term variability	++	−	−
Assessment of long-term variability	++	++	+
Association with preclinical organ damage	+++	+	+++
Assessment of arterial stiffness	−	−	++ (AASI)
Assessment of treatment-induced changes in organ damage	++	+	+++
Association with cardiovascular events risk	+++	+	+++
Compliance with drug treatment	+++	+	+
Patients' preference	+++	+	+
Repeated monitoring in longitudinal trials	+++	++	+
Cost	+++	++	+

BP blood pressure, *HBP* home BP, *OBP* office BP, *ABP* ambulatory BP, *AASI* ambulatory arterial stiffness index, +++ superior, − inferior

devoid of several major deficiencies of the conventional office measurements, including white coat effect (WCE), masked hypertension effect, the placebo effect, and observer prejudice and bias (when using automated electronic devices for home monitoring) [1, 2].

Because of the above mentioned advantages, HBPM has superior diagnostic accuracy and reproducibility than office measurements, with the standard deviation of the mean difference between two measurements being much lower than that achieved with casual office measurements (Fig. 19.1) [3]. More importantly,

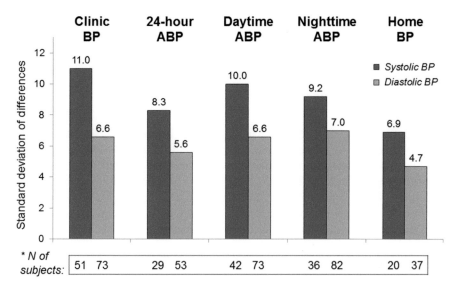

Fig. 19.1 Reproducibility of clinic, ambulatory, and home blood pressure, and sample size required for a comparative parallel design clinical trial of two antihypertensive drugs using each method (modified from [3]). *BP* blood pressure, *ABP* ambulatory BP, *N* number, *Asterisk,* required for a trial aiming to detect a difference in the effect of two drugs of 10 mmHg systolic or 5 mmHg diastolic BP with 0.90 power and 0.05 significance level

HBPM provides reliable predictive information, with strong associations with indices of preclinical organ damage and risk of cardiovascular events, which are superior to those obtained by office measurements and similar to those by ABPM [4–6].

Another advantage of HBPM is that it entails less discomfort and minimal restriction of daily activities and sleep, and therefore is more acceptable by patients than ambulatory monitoring [7, 8]. Thus, HBPM appears to be the optimal method for long-term follow-up of treated hypertension and has been shown to improve compliance with drug treatment and thereby hypertension control rates [9]. Last but not the least, HBPM not only can provide reliable guidance in treatment initiation and adjustment, but it can also be a more affordable choice for hypertension management in the community, since the cost of applying the method for treatment decision, titration, and follow-up appears to be lower than when using conventional office measurements complemented by ABPM [2, 10–13].

Self-Home Blood Pressure Monitoring in Clinical Research

The advantages of HBPM compared to conventional office measurements have important implications in clinical research. HBPM improves the sensitivity and accuracy of clinical trials and allows for the evaluation of additional aspects of the blood pressure profile and behavior at baseline and in response to blood pressure lowering interventions.

Subject Selection for Clinical Trials

The selection of appropriate study participants with homogenous characteristics is of vital importance for clinical research. By using HBPM instead of office measurements, a hypertension phenotype is accurately defined and subjects with intermediate phenotypes, such as white coat or masked hypertension, can be identified and excluded [14–16]. Subjects with white coat hypertension (WCH) show minimal response to antihypertensive drug treatment compared to sustained hypertensives [17] and may create diluting effects in the assessment of reductions in blood pressure.

Studies of resistant hypertension, defined as uncontrolled blood pressure on triple antihypertensive drug therapy, demonstrated the importance of using ABPM or HBPM for the exclusion of the WCH, which is common even among treated subjects [18]. Recent studies assessing the effectiveness of renal denervation have clearly demonstrated the importance of out-of-office blood pressure monitoring for the reliable diagnosis of resistant hypertension [19].

Moreover, because of its superior reproducibility, HBPM as well as ABPM provides a more accurate classification of the true baseline blood pressure of an individual.

Sample Size and Study Power

The reproducibility of a blood pressure measurement method, expressed as the standard deviation of differences, is an important factor in the calculation of the sample size required for a clinical trial. Because of its superior reproducibility (Fig. 19.1), HBPM as well as ABPM when used in a clinical trial comparing the antihypertensive efficacy of two drugs allow the same difference in blood pressure lowering effect to be identified with higher precision [3]. Alternatively, HBPM and ABPM allow a smaller sample size to be recruited in order to identify a difference in the blood pressure lowering effect of two drugs with the same study power (Fig. 19.1) [20–23].

The power curves of a randomized cross-over clinical trial comparing the antihypertensive efficacy of two drugs using clinic, ambulatory, or home blood pressure measurements are shown in Fig. 19.2 [24]. According to these data, for a trial aiming to detect a difference in the hypotensive effect of the drugs of 10 mmHg for systolic blood pressure, 5 mmHg for diastolic, or 3 mmHg for pulse pressure, the study power is much higher when using HBPM and ABPM instead of office measurements (Fig. 19.2) [24].

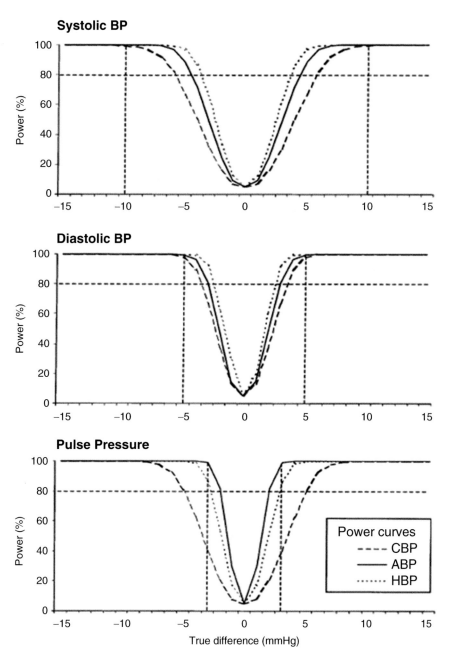

Fig. 19.2 Study power curves of a randomized crossover clinical trial comparing the efficacy of two antihypertensive drugs using blood pressure measurements in the clinic, at home, and with ambulatory monitoring (from [24]). *BP* blood pressure, *CBP* clinic BP, *ABP* 24-h ambulatory BP, *HBP* home BP, *Horizontal dotted lines* indicate 80 % power to detect a difference in the hypotensive effect of the drugs of 10 mmHg for systolic, 5 mmHg for diastolic BP, or 3 mmHg for pulse pressure (*vertical dotted lines*)

Assessment of Magnitude of Antihypertensive Drug Action

Because of its superior reproducibility, HBPM allows for the identification of anti-hypertensive drug treatment-induced blood pressure changes with greater precision and without the placebo effect, which largely affect clinical trials using clinic blood pressure measurements [25]. A randomized parallel design-controlled study, which evaluated the antihypertensive efficacy of the angiotensin converting enzyme inhibitor trandolapril versus placebo, showed no difference in blood pressure lowering effect compared to placebo when clinic measurements were used [26]. However, a significant placebo-corrected blood pressure lowering effect was observed when HBPM was employed (Fig. 19.3) [26]. Another randomized parallel design clinical trial comparing the beta-blocker bisoprolol with the calcium channel blocker nitrendipine found no difference in the antihypertensive effect of these two drugs when clinic or daytime ambulatory blood pressure was used, whereas self-home and daytime ambulatory blood pressure measurements demonstrated a significantly larger effect with bisoprolol (Fig. 19.4) [21]. For this particular study to have the sensitivity to identify a 10 mmHg difference between the effects of the two drugs on systolic blood pressure, at total of 118 subjects would be required if clinic blood pressure measurement were used, compared to 70 with ABPM and 56 with HBPM [21].

Another randomized cross-over clinical trial comparing the antihypertensive efficacy of the angiotensin converting enzyme inhibitor lisinopril with the angiotensin receptor blocker losartan showed that although all the blood pressure measurement methods (clinic, ambulatory, and home) suggested that lisinopril was more effective (Fig. 19.5), the difference between the two drugs was demonstrated with greater precision using HBPM ($p < 0.001$) than 24-h ABPM ($p < 0.01$), and the poorest precision for demonstrating this difference was provided by clinic measurements

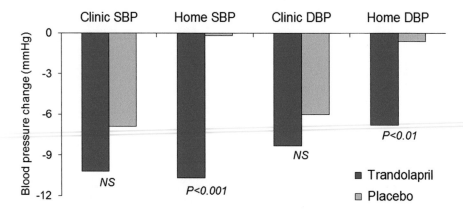

Fig. 19.3 Evaluation of the antihypertensive efficacy of a drug in a parallel design placebo controlled clinical trial using clinic or home systolic (SBP) and diastolic blood pressure (DBP) measurements (modified from [26])

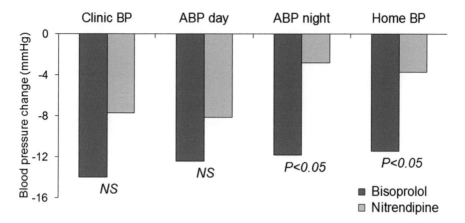

Fig. 19.4 Comparison of the antihypertensive efficacy of two drugs in a parallel design clinical trial using clinic, ambulatory, and home blood pressure measurements (modified from [21]). *BP* blood pressure, *ABP* ambulatory BP

($p<0.05$) [24]. Lisinopril was also found to be more effective in reducing home pulse pressure ($p<0.01$) and 24-h ambulatory pulse pressure ($p<0.03$), whereas no such difference was detected using clinic measurements (Fig. 19.5) [24].

These data clearly demonstrate that the use of HBPM increases the sensitivity and precision of clinical trials assessing the efficacy of antihypertensive drug action. The benefits of HBPM are attributed to its superior reproducibility, the absence of the placebo effect, the regression dilution bias (regression to the mean), and the observer prejudice and bias (when electronic devices with automated memory are used), all of which limit the reliability of clinical trials based on clinic blood pressure measurements.

Assessment of Duration of Antihypertensive Drug Action

The duration of antihypertensive action and 24-h coverage are usually assessed using the trough-to-peak ratio (T/P), which is based on 24-h ambulatory or on clinic blood pressure measurements [27]. The morning-to-evening (M/E) home blood pressure ratio assessed by self-monitoring can provide information of the "trough" effect of the drug by obtaining morning measurements before drug intake and the "plateau" effect in the evening [28]. Studies have shown that the M/E home blood pressure ratio might be a useful alternative to the T/P ambulatory blood pressure ratio for assessing the duration of antihypertensive drug action [29–31]. A randomized clinical trial that compared the duration of the antihypertensive drug action of the angiotensin converting enzyme inhibitor lisinopril with the angiotensin receptor blocker losartan showed higher T/P and M/E blood pressure ratios (evaluated by ABPM and HBPM respectively) with lisinopril, which was consistent when the

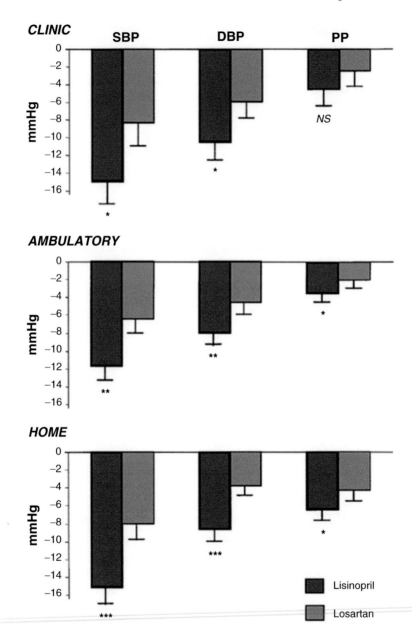

Fig. 19.5 Randomized crossover comparative clinical trial of the effects of two antihypertensive drugs on clinic, 24-h ambulatory, and home blood pressure (from [24]). SBP, systolic blood pressure; DBP, diastolic blood pressure; PP, pulse pressure; *, $p < 0.05$; **, $p < 0.01$; ***, $p < 0.001$ for differences between the two drugs)

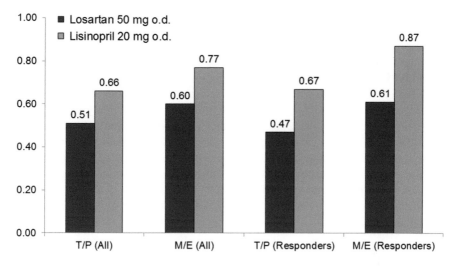

Fig. 19.6 Morning-to-evening (M/E) home blood pressure ratio versus trough-to-peak (T/P) ambulatory blood pressure ratio for assessing the duration of antihypertensive effect of two drugs in all study subjects and in those who responded to treatment (modified from [29])

analysis was restricted to subjects with significant blood pressure response to treatment (Fig. 19.6) [29].

A similar mathematical expression is the difference between morning and evening home blood pressure values (morning-evening difference), which has been shown to be a significant determinant of echocardiographic left ventricular hypertrophy (LVH), geometry, and diastolic function [32]. It should be mentioned, however, that the M/E home blood pressure ratio does not provide information on the peak effect of treatment and might therefore fail to identify an excessive hypotensive effect at peak.

Evaluation of Nocturnal Blood Pressure and Detection of Non-dippers

ABPM is regarded as a unique tool, because it allows the evaluation of blood pressure during nighttime sleep and thereby the detection of non-dippers. This advantage appears to have major clinical relevance because of the accumulating evidence suggesting that, compared to other aspects of the blood pressure profile, nocturnal blood pressure is the strongest predictor of cardiovascular risk. Non-dippers have demonstrated a higher risk of preclinical organ damage and cardiovascular events than dippers [33].

Advancement in technology of automated home blood pressure monitors provided the ability to obtain automated readings throughout nighttime sleep [34].

There is evidence that nocturnal home monitoring gives reproducible blood pressure values [34]. A cross-sectional study showed similar daytime and nighttime blood pressure levels assessed with home and ambulatory blood pressure and good agreement between the two methods in diagnosing non-dippers [35]. More importantly, these devices can provide nocturnal blood pressure evaluation for more than a single 24-h period, which is the case with ambulatory monitoring. The Japan Morning Surge—Home Blood Pressure (J-HOP) Study showed that automated asleep home blood pressure evaluated three times per night for at least two (average 9) nights gave comparable blood pressure values with nighttime ambulatory blood pressure [36]. More importantly, nocturnal systolic home blood pressure was more closely associated with indices of cardiac and renal organ damage than nocturnal ambulatory blood pressure [36]. Ishikawa et al. also reported significant association of nighttime home blood pressure with hypertensive target organ damage [37].

Thus, HBPM appears to be a useful alternative to ABPM even for the evaluation of nocturnal hypertension and might be more appropriate for the evaluation of treatment-induced changes in nocturnal blood pressure in clinical trials, because it can provide multiple assessments on different days and at lower cost.

Assessment of Treatment-Induced Effects on Blood Pressure Variability

HBPM is a useful tool for the evaluation of the effect of antihypertensive treatment on mid-term, day-by-day blood pressure variability. Analysis of the variation of home measurements allows the evaluation of differential effects of antihypertensive drugs on day-by-day blood pressure variability. More specifically, studies based on self-home measurements have shown that treatment with beta-blockers leads to greater home blood pressure variability, whereas alpha-blockers lower the variability [38]. Another study suggested that treatment with an angiotensin receptor blocker was associated with higher systolic home blood pressure variability compared to treatment with a calcium channel blocker [39]. Moreover, the addition of a calcium channel blocker on an angiotensin receptor blocker was shown to decrease home blood pressure variability to a greater extent than the addition of a thiazide [40]. In addition, self-home monitoring explores blood pressure behavior over time, by assessing the mid- and long-term aspects of blood pressure variability, which are currently suggested to provide additional information, independently associated with common study endpoints such as indices of subclinical target organ damage or cardiovascular events and mortality [38, 41–43].

Treatment-induced changes in home blood pressure variability have been suggested to independently correlate with regression of organ damage. Matsui et al. reported that a 6-month change in pulse wave velocity achieved using a two-drug combination treatment (angiotensin receptor blocker and calcium channel blocker) was independently associated with the corresponding change in systolic home blood pressure variability [40], whereas another study showed that the decrease in urinary albumin excretion was not associated with that of home blood pressure variability after 6-month treatment with a combination of an angiotensin receptor blocker with a thiazide diuretic [44].

Assessment of Treatment-Induced Effects on Organ Damage and Events

Several studies have shown that self-home blood pressure measurements are superior to office measurement and as good as ambulatory monitoring in terms of their association with several indices of preclinical target organ damage [6]. Clinical trials designed to investigate treatment-induced regression of target organ damage in association with blood pressure changes require long-term follow-up in order to observe the beneficial effects on the heart, arteries, and kidneys. In such conditions, HBPM appears to be a reliable and convenient tool to track blood pressure changes. A study in 116 hypertensives with 13.4 months follow-up showed that treatment-induced changes in self-home or ambulatory blood pressure were more closely related than office measurements with treatment-induced changes in organ damage (echocardiographic left ventricular mass index, pulse wave velocity, albuminuria) [45]. The Study on Ambulatory Monitoring of Blood Pressure and Lisinopril Evaluation (SAMPLE) in 206 hypertensives followed for 12 months reported that treatment-induced regression in LVH was more closely associated with treatment-induced changes in ambulatory than in clinic or home blood pressure measurements [46]. However, only two home readings were obtained, which has considerably limited the reliability of the method.

A more ambitious approach for exploring long-term treatment effects by HBPM is the investigation of more complex endpoints, including cardiovascular events. The Home blood pressure measurement with Olmesartan Naive patients to Establish Standard Target blood pressure (HONEST) study established the prognostic value of home blood pressure by identifying its threshold for the risk of major cardiovascular events over 2 years of treatment with an angiotensin receptor blocker-based regimen (olmesartan) even in subjects with controlled office blood pressure [47].

Assessment of Other Aspects of the Blood Pressure Profile and Behavior

There is increasing interest on morning hypertension which appears to be related with morning blood pressure surge or follows a non-dipping status or nocturnal hypertension [48–50]. Studies have shown that morning hypertension has independent prognostic significance for target organ damage and stroke [49]. There is evidence that morning HBPM and ABPM have considerable similarity and diagnostic agreement and therefore appear to be interchangeable methods for the assessment of morning hypertension [50]. An important advantage of morning home compared to ambulatory blood pressure measurement is that morning readings at home are taken under more standardized conditions of environment, activity, and posture (seated at home). In addition, they are based on measurements taken over several days, compared to a single day with ambulatory monitoring. Since treated patients' measurements are taken before drug intake, they are truly trough measurements [48]. Therefore, recent studies attempted to test treatment-induced effects on elevated morning blood pressure levels by using self-home monitoring. Redon et al. reported that telmisartan alone or with hydrochlorothiazide improved morning home blood pressure control and maintained a smooth home blood pressure profile throughout the day [51]. Similar results were obtained by Kario et al. in the HONEST Study using an olmesartan-based regimen [52].

HBPM has also been used in chronotherapy studies, which explored the optimal time of drug administration in relation to blood pressure levels, organ damage, and adverse effects [53–55]. Mori et al. showed that olmesartan effectively decreased morning home blood pressure and urinary albumin-to-creatinine ratio, regardless of whether the drug was administered in the morning or in the evening [53]. Moreover, Mengden et al. found that the time of once-a-day amlodipine administration did not influence its efficacy for 24-h blood pressure control assessed by home monitoring [55]. In contrast, Hashimotto et al. reported that bedtime administration of the centrally acting alpha$_2$-agonists effectively suppressed elevated morning blood pressure in treated hypertensives [54].

Another research question investigated by HBPM is the time of maximum antihypertensive effect, which was evaluated by determining the velocity of hypotensive effect using exponential decay function analysis based on serial home blood pressure measurements [56, 57].

Since HBPM is well-accepted by hypertensive patients for repeated long-term use and preferred to ABPM, this method appears to be appropriate for long-term follow-up of blood pressure changes in longitudinal hypertension outcome trials [7, 8]. Thus, the need for frequent office visits can be reduced, which is convenient for both patients and researchers and is potentially more cost-effective. This application is also supported by evidence showing improvement of patients' compliance with drug treatment when using HBPM [9].

Limitations of Self-Home Blood Pressure Monitoring

Although HBPM overcomes certain important limitations of office and ABPM, a major drawback that is often neglected is the "reporting bias" (over- or under-reporting of self-measurements by patients), which has been characterized as the

"Achilles's heel" of the method [58]. Several studies have documented that the reporting bias of self-home measurements is common and can lead to under- and overdiagnosis of hypertension. Unless this bias is prevented, home measurement should not be used as endpoints in hypertension research. The use of validated electronic home monitors with automated memory and capacity to export the readings, or of home blood pressure tele-monitoring systems, can prevent this bias. Another problem of self-home monitoring is due to the spontaneous blood pressure variability, which can cause anxiety to some individuals and lead to self-modification of treatment and study protocol violation. Most of these cases can be prevented or efficiently managed with careful training and consultation with the clinical researcher.

Home Blood Pressure Tele-monitoring

Current technological advances and increasing use of tele-communications make home-blood pressure tele-monitoring a promising twenty-first century solution, which allows prompt collection and unbiased assessment of blood pressure data, especially in remote or special populations, or high-risk populations with a need for closer and more regular blood pressure monitoring and tight control of hypertension. Home blood pressure tele-monitoring is also ideal for long-term in-treatment follow-up of antihypertensive drug trials and has been shown to be more expensive, yet a more cost-effective strategy for blood pressure monitoring [59]. Tele-medicine systems based on home measurements have been used in clinical trials comparing the effects of antihypertensive drugs on the diurnal variation and blood pressure variability of home blood pressure [60].

Conclusions

The use of HBPM has important advantages in clinical hypertension research. Its application improves the sensitivity and precision of clinical trials of antihypertensive drug efficacy and increases the study power or decreases the sample size required. Moreover, self-home monitoring allows for the investigation of additional research aspects of the blood pressure profile and behavior, such as the duration of antihypertensive drug effect, morning and nocturnal hypertension, blood pressure variability, treatment-induced changes in organ damage, and cardiovascular risk. Furthermore, home blood pressure tele-monitoring provides a modern and reliable solution for the unbiased evaluation of long-term treatment-induced blood pressure changes.

References

1. Parati G, Stergiou GS, Asmar R, et al.; ESH Working Group on Blood Pressure Monitoring. European Society of Hypertension guidelines for blood pressure monitoring at home: a summary report of the Second International Consensus Conference on Home Blood Pressure Monitoring. J Hypertens. 2008;26:1505–26.
2. Stergiou GS, Kollias A, Zeniodi M, Karpettas N, Ntineri A. Home blood pressure monitoring: primary role in hypertension management. Curr Hypertens Rep. 2014;16:462.
3. Stergiou GS, Baibas NM, Gantzarou AP, et al. Reproducibility of home, ambulatory, and clinic blood pressure: implications for the design of trials for the assessment of antihypertensive drug efficacy. Am J Hypertens. 2002;15:101–4.
4. Stergiou GS, Siontis KC, Ioannidis JP. Home blood pressure as a cardiovascular outcome predictor: it's time to take this method seriously. Hypertension. 2010;55:1301–3.
5. Ward AM, Takahashi O, Stevens R, Heneghan C. Home measurement of blood pressure and cardiovascular disease: systematic review and meta-analysis of prospective studies. J Hypertens. 2012;30:449–56.
6. Bliziotis IA, Destounis A, Stergiou GS. Home versus ambulatory and office blood pressure in predicting target organ damage in hypertension: a systematic review and meta-analysis. J Hypertens. 2012;30:1289–99.
7. Nasothimiou EG, Karpettas N, Dafni MG, Stergiou GS. Patients' preference for ambulatory versus home blood pressure monitoring. J Hum Hypertens. 2014;28:224–9.
8. Little P, Barnett J, Barnsley L, Marjoram J, Fitzgerald-Barron A, Mant D. Comparison of acceptability of and preferences for different methods of measuring blood pressure in primary care. Br Med J. 2002;325:358–9.
9. Ogedegbe G, Schoenthaler A. A systematic review of the effects of home blood pressure monitoring on medication adherence. J Clin Hypertens (Greenwich). 2006;8:174–80.
10. Stergiou GS, Karpettas N, Destounis A, et al. Home blood pressure monitoring alone vs. combined clinic and ambulatory measurements in following treatment-induced changes in blood pressure and organ damage. Am J Hypertens. 2014;27:184–92.
11. Asayama K, Ohkubo T, Metoki H, et al.; Hypertension Objective Treatment Based on Measurement by Electrical Devices of Blood Pressure (HOMED-BP). Cardiovascular outcomes in the first trial of antihypertensive therapy guided by self-measured home blood pressure. Hypertens Res. 2012;35:1102–10.
12. Staessen JA, Den Hond E, Celis H, et al.; Treatment of Hypertension Based on Home or Office Blood Pressure (THOP) Trial Investigators. Antihypertensive treatment based on blood pressure measurement at home or in the physician's office: a randomized controlled trial. JAMA. 2004;291:955–64.
13. Boubouchairopoulou N, Karpettas N, Athanasakis K, et al. Cost estimation of hypertension management based on home blood pressure monitoring alone or combined office and ambulatory blood pressure measurements. J Am Soc Hypertens. 2014;8:732–8.
14. Nasothimiou EG, Tzamouranis D, Rarra V, Roussias LG, Stergiou GS. Diagnostic accuracy of home vs. ambulatory blood pressure monitoring in untreated and treated hypertension. Hypertens Res. 2012;35:750–5.
15. Stergiou GS, Zourbaki AS, Skeva II, Mountokalakis TD. White coat effect detected using self-monitoring of blood pressure at home: comparison with ambulatory blood pressure. Am J Hypertens. 1998;11:820–7.
16. Stergiou GS, Efstathiou SP, Argyraki CK, Roussias LG, Mountokalakis TD. White coat effect in treated versus untreated hypertensive individuals: a case-control study using ambulatory and home blood pressure monitoring. Am J Hypertens. 2004;17:124–8.
17. Mancia G, Facchetti R, Parati G, Zanchetti A. Effect of long-term antihypertensive treatment on white-coat hypertension. Hypertension. 2014;64:1388–98.
18. Nasothimiou EG, Tzamouranis D, Roussias LG, Stergiou GS. Home versus ambulatory blood pressure monitoring in the diagnosis of clinic resistant and true resistant hypertension. J Hum Hypertens. 2012;26:696–700.

19. Bhatt DL, Kandzari DE, O'Neill WW, et al.; SYMPLICITY HTN-3 Investigators. A controlled trial of renal denervation for resistant hypertension. N Engl J Med. 2014;370:1393–401.
20. Altman DG. Statistics and ethics in medical research: how large a sample? Br Med J. 1980;281:1336–8.
21. Mengden T, Binswanger B, Weisser B, Vetter W. An evaluation of self-measured blood pressure in a study with a calcium-channel antagonist versus a beta-blocker. Am J Hypertens. 1992;5:154–60.
22. Mengden T, Battig B, Vetter W. Self-measurement of blood pressure improves the accuracy and reduces the number of subjects in clinical trials. J Hypertens. 1991;9(suppl 6): S336–7.
23. Stergiou GS, Efstathiou SP, Argyraki CK, Gantzarou AP, Roussias LG, Mountokalakis TD. Clinic, home and ambulatory pulse pressure: comparison and reproducibility. J Hypertens. 2002;20:1987–93.
24. Stergiou GS, Efstathiou SP, Skeva II, Baibas NM, Kalkana CB, Mountokalakis TD. Assessment of drug effects on blood pressure and pulse pressure using clinic, home and ambulatory measurements. J Hum Hypertens. 2002;16:729–35.
25. Chatellier G, Day M, Bobrie G, Menard J. Feasibility study of N-of-1 trials with blood pressure self-monitoring in hypertension. Hypertension. 1995;25:294–301.
26. Vaur L, Dubroca II, Dutrey-Dupagne C, et al. Superiority of home blood pressure measurements over office measurements for testing antihypertensive drugs. Blood Press Monit. 1998;3:107–14.
27. Meredith PA. How to evaluate the duration of blood pressure control: the trough:peak ratio and 24-hour monitoring. J Cardiovasc Pharmacol. 1998;31(suppl 2):S17–21.
28. Menard J, Chatellier G, Day M, Vaur L. Self-measurement of blood pressure at home to evaluate drug effects by the trough:peak ratio. J Hypertens Suppl. 1994;12:S21–5.
29. Stergiou GS, Efstathiou SP, Skeva II, Baibas NM, Roussias LG, Mountokalakis TD. Comparison of the smoothness index, the trough:peak ratio and the morning:evening ratio in assessing the features of the antihypertensive drug effect. J Hypertens. 2003;21:913–20.
30. Zannad F, Vaur L, Dutrey-Dupagne C, et al. Assessment of drug efficacy using home self-blood pressure measurement: the SMART study. Self Measurement for the Assessment of the Response to Trandolapril. J Hum Hypertens. 1996;10:341–7.
31. Nishimura T, Hashimoto J, Ohkubo T, et al. Efficacy and duration of action of the four selective angiotensin II subtype 1 receptor blockers, losartan, candesartan, valsartan and telmisartan, in patients with essential hypertension determined by home blood pressure measurements. Clin Exp Hypertens. 2005;27:477–89.
32. Matsui Y, Eguchi K, Shibasaki S, et al. Association between the morning-evening difference in home blood pressure and cardiac damage in untreated hypertensive patients. J Hypertens. 2009;27:712–20.
33. Hansen TW, Li Y, Boggia J, Thijs L, Richart T, Staessen JA. Predictive role of the night-time blood pressure. Hypertension. 2011;57:3–10.
34. Hosohata K, Kikuya M, Ohkubo T, et al. Reproducibility of nocturnal blood pressure assessed by self-measurement of blood pressure at home. Hypertens Res. 2007;30:707–12.
35. Stergiou GS, Nasothimiou EG, Destounis A, Poulidakis E, Evagelou I, Tzamouranis D. Assessment of the diurnal blood pressure profile and detection of non-dippers based on home or ambulatory monitoring. Am J Hypertens. 2012;25:974–8.
36. Hoshide S, Kario K, Yano Y, et al. J-HOP Study Group. Association of morning and evening blood pressure at home with asymptomatic organ damage in the J-HOP Study. Am J Hypertens. 2014;27:939–47.
37. Ishikawa J, Hoshide S, Eguchi K, Ishikawa S, Shimada K, Kario K. Nighttime home blood pressure and the risk of hypertensive target organ damage. Hypertension. 2012;60: 921–8.
38. Stergiou GS, Ntineri A, Kollias A, Ohkubo T, Imai Y, Parati G. Blood pressure variability assessed by home measurements: a systematic review. Hypertens Res. 2014;37: 565–72.

39. Ishikura K, Obara T, Kato T, et al. J-HOME-Morning Study Group. Associations between day-by-day variability in blood pressure measured at home and antihypertensive drugs: the J-HOME-Morning study. Clin Exp Hypertens. 2012;34:297–304.
40. Matsui Y, O'Rourke MF, Hoshide S, Ishikawa J, Shimada K, Kario K. Combined effect of angiotensin II receptor blocker and either a calcium channel blocker or diuretic on day-by-day variability of home blood pressure: the Japan Combined Treatment With Olmesartan and a Calcium-Channel Blocker Versus Olmesartan and Diuretics Randomized Efficacy Study. Hypertension. 2012;59:1132–8.
41. Asayama K, Kikuya M, Schutte R, et al. Home blood pressure variability as cardiovascular risk factor in the population of Ohasama. Hypertension. 2013;61:61–9.
42. Okada T, Matsumoto H, Nagaoka Y, Nakao T. Association of home blood pressure variability with progression of chronic kidney disease. Blood Press Monit. 2012;17:1–7.
43. Johansson JK, Niiranen TJ, Puukka PJ, Jula AM. Prognostic value of the variability in home-measured blood pressure and heart rate: the Finn-Home Study. Hypertension. 2012;59: 212–8.
44. Hoshide S, Yano Y, Shimizu M, Eguchi K, Ishikawa J, Kario K. Is home blood pressure variability itself an interventional target beyond lowering mean home blood pressure during anti-hypertensive treatment? Hypertens Res. 2012;35:862–6.
45. Karpettas N, Destounis A, Kollias A, Nasothimiou E, Moyssakis I, Stergiou GS. Prediction of treatment-induced changes in target-organ damage using changes in clinic, home and ambula-tory blood pressure. Hypertens Res. 2014;37:543–7.
46. Mancia G, Zanchetti A, Agabiti-Rosei E, et al. Ambulatory blood pressure is superior to clinic blood pressure in predicting treatment-induced regression of left ventricular hypertrophy. SAMPLE Study Group. Study on Ambulatory Monitoring of Blood Pressure and Lisinopril Evaluation. Circulation. 1997;95:1464–70.
47. Kario K, Saito I, Kushiro T, et al. Home blood pressure and cardiovascular outcomes in patients during antihypertensive therapy: primary results of HONEST, a large-scale prospec-tive, real-world observational study. Hypertension. 2014;64:989–96.
48. Stergiou G, Parati G. Further insights into the 24-h blood pressure profile by home blood pres-sure monitoring: the issue of morning hypertension. J Hypertens. 2009;27:696–9.
49. Asayama K, Ohkubo T, Kikuya M, et al. Prediction of stroke by home "morning" versus "eve-ning" blood pressure values: the Ohasama study. Hypertension. 2006;48:737–43.
50. Stergiou GS, Nasothimiou EG, Roussias LG. Morning hypertension assessed by home or ambulatory monitoring: different aspects of the same phenomenon? J Hypertens. 2010;28: 1846–53.
51. Redon J, Bilo G, Parati G. Surge Steering Committee. The effects of telmisartan alone or in combination with hydrochlorothiazide on morning home blood pressure control: the SURGE 2 practice-based study. Blood Press. 2013;22:377–85.
52. Kario K, Saito I, Kushiro T, et al. Effect of the angiotensin II receptor antagonist olmesartan on morning home blood pressure in hypertension: HONEST study at 16 weeks. J Hum Hypertens. 2013;27:721–8.
53. Mori H, Yamamoto H, Ukai H, et al. COMPATIBLE Study Group. Comparison of effects of angiotensin II receptor blocker on morning home blood pressure and cardiorenal protection between morning administration and evening administration in hypertensive patients: the COMPATIBLE study. Hypertens Res. 2013;36:202–7.
54. Hashimoto J, Chonan K, Aoki Y, et al. Therapeutic effects of evening administration of guana-benz and clonidine on morning hypertension: evaluation using home-based blood pressure measurements. J Hypertens. 2003;21:805–11.
55. Mengden T, Binswanger B, Spühler T, Weisser B, Vetter W. The use of self-measured blood pressure determinations in assessing dynamics of drug compliance in a study with amlodipine once a day, morning versus evening. J Hypertens. 1993;11:1403–11.
56. Metoki H, Ohkubo T, Kikuya M, et al. J-HOME-AI Study group. The velocity of antihyper-tensive effect of losartan/hydrochlorothiazide and angiotensin II receptor blocker. J Hypertens. 2012;30:1478–86.

57. Mashima K, Nakatsu T, Murakami T, et al. Exponential-exponential cosine fitting of blood pressure decay induced by a long-acting calcium blocker, amlodipine, using home blood pressure measurement. Clin Exp Hypertens. 2003;25:145–54.
58. Myers MG, Stergiou GS. Reporting bias: Achilles' heel of home blood pressure monitoring. J Am Soc Hypertens. 2014;8:350–7.
59. Stoddart A, Hanley J, Wild S, et al. Telemonitoring-based service redesign for the management of uncontrolled hypertension (HITS): cost and cost-effectiveness analysis of a randomised controlled trial. BMJ Open. 2013;3:e002681.
60. Nakamoto H, Nishida E, Ryuzaki M, et al. Effect of telmisartan and amlodipine on home blood pressure by monitoring newly developed telemedicine system: monitoring test by using telemedicine. Telmisartans effect on home blood pressure (TelTelbosu). Clin Exp Hypertens. 2008;30:57–67.

Chapter 20
Ambulatory Blood Pressure Monitoring in Clinical Trials of Drugs and Devices

William B. White and Line Malha

Introduction

The utilization of 24-h ambulatory blood pressure (BP) monitoring to assess new drugs and devices for hypertension has markedly increased over the past two decades. The determination of dosage and comparative efficacy of antihypertensive regimens has been guided by ambulatory BP monitoring in diverse patient populations with hypertension. More recently, studies of renal denervation devices have also used ambulatory BP measurements to determine more precise effects of partially interrupting the sympathetic nervous system.

Several specific attributes have made ambulatory monitoring of BP important in clinical trials involving the assessment of antihypertensive therapies [1–4]. Some of these benefits include removal of observer bias or error [5], better short- and long-term BP reproducibility [6], elimination of the white coat effect during patient selection [7, 8], and the ability to assess the effects of therapy on diurnal and nocturnal BP variability [9]. Furthermore, recent data have demonstrated that ambulatory BP is a superior predictor of hemodynamic abnormalities in the hypertensive patient [10], hypertensive target organ involvement [11, 12], and prognostic outcomes, including myocardial infarction, stroke, and other types of cardiovascular morbidity [13–19].

In this chapter, an overview of the utility of ambulatory BP monitoring in clinical pharmacology and medical device research will be provided with several examples

W.B. White, M.D. (✉)
Calhoun Cardiology Center, University of Connecticut School of Medicine,
263 Farmington Avenue, Farmington, CT 06030-3940, USA
e-mail: wwhite@uchc.edu

L. Malha, M.D.
NYU School of Medicine, New York, NY, USA

© Springer International Publishing Switzerland 2016
W.B. White (ed.), *Blood Pressure Monitoring in Cardiovascular Medicine
and Therapeutics*, Clinical Hypertension and Vascular Diseases,
DOI 10.1007/978-3-319-22771-9_20

using data from randomized, controlled, or comparator trials. Furthermore, examples that show the utility of ambulatory monitoring for the assessment of treated patients in clinical practice will also be discussed.

Impact of Blood Pressure Variability on the Reproducibility of Office vs. Ambulatory Blood Pressure as it Relates to Drug Development

The typical reduction in systolic or diastolic BP observed in a clinical trial of an antihypertensive drug (generally in the range of 5–20 %) must be viewed in light of the magnitude of the relatively large variability of office BP from one visit to the next (12–18 %). Studies that have examined the repeatability of office and ambulatory BP in patients with hypertension have consistently demonstrated much less variance with ambulatory BP [20–22].

Many years ago, Conway et al. [20] recorded the diastolic BP of 75 hypertensive subjects on two occasions, 1 month apart, while they were being administered placebo. With clinic measurements, the mean difference in diastolic BP was 1.7 mmHg and the standard deviation of this difference was 12.3 mmHg. In contrast, the daytime ambulatory BP fell by 0.9 mmHg and the standard deviation of the difference was halved to 6.3 mmHg. The implications of this marked reduction in BP variability with ambulatory BP recordings compared to the clinic pressure are that it will double the precision of a short-term trial and allow as much as a fourfold reduction in the number of patients required to achieve an accurate result.

Similarly, the long-term reproducibility of ambulatory BP is also superior to office BP [21]. Patients with hypertension were studied under the same therapeutic and environmental conditions and their blood pressure was measured twice, 2 years apart. The standard deviation of the differences in blood pressure was significantly lower and the correlation coefficients significantly higher for ambulatory BP than for office BP (Table 20.1). The improved reproducibility of ambulatory over office BP continued to be present when the data were divided into awake and sleep periods. These data suggest that clinical trials involving ambulatory BP over long periods would also

Table 20.1 Reproducibility of clinic and ambulatory blood pressure studies separated by up to 2 years in patients with hypertension

Blood pressure measure	Systolic			Diastolic		
	R-value	SDD	CV	R-value	SDD	CV
Office	0.48	17.0	11.0	0.31	10.0	10.0
24-h mean	0.87[a]	9.8[a]	7.0	0.90[a]	4.7[a]	5.6
Awake	0.86[a]	10.7[a]	7.4	0.88[a]	5.8[a]	6.5
Sleep	0.92[a]	7.7	6.3	0.88[a]	5.2	7.1

R-value, correlation coefficient; SDD standard deviation of the differences, CV coefficient of variation
[a]Significantly different from the office blood pressure correlation coefficients, SDD, and CV. From [21]

require smaller sample sizes than similarly designed trials in which the statistical power is based on the ability to show changes in a more highly variable clinic BP.

In contrast, there may be little advantage of ambulatory BP over clinic pressure in clinical trials when the measure of interest is a small block of time, such as 1 or 2 h. In an evaluation of a group of hypertensives using both noninvasive and intra-arterial BP over 24 h, Mancia et al. [23] showed that the standard deviation of the differences for 24-h mean BP values was similar for the two methodologies. However, despite the much larger number of BP values obtained in an intra-arterial study, the hourly BP reproducibility was no different for the direct measurements than it was for noninvasive BP monitoring. Thus, unlike the larger blocks of time (e.g., 24 h, the awake period, or the sleep period), the reproducibility of hourly ambulatory BP data has not been shown to be superior to that of office BP measurements [23]. Hence, ambulatory BP recordings will not allow a reduction in sample sizes if the end point is for short periods of time. This increased variability in hourly BP levels is probably secondary to differences in the activities of patients monitored on two different days. Because controlling for hourly physical and mental activities is nearly impossible in free-ranging subjects, longer periods of time (e.g., 4 h) will remain statistically and practically appropriate for clinical trials involving ambulatory BP monitoring.

The benefits of ambulatory monitoring of the BP over clinic BP with regard to sample size requirements in clinical trials of the elderly may be substantially reduced, however. One report in elderly hypertensive patients with isolated systolic hypertension suggests that there would not be improvement in reproducibility for ambulatory BP over clinic BP measurements, as the between-subject variance was not much different for the two methods [24]. Staessen et al. reported that 60 subjects with isolated systolic hypertension would be required to detect a 10-mmHg difference in systolic BP between two treatments in a parallel design using clinic readings, whereas if ambulatory BP monitoring was used, the number would only fall to 54. In contrast, if a crossover design was used, the number of subjects needed to show the same systolic BP difference would be 18 and 14, respectively, for clinic vs ambulatory BP measurements.

Ambulatory Blood Pressure for Evaluating Patients for Clinical Trial Entry

At the recruitment and enrollment phases of a clinical hypertension trial, current antihypertensive medication is discontinued, and baseline BPs and heart rates are obtained during a single-blind placebo period that generally lasts for 2–4 weeks. Conventional inclusion criteria for these trials have been based on the seated clinic systolic or diastolic BPs at the end of the single-blind placebo period. In recent years, many protocols have also included ambulatory BP values as primary or secondary criteria for inclusion into the study. For example, it is not uncommon to

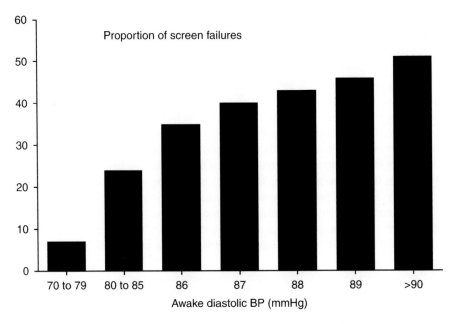

Fig. 20.1 Effects of patient recruitment using an office diastolic blood pressure >90 mmHg and various awake ambulatory diastolic blood pressures as the selection criteria in antihypertensive drug trials (Modified from [1])

require that the seated diastolic BP in the clinic exceed 90 or 95 mmHg and that the awake (or daytime) ambulatory BP exceed 85 or 90 mmHg [1]. The impact of various awake ambulatory BP values for exclusion of patients during the screening process can be fairly dramatic when the requirement for the office diastolic BP is 90 mmHg or greater.

An example of this is shown in an analysis from a multicenter US clinical trial (Fig. 20.1). In this study, a seated clinic diastolic BP of >95 and <115 mmHg was used as the criterion for entering and remaining in the single-blind portion of the trial. To progress into the double-blind randomized portion of the study, ambulatory BP values at certain thresholds were used. However, when using an ambulatory awake BP cutoff value of 85 mmHg, nearly 30 % of the study group was excluded from randomization into the double-blind part of the trial.

When 90 mmHg was the cutoff value for ambulatory diastolic pressure, more than 50 % of the group was excluded from randomization. The major reason for the high exclusion rate based on the ambulatory BP values compared to the office pressure is that a relatively high percentage of patients entering these trials experience a white coat effect [3, 7, 25, 26]. There has always been substantial controversy as to whether patients with white coat hypertension should be included or excluded from participation in clinical trials of antihypertensive drugs. The viewpoint of those favoring inclusion of white coat hypertensive patients is that it is relevant to study their hemodynamic response to the new drug because it is likely that many patients with the white coat syndrome will have therapy prescribed by physicians who base treatment decisions solely on office BP measurements. Although not an unreasonable concern, a number of studies have demonstrated that patients with white coat hypertension exhibit few changes in ambulatory BP following antihypertensive therapy [27, 28]. The typical compromise in recent years has been to include an intermediate cutoff BP entry value for ambulatory BP that is lower than the office BP entry criteria. By using the ambulatory BP criteria, fewer patients will be required in the randomized portion of the study, but the number of individuals screened in the single-blind period is typically increased [9, 20, 21]. Even in 2015, it remains commonplace to recruit about 130–140 % of the required final number of patients who can be evaluated to assure that the statistical power required to show the desired changes from baseline will be achieved.

Multicenter Trials to Evaluate Antihypertensive Therapy

A multicenter trial is a clinical trial conducted simultaneously by several investigators working in different institutions, but using the same protocol and identical methods in order to pool the data collected and analyze them together [29, 30]. Two key reasons for conducting multicenter studies rather than single-center studies is to enhance patient recruitment and to make the study group more "representative" of the entire patient population, as there may be unique or homogeneous local population characteristics from a single center.

Analyses of Multicenter Hypertension Trials: Relevant Problems for Ambulatory Blood Pressure Recordings

There are several problems specific to multicenter hypertension trials, including those utilizing ambulatory BP measurements. First, there is the "center" factor: incorporation of the center factor into the analysis improves the power of comparison of treatments. One can assess the variability among centers from the residual variability in order to improve the sensitivity in detecting differences between treatments. However, in the extreme situation of 1–2 patients in a center, it is not possible to differentiate between a center-related effect and one related to the treatments. In such cases, the smallest centers should be pooled to serve as a larger "center" in the statistical model.

Second, it is important to evaluate whether the differences between treatment modalities vary outside of random fluctuations across all centers. If a major difference does exist, it may be proven statistically by performing a test of treatment by center interaction.

Table 20.2 Causes of treatment-by-center interactions in multicenter clinical trials

Differences in patient features from one center to another
Abnormal frequency of protocol violations, losses to follow-up, or noncompliance in one or more centers
Outlier center (small number of "doubtful" cases)
Real variations of differences between treatments according to centers

From [32]

It is relevant to evaluate the causes of treatment by center interactions because they may invalidate the principal findings of a study [31], including those using ambulatory BP monitoring. Some of the causes of treatment-by-center interactions are listed in Table 20.2. An abnormal or unusual frequency of protocol violations, losses to follow-up, or noncompliant patients may occur in one or more centers. When this occurs, it may reflect poor adherence to the protocol or insufficient motivation of the investigators or study coordinators at these centers. For example, when a center has inexperienced or apathetic personnel involved in an ambulatory BP monitoring protocol, there may be excessive data loss during the recording period, poor correlation between cuff and device measurements, or inaccuracy with regard to drug dosing and recorder hookup times [3, 7, 32].

Outlier centers, possibly because of a small number of doubtful cases, may decrease credibility concerning these data and may also cause a center effect. However, tests for outliers may be misleading in a large clinical trial. For example, if three or four centers are identified as outliers, it is possible that these are the clinics that are doing a good job while the others are not. Thus, statistical tests for outliers, which are essentially tests of homogeneity, must be used carefully and intelligently by the statisticians in charge of the final analyses. Finally, real variations of differences between treatments according to centers may occur and restrict the general applicability of the results.

Bias in a Multicenter Trial Using Ambulatory Blood Pressure Monitoring

Bias enters into a multicenter trial through two primary mechanisms: selection bias and misclassification bias. An example of selection bias in an antihypertensive drug trial involving ambulatory BP monitoring might be recruiting a more severely hypertensive population to avoid inclusion of white coat hypertensives. Many investigators have learned to avoid screen failures (Fig. 20.1), which has a possible financial impact on the center, so they will enroll either a patient with higher clinic pressures or one who has a "known" ambulatory BP from a previous trial. Misclassification bias in the multicenter trial is exemplified by clinic BP measurement error (e.g., using improper methodology for measurement) and may induce a center effect if untrained or inexperienced personnel are used. Misclassification bias is probably uncommon in studies using experienced investigators and coordinators, but in recent multinational, multicenter trials, the use of centers inexperienced in performing clinical research and measurement errors have become more prevalent.

Practical Concerns in the Conduct of Multicenter Trials That Use Ambulatory Blood Pressure Recorders

The use of ambulatory BP monitors in a clinical trial requires the availability of skilled, trained technicians. Multiple devices are necessary in order to complete a clinical trial in a timely fashion, to facilitate the scheduling of large numbers of participants and to minimize the impact of mechanical problems when they occur. These requirements increase study costs, but are critical to the success of the trial. An additional concern is the possibility that the data for some individuals may be excluded from analyses because of the poor quality of an ambulatory BP recording or mechanical difficulty [33]. Rarely, the use of ambulatory BP monitoring may hinder recruitment efforts because certain individuals may decline participation in a trial as a result of the perceived burden of wearing and returning a recorder. Appel et al. [33] have reported that patient recruitment efforts improve when the technique is presented as a standard part of the study. Then the expectation is that the ambulatory BP data collection is a primary part of the study [34] as opposed to an optional or ancillary procedure.

Importance of the Placebo Effect in Clinic vs. Ambulatory Blood Pressure

It remains standard practice to include a placebo group in clinical trials involving antihypertensive therapy, especially studies that are considered dose ranging or "pivotal" during the earlier phases of drug development. Because of the marked variability of office BP, most investigators have found it necessary to distinguish true drug effect from placebo effect in BP trials. Several factors might create a reduction in BP on placebo, including regression to the mean [34], the presence of a pressor response in the doctor's office that resolves the white coat effect [35, 36], and expectations of the patient and the clinical observer [5]. Unfortunately, surreptitious readings may also play a role in BP reductions on placebo.

In contrast to studies that employ clinic pressure as the primary means to obtain the primary study end point, the placebo effect is either minimal or absent when ambulatory BP monitoring is used in antihypertensive drug trials [37–39]. The lack of observed placebo effect on ambulatory BP is probably secondary to both the lack of observer bias and the increased number of BP values obtained over a 24-h study period. In contrast, ambulatory BP monitoring probably would not remove regression to the mean or other potential patient factors that contribute to the placebo effect. In fact, it is somewhat difficult to separate the regression to the mean effect from the placebo effect and the decrease in a white coat effect over time. This phenomenon of regression to the mean in an ambulatory BP monitoring study has been shown quite clearly in a study by White et al. [40]. In this trial, patients with hypertension were randomized to receive either placebo or controlled-onset extended-release (COER) verapamil for 8 weeks after a 3–4-week single-blind placebo baseline period. The patients were then divided into those with BP fall by >10 % during sleep compared to their awake values (dippers) and those with BP falls by <10 % during sleep (non-dippers). In the non-dipper patients randomized to receive placebo, nocturnal systolic BP fell by 4 mmHg compared to the first baseline study (also on placebo but during the single-blind period). In the dipper patients randomized to receive placebo, nocturnal systolic BP increased by about 4 mmHg compared to the baseline BP. Thus, the spread between the two types of patients in the placebo group for nocturnal pressure was nearly 8 mmHg (Fig. 20.2).

The changes in nocturnal BP on active drug were also consistently greater across all doses and greater in non-dippers compared to dippers. Thus, if this substantial regression to the mean on placebo had not been accounted for, the response to active treatment with COER verapamil in the dippers would have been underestimated and the response in the non-dippers would have been overestimated.

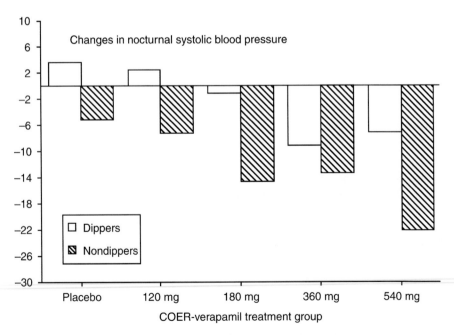

Fig. 20.2 Changes in nocturnal (10 PM to 5 AM) blood pressure (BP) from baseline measured by ambulatory BP monitoring in dippers (decline in mean BP from the daytime period to the nocturnal period was >10 %) contrasted with changes in nocturnal BP in non-dippers (<10 % decline in nocturnal BP) on placebo and four doses of controlled-onset extended-release (COER) verapamil (Modified from [40])

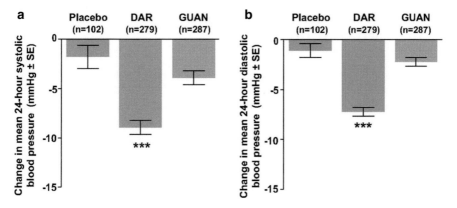

Fig. 20.3 Difference in mean 24-h ambulatory systolic (**a**) and diastolic (**b**) BP after 14 weeks of treatment with placebo, darusentan, and guanfacine. ***$p < 0.001$ as compared with placebo or guanfacine (From [41])

More recently, Bakris et al. [41] randomized 849 patients with resistant hypertension to darusentan (a selective endothelin-A receptor antagonist), placebo, and guanfacine (central α-2 agonist). At 14 weeks, the systolic BP in the placebo group decreased by 14 ± 14 mmHg in the office measurements, while the mean 24-h systolic BP only decreased by 2 ± 12 mmHg. Hence, when mean 24-h BP is taken into account, the placebo effect is dramatically attenuated. While the drop in clinic systolic BP at 14 weeks with darusentan was not significantly different from placebo, the mean 24-h systolic BP was lower for darusentan group ($p < 0.001$) (Fig. 20.3).

A study by Mutti et al. [39] reported a significant $10/3 \pm 3/2$ mmHg fall in office BP after 4 weeks of placebo, whereas the overall 24-h BP was unchanged. However, the ambulatory BP did fall slightly during the first 8 h of placebo administration, which the authors attributed to the white coat effect. Of note is that this initial fall did not have a statistical effect on the overall mean BP and thus ambulatory BP monitoring still allowed for better characterization of the placebo effect.

In a much longer-term study by Staessen et al. [42] in older patients with isolated systolic hypertension, one treatment arm was randomized to placebo for 1 year. Compared to the baseline period, the clinic systolic BP fell by 7 ± 16 mmHg on placebo and the 24-h systolic BP fell by just 2 ± 11 mmHg. Because the ambulatory BP has a superior repeatability index compared to the clinic pressure, the changes in 24-h systolic BP met statistical significance, whereas the larger mean reduction in clinic BP showed only a trend ($p = 0.06$). Because this was a patient population with normal diastolic BP, there were no statistically significant changes in clinic or ambulatory diastolic BP on placebo therapy during this study. The authors also noted that the 24-h systolic BP was more likely to decrease on placebo if it was higher at baseline and if the follow-up was longer. The authors discounted regression to the mean or the white coat effect as having an impact on these placebo effects and recommended that long-term studies in older patients using noninvasive ambulatory BP monitoring require a placebo-controlled design.

Analysis of Ambulatory Blood Pressure Data in Antihypertensive Drug Trials

Data from ambulatory BP studies in hypertension trials can be analyzed in a number of ways (Table 20.3). Features of any method of analysis for ambulatory BP data should include the statistical ease of calculation, clinical relevance of the measure, and relationship of the parameter to the hypertensive disease process. The most popular methods remain the change from baseline in the 24-h systolic and diastolic BP and the visual assessment of the hourly curves over 24 h. However, the use of daytime and nighttime means (or preferably awake and sleep values), blood pressure loads (the proportion of values above a cutoff value during wakefulness [>140/90 mmHg] or sleep [>120/80 mmHg] divided by the total number of BP readings), area under the 24-h BP curve (AUC), and smoothing techniques designed to remove some of the variability from the raw BP data analysis are also among the utilized methods of analysis [1–4, 9, 10].

The 24-h mean BP remains an important parameter for evaluation in antihypertensive drug trials because it appears to be a strong predictor of hypertensive target organ disease [2], is easy to calculate, utilizes all of the ambulatory BP data, and as previously mentioned, is remarkably reproducible in both short-term [6] and long-term [21] studies.

The blood pressure load has been used as a simple method of analysis in evaluating the effects of antihypertensive drugs. Blood pressure load has been defined as the percentage of BPs exceeding 140/90 mmHg while the patient is awake plus the percentage of BPs exceeding 120/80 mmHg during sleep [43]. A number of years ago, we evaluated the relationship between this BP load and cardiac target organ indexes in previously untreated hypertensives. At a 40 % diastolic BP load, the incidence of LVH was nearly 80 %, but below a 40 % diastolic BP load, the prevalence of LVH fell to about 8 %. In contrast, the office BP and even the 24-h average BP were not as discriminating in predicting LVH in this group of previously untreated patients. Thus, in mild to moderately hypertensive patients, one would desire a low (conservatively <30 %) BP load while being treated with antihypertensive drug therapy.

Table 20.3 Methods for evaluating ambulatory blood pressure data in clinical trials

24-h means (and standard deviation as a measure of variability)
Awake and sleep means based on patient diaries or activity recorders
Hourly means
Blood pressure load (proportion method)
Area under the blood pressure curve
Placebo-subtracted curves showing hourly means
Various data smoothing techniques (including cosinor analyses or fast Fourier transformation)
Modeling of 24-h curves
Trough-to-peak ratio (for once or twice daily drugs)

In studies in which the patient population has a greater range in BP, the proportional (or percentage) BP load becomes less useful. Because the upper limit of the BP load is 100 %, this value may represent a substantial number of individuals with broad ranges of moderate to severe hypertension. To overcome this problem, we devised a method to integrate the area under the ambulatory BP curve and relate its values to predicting hemodynamic indices in untreated essential hypertensives [10]. Areas under the BP curve were computed separately for periods of wakefulness and sleep and combined to form the 24-h AUC. Threshold values were used to calculate AUC such as 135 or 140 mmHg systolic while awake and 85 or 90 mmHg diastolic while awake. Values during sleep were reduced to 115 and 120 mmHg systolic and 75 and 80 mmHg diastolic.

Smoothing of ambulatory BP data may be used to aid in the identification of the peak and trough effects of an antihypertensive drug. The extent of variability in an individual's BP curve may be large as a result of both mental and physical activity; thus, evaluating the peak antihypertensive effect of a short- or intermediate-acting drug may be difficult. Other than the benefits associated with examining pharmacodynamic effects of new antihypertensive drugs, data and curve smoothing for 24-h BP monitoring appear to have little clinical relevance. Furthermore, editing protocols are not uniform in the literature, and missing data may alter the balance of mean values for shorter periods of time. To avoid excessive data reduction in a clinical trial, one statistical expert suggested that data smoothing should be performed on individual BP profiles rather than on group means [44].

Situations in Which Ambulatory Blood Pressure Monitoring Has Been Useful in Antihypertensive Drug Trials

Treating the White-Coat Hypertensive Patient

The inclusion of white coat hypertensive patients in an antihypertensive drug trial that uses only clinic BP criteria for study entry will have a potentially confounding effect on efficacy, because these patients are not hypertensive outside of the medical care environment [7, 8, 11, 13]. Furthermore, patients may develop excessive drug-induced side effects without much change in BP, especially if titration of the dose is based on office pressures.

In a study by Weber et al. [28], a sustained fall in BP was found across a study group taking a long-acting form of diltiazem. In a subset of six patients who had hypertensive office BP readings but whose ambulatory BPs were normotensive (i.e., a white coat hypertensive group), no significant ambulatory BP changes from placebo baseline (0/1 mmHg) were observed. In contrast, the diltiazem therapy decreased 24-h BPs by 18/13 mmHg in the subgroup of nine patients who were hypertensive by both office and ambulatory BP. Thus, treating white coat hypertensive patients may be of little to no benefit if the only place where BP reduction is observed is in the medical care environment.

Utility of Ambulatory Blood Pressure Monitoring in Dose-Finding Studies

Since the early 1990s, numerous studies have been performed with ambulatory BP monitoring to fully assess the efficacy of a wide range of doses of new antihypertensive agents. The advantage of ambulatory BP monitoring in dose-finding studies is the ability to discern differences among the doses with smaller numbers of study participants compared to the sample size requirements when clinic pressures are used.

Examples are shown next.

Eplerenone

The efficacy of eplerenone, a novel selective aldosterone receptor antagonist, was studied in patients with essential hypertension using a multicenter, randomized, placebo-controlled design [45]. In this trial, the drug was assessed using a once-daily dosing regimen of either 25 or 200 mg. Clinic and ambulatory BPs were compared to both baseline values and the effects of placebo. As shown in Fig. 20.4, there was a dose-related reduction in BP at the trough for both clinic and ambulatory BP. The ambulatory BP values were better at delineating the dose–response than the clinic BP readings.

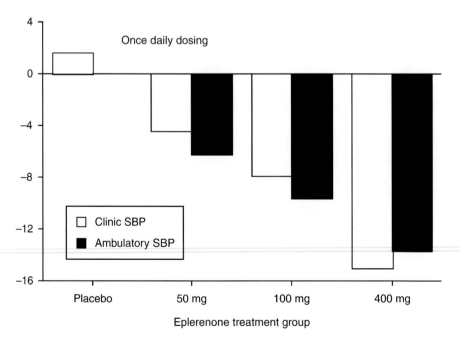

Fig. 20.4 Changes from baseline in ambulatory vs clinic systolic blood pressure in a dose-ranging trial with a selective aldosterone antagonist, eplerenone (Data from [45])

Utility of Ambulatory Blood Pressure Monitoring in Comparator Trials

Ambulatory BP monitoring has been very helpful in comparing antihypertensive drugs, especially when assessing duration of action. Numerous examples in the literature illustrate this benefit, including the superiority of ambulatory BP over clinic BP in assessing the trough-to-peak ratio of various agents [46].

Comparisons Within the Same Class

In a multicenter study, Neutel et al. [47] compared the β-blockers bisoprolol and atenolol in 606 patients using both clinic and ambulatory BP. Following therapy, trough BP in the clinic was reduced 12/12 mmHg by bisoprolol and 11/12 mmHg by atenolol. Although these changes were significantly different from baseline therapy, there were no differences when comparing the effects of each drug. In contrast, daytime systolic and diastolic BPs (6 AM to 10 PM) and the last 4 h of the dosing interval (6–10 AM) were lowered significantly more by bisoprolol than by atenolol. This finding was present whether the assessment was made by examination of the overall means, area under the curve, or BP loads. These data demonstrated that despite there being no difference in office BP, bisoprolol had significant differences in efficacy and duration of action compared with atenolol when assessed by 24-h BP monitoring.

The antihypertensive efficacy of the selective angiotensin II receptor antagonists azilsartan medoxomil, valsartan, and olmesartan medoxomil was compared with placebo in a randomized, multicenter, parallel group, double-blind trial of 1291 patients with hypertension [48]. Azilsartan medoxomil is metabolized to azilsartan, an active metabolite with potent angiotensin II type 1 receptor antagonist properties. After 2 weeks of single-blind placebo baseline treatment, patients were randomized to receive 160 mg valsartan, 20 mg of olmesartan, 20 or 40 mg azilsartan medoxomil or placebo once daily. The doses were up-titrated to double the initial dose after 2 weeks and maintained until week 6 after randomization. Based on placebo-adjusted 24-h BP measurements, the reductions in systolic BP were -14.3 mmHg for azilsartan, -11.7 mmHg for olmesartan, and -10.0 mmHg for valsartan. Changes in BP induced by azilsartan were significantly greater than the reductions in BP observed with olmesartan ($p = 0.009$) and valsartan ($p < 0.001$) (Fig. 20.5). The decreases in blood pressure measured in the office using digital devices were consistent with the changes from baseline in the mean 24-h BP measurements in this study. This contrasts with prior findings by Mallion et al. [49] where office BP did not demonstrate a blood pressure difference between telmisartan and losartan, while ambulatory BP monitoring was able to identify a more drop of systolic BP for the telmisartan group compared to the losartan group at 18–24-h after the dose was administered.

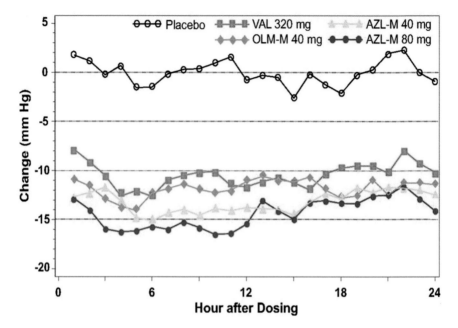

Fig. 20.5 Change in systolic BP from baseline after 6 weeks of treatment with placebo, 40 or 80 mg of azilsartan medoxomil (AZL-M), 320 mg of valsartan (VAL), and 40 mg of olmesartan (OLM-M) (Modified from [48])

Comparisons of Drugs in Different Classes

The Anglo-Scandinavian Cardiac Outcomes Trial-Blood Pressure Lowering Arm (ASCOT-BPLA) compared the prevention of cardiovascular events from an antihypertensive regimen based on a calcium channel blocker (amlodipine 5–10 mg once daily) in combination with an angiotensin-converting enzyme inhibitor (perindopril 4–8 mg once daily) to a combination of a beta blocker (atenolol 50–100 mg once daily) and a thiazide diuretic (bendroflumethiazide 1.25–2.5 mg once daily) [50]. In a substudy of the ASCOT-BPLA, Dolan et al. compared the ability of ambulatory BP versus office BP to predict cardiovascular events [51]. The substudy randomized 1905 patients to either amlodipine-peridopril or atenolol-thiazide regimens. Both ambulatory and office BP were correlated with cardiovascular events, but the ambulatory BP monitor demonstrated that nocturnal BP was reduced to a greater extent by amlodipine-perindopril versus atenolol-thiazide therapy.

The ASCOT BPLA substudy also demonstrated a lower risk for cardiovascular events in the amlodipine-perindopril group. The hazard ratio was further strengthened when integrating nighttime systolic BP values with accumulated mean office BP in a multivariate model. These data suggested that the addition of ambulatory BP allowed for improved characterization of the prognostic implications of different drug regimens in a clinical outcome trial [50].

Use of Ambulatory Monitoring to Assess the Effects of Dosing Time

In general, when antihypertensive therapies are administered, there is an attempt to match the effects of a drug to the timing of the BP variability [52–54]. In the case of hypertension and coronary artery disease, this imparts a great deal of clinical relevance because BP and heart rate have distinct, reproducible circadian rhythms. In most patients, the BP and heart rate are lowest during sleep and highest during the day. As noted previously by several authors in this volume, most cardiovascular diseases, including myocardial infarction [55]), angina and myocardial ischemia [56], and stroke [57], have circadian patterns that are all characterized by the highest incidences in the early morning hours.

Timing of Drug Administration

Several authors have made attempts to alter the effects of conventional drugs by dosing them prior to sleep vs upon arising [58–65]. In one of these studies [64], the angiotensin-converting enzyme inhibitor (ACE) quinapril was dosed in the early morning vs at bedtime in 18 moderately hypertensive patients. The study was conducted in a double-blind crossover design with quinapril dosed at either 8 AM or 10 PM for 4 weeks in each period. Ambulatory BP monitoring was carried out before and at the end of each 4-weeks double-blind period. Daytime BP was reduced similarly by both dosing regimens. In contrast, nighttime systolic and diastolic BP was decreased to a significantly greater extent with the evening administration of quinapril. Measurement of ACE activity showed that evening administration of quinapril induced a more sustained decline in plasma ACE but not a more pronounced change. The findings in this study are of substantial interest because nocturnal BP has largely been ignored in the past [63], and in many types of hypertensive patients the BP during sleep may remain elevated despite "normal" BP measurement in the doctor's office.

The MAPEC (Monitoración Ambulatoria para Predicción de Eveventos Cardiovasculares) study [59] from Spain randomized 2156 participants with hypertension and instructed them to ingest all their antihypertensive medications upon awakening versus taking one or more at bedtime. The bedtime medication group had improvement in ambulatory BP control, reduction in the occurrence of non-dipping pattern, and a lower risk (relative risk 0.39, $p < 0.001$) for cardiovascular events (median time = 5.6 years). Cardiovascular events were defined in terms of all cause mortality and morbidity including: angina, coronary artery disease (myocardial infarction or coronary revascularization), heart failure, peripheral vascular disease (lower extremity or retinal arterial occlusions), aortic aneurysmal rupture, and stroke (hemorrhagic, ischemic, and transient ischemic attack). Further studies from the same research group had reproducible results with benefit of bedtime dosing of antihypertensive medication on cardiovascular morbidity and mortality [61].

Other studies [66–68] show that little change in BP or heart rate occurs by altering the dosing time of these long-acting agents to nighttime. However, most of the studies have small sample sizes and had low statistical power to show changes less than 5–10 mmHg in ambulatory BP. Thus, whether or not altering the dosing time of a long-acting antihypertensive agent truly changes the level of ambulatory BP has not been shown with any great degree of confidence.

Situations in Which Ambulatory Blood Pressure Monitoring Has Been Useful in Antihypertensive Device Trials

Utility of Ambulatory Blood Pressure Monitoring in Evaluation of Treatment Efficacy of Renal Sympathetic Denervation

Renal sympathetic denervation by radiofrequency ablation is an emerging technique to treat severe and drug-resistant hypertension. The goal of the procedure is to disrupt the sympathetic nerves overlying the renal artery and attenuate the release of catecholamines [69, 70]. The first randomized, controlled trial using this technology (SYMPLICITY HTN-3) [71] evaluated the change in ambulatory systolic BP at 6 months with renal denervation as compared to a sham procedure. The trial randomized 535 patients with drug-resistant hypertension, but failed to demonstrate a benefit of renal sympathetic denervation on changes in office BP. Bakris et al. [72] later published the ambulatory BP monitoring results from SYMPLICITY-3. There was no difference in the change from baseline in 24 h ambulatory BP between treatment groups; the nocturnal systolic BP trended to be lower following renal denervation (-3.3 mmHg, $p = 0.06$, versus sham procedure). Still it is unknown whether reductions in sympathetic nervous system activation may modulate beneficial effects on nighttime BP control, a key factor in cardiovascular risk prevention.

The findings of SYMPLICITY-3 [71] contrast with results from prior uncontrolled and unblinded studies [73, 74]. These open-label studies demonstrated large reductions in clinic BP and much more modest reductions in ambulatory BP, 3–6 months after renal denervation. However, with lack of blinding and sham-control, the strength of evidence in these prior studies is limited.

Mahfoud et al. [73] pooled data from a series of 346 renal denervation patients who had had uncontrolled hypertension by office measurements and divided them into true and pseudo-resistant hypertension based on the ambulatory systolic BP. If the 24-h mean systolic BP was <130 mmHg, they were considered pseudo-resistant. In patients with true resistant hypertension, renal denervation significantly decreased the 24-h systolic and diastolic BP by $-11.7/-7.4$ mmHg ($p < 0.007$) at 12 months. However, renal denervation did not significantly decrease ambulatory BP in the pseudo-resistant hypertension group despite a large reduction in office BP (Fig. 20.6).

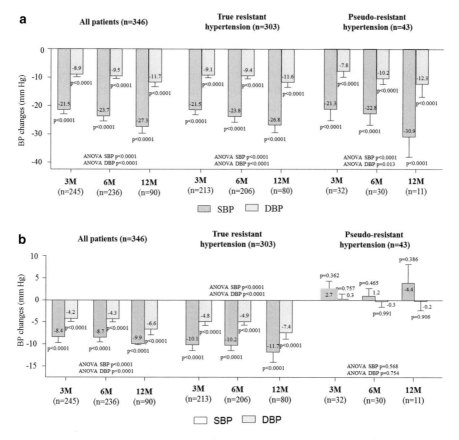

Fig. 20.6 Systolic blood pressure (SBP) and diastolic blood pressure changes (compared to baseline BP) in all patients, in patients with true and with pseudo-resistant hypertension at 3 months (3M), 6 months (6M), and 12 months (12M) after renal denervation. Panel A represents office blood pressure measurement and panel B represents 24-h mean BP by ambulatory BP monitoring. Adapted from [73]

These results demonstrated that ambulatory BP was a superior means to assess blood pressure responses in patients undergoing renal denervation. The differential response of ambulatory and office blood pressures to renal denervation can be explained in part by observer bias, white coat effect, and perhaps disparities in the physiologic basis for true resistant hypertension versus pseudo-resistant hypertension [41, 73].

While the efficacy of renal denervation in the first sham-procedure trial was not significant, numerous issues related to the lack of effectiveness have been identified [75] and it is expected that numerous newly designed device trials will be initiated as technological advances occur [76, 77].

Ambulatory Blood Pressure Monitoring in Community-Based Trials

Traditional clinical trials in hypertension measure the efficacy of anti-hypertensive drugs, but may not fully assess their effectiveness in clinical practice. Thus, it was relevant to evaluate a community-based trial that could provide this information using an open-label design without being subject to observer bias. To meet this requirement, White et al. [78] (Fig. 20.7) used ambulatory BP monitoring to overcome these

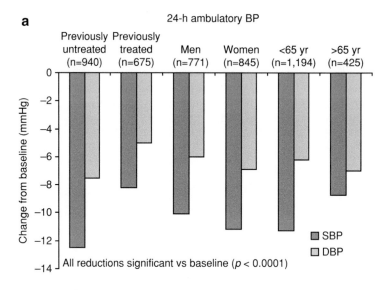

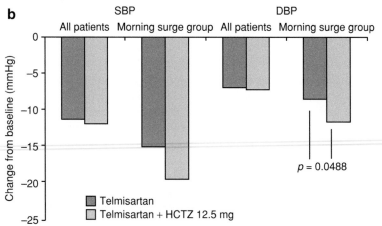

Fig. 20.7 Effects of telmisartan or telemisartan and hydrochlorothiazide on 24-h ambulatory BP (*upper panel*) and the last 4 h of the dosing interval (*lower panel*) from the MICCAT-2 trial. Patients were characterized as having a morning surge if their early morning BP exceeded the pre-awakening sleep BP by 30 mmHg systolic (Modified from [78])

shortcomings in a large community-based trial involving more than 600 medical practices in the United States. Patients with hypertension, either untreated or currently on treatment, were started on, or switched to, the angiotensin receptor blocker telmisartan 40 mg daily; after 2 weeks, if office BP remained >140/85 mmHg, the dose was increased to 80 mg and, if necessary, hydrochlorothiazide 12.5 mg added after a further 4 weeks and continued for the final 4-week period. Twenty-four-hour ABPM was performed at baseline and at the end of the treatment period. Baseline and treatment ambulatory BP measurements were completed in 940 previously untreated patients and 675 previously treated patients. The average reduction of the entire cohort was −10.7/−6.5 mmHg ($p>0.0001$; 24-h BP averages were reduced by 12/8 and 8/5 mmHg in untreated and previously treated patients, respectively). In contrast, the office BPs fell by an average of 23/12 and 17/10 mmHg in previously untreated and treated patients. In 401 patients whose baseline 24-h BP was >130/85 mmHg, the mean decrease in 24-h BP was 16.8/11.4 mmHg. Based on the ambulatory BP criteria, the BP was fully controlled (<130/85 mmHg) in 70 % of patients and, based on office measurement criteria (<140/90 mmHg), in 79 %. Thus, observer and measurement bias was substantially based on the changes from baseline by clinical measurements in contrast to ambulatory BP recordings. The successful use of this procedure in primary care research will create further opportunities to define the effectiveness of treatment in the environment in which it is customarily prescribed.

Conclusions

The data from the past 15–20 years of clinical trials now overwhelmingly support the usefulness of ambulatory BP monitoring in the assessment and development of new antihypertensive drugs. Numerous reports show that the ambulatory BP is a powerful, independent predictor of cardiovascular morbidity. Additionally, several studies also show that ambulatory BP monitoring has excellent potential as a tool to aid in the management of hypertension, including determining whether the initiation, adjustment, and withdrawal of antihypertensive treatment should be considered. Finally, based on most analyses, ambulatory monitoring of the BP is, at worst, cost-neutral and should become cost-effective in most countries when used for the appropriate clinical diagnoses and charged for at reasonable costs.

References

1. Mansoor GA, White WB. Contribution of ambulatory blood pressure monitoring to the design and analysis of antihypertensive therapy trials. J Cardiovasc Risk. 1994;1(2):136–42.
2. Mansoor GA, White WB. Ambulatory blood pressure monitoring in current clinical practice and research. Curr Opin Nephrol Hypertens. 1995;4(6):531–7.
3. White WB, Morganroth J. Usefulness of ambulatory monitoring of blood pressure in assessing antihypertensive therapy. Am J Cardiol. 1989;63(1):94–8.

4. White WB. The role of ambulatory monitoring of the blood pressure for assessment of antihypertensive agents. J Clin Pharmacol. 1992;32(6):524–8.
5. Bruce NG, Shaper AG, Walker M, Wannamethee G. Observer bias in blood pressure studies. J Hypertens. 1988;6(5):375–80.
6. James GD, Pickering TG, Yee LS, Harshfield GA, Riva S, Laragh JH. The reproducibility of average ambulatory, home, and clinic pressures. Hypertension. 1988;11:545–9.
7. Pickering TG, James GD, Boddie C, Harshfield GA, Blank S, Laragh JH. How common is white coat hypertension? JAMA. 1988;259(2):225–8.
8. White WB. Assessment of patients with office hypertension by 24-hour noninvasive ambulatory blood pressure monitoring. Arch Intern Med. 1986;146(11):2196–9.
9. White WB. Methods of blood pressure determination to assess antihypertensive agents: are casual measurements enough? Clin Pharmacol Ther. 1989;45(6):581–6.
10. White WB, Lund-Johansen P, Weiss S, Omvik P, Indurkhya N. The relationships between casual and ambulatory blood pressure measurements and central hemodynamics in essential human hypertension. J Hypertens. 1994;12(9):1075–81.
11. White WB, Schulman P, McCabe EJ, Dey HM. Average daily blood pressure, not office blood pressure, determines cardiac function in patients with hypertension. JAMA. 1989;261(6):873–7.
12. Shimada K, Kawamoto A, Matsubayashi K, Ozawa T. Silent cerebrovascular disease in the elderly: correlation with ambulatory blood pressure. Hypertension. 1990;16(6):692–9.
13. Perloff D, Sokolow M, Cowan RM, Juster RP. Prognostic value of ambulatory blood pressure measurements: further analyses. J Hypertens. 1989;7(3):S3–10.
14. Redon J, Campos C, Narciso ML, Rodicio JL, Pascual JM, Ruilope LM. Prognostic value of ambulatory blood pressure monitoring in refractory hypertension: a prospective study. Hypertension. 1998;31(2):712–8.
15. Verdecchia P, Angeli F, Cavallini C. Ambulatory blood pressure for cardiovascular risk stratification. Circulation. 2007;115(16):2091–3.
16. Verdecchia P, Porcellati C, Schillaci G, et al. Ambulatory blood pressure. An independent predictor of prognosis in essential hypertension. Hypertension. 1994;24(6):793–801.
17. Khattar RS, Senior R, Lahiri A. Cardiovascular outcome in white-coat versus sustained mild hypertension: a 10-year follow-up study. Circulation. 1998;98(18):1892–7.
18. Staessen JA, Thijs L, Fagard R, et al. Predicting cardiovascular risk using conventional vs ambulatory blood pressure in older patients with systolic hypertension. Systolic Hypertension in Europe Trial Investigators. JAMA. 1999;282(6):539–46.
19. Staessen JA, Thijs L, O'Brien ET, et al. Ambulatory pulse pressure as predictor of outcome in older patients with systolic hypertension. Am J Hypertens. 2002;15:835–43.
20. Conway J, Johnston J, Coats A, Somers V, Sleight P. The use of ambulatory blood pressure monitoring to improve the accuracy and reduce the numbers of subjects in clinical trials of antihypertensive agents. J Hypertens. 1988;6(2):111–6.
21. Mansoor GA, McCabe EJ, White WB. Long-term reproducibility of ambulatory blood pressure. J Hypertens. 1994;12(6):703–8.
22. Campbell P, Ghuman N, Wakefield D, Wolfson L, White WB. Long-term reproducibility of ambulatory blood pressure is superior to office blood pressure in the very elderly. J Hum Hypertens. 2010;24:749–54.
23. Mancia G, Omboni S, Parati G, Trazzi S, Mutti E. Limited reproducibility of hourly blood pressure values obtained by ambulatory blood pressure monitoring: implications for studies on antihypertensive drugs. J Hypertens. 1992;10(12):1531–5.
24. Staessen JA, Thijs L, Clement D, et al. Ambulatory pressure decreases on long-term placebo treatment in older patients with isolated systolic hypertension. Syst-Eur Investigators. J Hypertens. 1994;12(9):1035–9.
25. Gradman AH, Pangan P, Germain M. Lack of correlation between clinic and 24 hour ambulatory blood pressure in subjects participating in a therapeutic drug trial. J Clin Epidemiol. 1989;42(11):1049–54.
26. de la Sierra A, Segura J, Banegas JR, et al. Clinical features of 8295 patients with resistant hypertension classified on the basis of ambulatory blood pressure monitoring. Hypertension. 2011;57(5):898–902.

27. Myers MG, Reeves RA. White coat phenomenon in patients receiving antihypertensive therapy. Am J Hypertens. 1991;4:844–9.
28. Weber MA, Cheung DG, Graettinger WF, Lipson JL. Characterization of antihypertensive
therapy by whole-day blood pressure monitoring. JAMA. 1988;259(22):3281–5.
29. Meinert CL. Toward more definitive clinical trials. Control Clin Trials. 1980;1(3):249–61.
30. Sylvester RJ, Pinedo HM, De Pauw M, et al. Quality of institutional participation in multicenter
clinical trials. N Engl J Med. 1981;305(15):852–5.
31. Spriet A, Dupin-Spriet T, Simon P. Methodology of clinical drug trials. 2nd ed. Basel: Karger; 1994.
32. White WB, Walsh SJ. Ambulatory monitoring of the blood pressure in multicenter clinical
trials. Blood Press Monit. 1996;1(3):227–9.
33. Appel LJ, Marwaha S, Whelton PK, Patel M. The impact of automated blood pressure devices
on the efficiency of clinical trials. Control Clin Trials. 1992;13(3):240–7.
34. McDonald CJ, Mazzuca SA, McCabe Jr GP. How much of the placebo 'effect' is really
statistical regression? Stat Med. 1983;2(4):417–27.
35. Mancia G, Bertinieri G, Grassi G, et al. Effects of blood-pressure measurement by the doctor
on patient's blood pressure and heart rate. Lancet. 1983;2(8352):695–8.
36. Mansoor GA, McCabe EJ, White WB. Determinants of the white-coat effect in hypertensive
subjects. J Hum Hypertens. 1996;10(2):87–92.
37. Bottini PB, Carr AA, Rhoades RB, Prisant LM. Variability of indirect methods used to
determine blood pressure. Office vs mean 24-hour automated blood pressures. Arch Intern
Med. 1992;152(1):139–44.
38. Dupont AG, Van der Niepen P, Six RO. Placebo does not lower ambulatory blood pressure. Br
J Clin Pharmacol. 1987;24(1):106–9.
39. Mutti E, Trazzi S, Omboni S, Parati G, Mancia G. Effect of placebo on 24-h non-invasive
ambulatory blood pressure. J Hypertens. 1991;9(4):361–4.
40. White WB, Mehrotra DV, Black HR, Fakouhi TD. Effects of controlled-onset extended-release
verapamil on nocturnal blood pressure (dippers versus nondippers). COER-Verapamil Study
Group. Am J Cardiol. 1997;80(4):469–74.
41. Bakris GL, Lindholm LH, Black HR, et al. Divergent results using clinic and ambulatory blood
pressures: report of a darusentan-resistant hypertension trial. Hypertension. 2010;56(5):824–30.
42. Staessen JA, Thijs L, Mancia G, Parati G, O'Brien ET. Clinical trials with ambulatory blood pressure monitoring: fewer patients needed? Syst-Eur Investigators. Lancet. 1994;344(8936):1552–6.
43. White WB, Dey HM, Schulman P. Assessment of the daily blood pressure load as a determinant of
cardiac function in patients with mild-to-moderate hypertension. Am Heart J. 1989;118(4):782–95.
44. Dickson D, Hasford J. 24-hour blood pressure measurement in antihypertensive drug trials:
data requirements and methods of analysis. Stat Med. 1992;11(16):2147–58.
45. White WB, Carr AA, Krause S, Jordan R, Roniker B, Oigman W. Assessment of the novel
selective aldosterone blocker eplerenone using ambulatory and clinical blood pressure in
patients with systemic hypertension. Am J Cardiol. 2003;92(1):38–42.
46. White WB. Relevance of the trough-to-peak ratio to the 24 h blood pressure load. Am
J Hypertens. 1996;9(10 Pt 2):91S–6S.
47. Neutel JM, Smith DH, Ram CV, et al. Application of ambulatory blood pressure monitoring in
differentiating between antihypertensive agents. Am J Med. 1993;94(2):181–7.
48. White WB, Weber MA, Sica D, et al. Effects of the angiotensin receptor blocker azilsartan
medoxomil versus olmesartan and valsartan on ambulatory and clinic blood pressure in
patients with stages 1 and 2 hypertension. Hypertension. 2011;57(3):413–20.
49. Mallion J, Siche J, Lacourciere Y. ABPM comparison of the antihypertensive profiles of the
selective angiotensin II receptor antagonists telmisartan and losartan in patients with mild-
to-moderate hypertension. J Hum Hypertens. 1999;13(10):657–64.
50. Dahlof B, Sever PS, Poulter NR, et al. Prevention of cardiovascular events with an
antihypertensive regimen of amlodipine adding perindopril as required versus atenolol adding
bendroflumethiazide as required, in the Anglo-Scandinavian Cardiac Outcomes Trial-Blood
Pressure Lowering Arm (ASCOT-BPLA): a multicentre randomised controlled trial. Lancet.
2005;366(9489):895–906.

51. Dolan E, Stanton AV, Thom S, et al. Ambulatory blood pressure monitoring predicts cardiovascular events in treated hypertensive patients—an Anglo-Scandinavian cardiac outcomes trial substudy. J Hypertens. 2009;27(4):876–85.
52. Smolensky MH, D'Alonzo GE. Medical chronobiology: concepts and applications. Am Rev Respir Dis. 1993;147(6 Pt 2):S2–19.
53. Straka RJ, Benson SR. Chronopharmacologic considerations when treating the patient with hypertension: a review. J Clin Pharmacol. 1996;36(9):771–82.
54. White WB. A chronotherapeutic approach to the management of hypertension. Am J Hypertens. 1996;9(4 Pt 3):29–33.
55. Muller JE, Tofler GH, Stone PH. Circadian variation and triggers of onset of acute cardiovascular disease. Circulation. 1989;79(4):733–43.
56. Waters DD, Miller DD, Bouchard A, Bosch X, Theroux P. Circadian variation in variant angina. Am J Cardiol. 1984;54(1):61–4.
57. Marler JR, Price TR, Clark GL, et al. Morning increase in onset of ischemic stroke. Stroke. 1989;20(4):473–6.
58. Hermida RC, Ayala DE, Mojon A, et al. Comparison of the effects on ambulatory blood pressure of awakening versus bedtime administration of torasemide in essential hypertension. Chronobiol Int. 2008;25(6):950–70.
59. Hermida RC, Ayala DE, Mojon A, Fernandez JR. Influence of circadian time of hypertension treatment on cardiovascular risk: results of the MAPEC study. Chronobiol Int. 2010;27(8):1629–51.
60. Hermida RC, Ayala DE, Mojon A, Fontao MJ, Fernandez JR. Chronotherapy with valsartan/hydrochlorothiazide combination in essential hypertension: improved sleep-time blood pressure control with bedtime dosing. Chronobiol Int. 2011;28(7):601–10.
61. Hermida RC, Rios MT, Crespo JJ, et al. Treatment-time regimen of hypertension medications significantly affects ambulatory blood pressure and clinical characteristics of patients with resistant hypertension. Chronobiol Int. 2013;30(1–2):192–206.
62. Moya A, Crespo JJ, Ayala DE, et al. Effects of time-of-day of hypertension treatment on ambulatory blood pressure and clinical characteristics of patients with type 2 diabetes. Chronobiol Int. 2013;30(1–2):116–31.
63. Lemmer B. Differential effects of antihypertensive drugs on circadian rhythm in blood pressure from the chronobiological point of view. Blood Press Monit. 1996;1(2):161–9.
64. Palatini P, Racioppa A, Raule G, Zaninotto M, Penzo M, Pessina AC. Effect of timing of administration on the plasma ACE inhibitory activity and the antihypertensive effect of quinapril. Clin Pharmacol Ther. 1992;52(4):378–83.
65. Mengden T, Binswanger B, Gruene S. Dynamics of drug compliance and 24 hour blood pressure control of once daily morning vs evening amlodipine. J Hypertens. 1992;10 Suppl 4:S136–S42.
66. Gillman MW, Kannel WB, Belanger A, D'Agostino RB. Influence of heart rate on mortality among persons with hypertension: the Framingham Study. Am Heart J. 1993;125(4):1148–54.
67. White WB, Mansoor GA, Pickering TG, et al. Differential effects of morning and evening dosing of nisoldipine ER on circadian blood pressure and heart rate. Am J Hypertens. 1999;12(8 Pt 1):806–14.
68. White WB, Mansoor GA, Tendler BE, Anwar YA. Nocturnal blood pressure epidemiology, determinants, and effects of antihypertensive therapy. Blood Press Monit. 1998;3(1):43–51.
69. Krum H, Schlaich M, Sobotka P. Renal sympathetic nerve ablation for treatment-resistant hypertension. Br J Clin Pharmacol. 2013;76(4):495–503.
70. Mahfoud F, Luscher TF, Andersson B, et al. Expert consensus document from the European Society of Cardiology on catheter-based renal denervation. Eur Heart J. 2013;34(28):2149–57.
71. Kandzari DE, Bhatt DL, Sobotka PA, et al. Catheter-based renal denervation for resistant hypertension: rationale and design of the SYMPLICITY HTN-3 trial. Clin Cardiol. 2012;35:528–35.
72. Bakris GL, Townsend RR, Liu M, et al. Impact of renal denervation on 24-hour ambulatory blood pressure: results from SYMPLICITY HTN-3. J Am Coll Cardiol. 2014;64(11):1071–8.
73. Mahfoud F, Ukena C, Schmieder RE, et al. Ambulatory blood pressure changes after renal sympathetic denervation in patients with resistant hypertension. Circulation. 2013;128:132–40.

74. Krum H, Schlaich M, Whitbourn R, et al. Catheter-based renal sympathetic denervation for resistant hypertension: a multicentre safety and proof-of-principle cohort study. Lancet. 2009;373:1275–81.
75. Kandzari DE, Bhatt DL, Brar S, et al. Predictors of blood pressure response in the SYMPLICITY HTN-3 trial. Eur Heart J. 2015;36(4):219–27.
76. Gulati V, White WB. Review of the state of renal nerve ablation for patients with severe and resistant hypertension. J Am Soc Hypertens. 2013;7(6):484–93.
77. White WB, Turner JR, Sica DA, et al. Detection, evaluation, and treatment of severe and resistant hypertension: proceedings from an American Society of Hypertension Interactive forum held in Bethesda, MD, U.S.A., October 10th 2013. J Am Soc Hypertens. 2014;8(10):743–57.
78. White WB, Giles T, Bakris GL, Neutel JM, Davidai G, Weber MA. Measuring the efficacy of antihypertensive therapy by ambulatory blood pressure monitoring in the primary care setting. Am Heart J. 2006;151(1):176–84.

Chapter 21
Out-of-Office Monitoring in Clinical Practice

Raymond R. Townsend

Introduction

Clinical undertaking of an ABPM program is no small endeavor. Current reimbursements are marginal and start up, as well as maintenance, costs are significant. A checklist for one's resolve in undertaking the establishment of 24-h ABPM might include the following:

- The purchase of software and of ABPM devices.
- Training of staff to initialize, manage, and enable draft ABPM reports.
- Education of patients while wearing the ABP monitor.
- Expectations of what constitutes an "adequate" ABPM recording.
- A plan to deal with phone calls while patients are wearing the ABP Monitor.
- What to do with the diary that patients bring back to the clinic?
- Recognition of patterns on ABPM and adequate expertise to comment on the clinical question that generated the ABPM request.

Reasons Why Out-of-Office Monitoring is Useful

Many chapters in this book review select aspects of either the circadian rhythm, or the value of Out-of-Office monitoring in a number of clinical circumstances. Table 21.1 provides at a glance some reasons for conducting ABPM studies in clinical practice as espoused by recent guidance documents on blood pressure monitoring in the US, Canada, and Europe with examples in this chapter.

R.R. Townsend, M.D. (✉)
Perelman School of Medicine, University of Pennsylvania,
122 Founders Building, 3400 Spruce Street, Philadelphia, PA 19104, USA
e-mail: townsend@upenn.edu

© Springer International Publishing Switzerland 2016
W.B. White (ed.), *Blood Pressure Monitoring in Cardiovascular Medicine and Therapeutics*, Clinical Hypertension and Vascular Diseases,
DOI 10.1007/978-3-319-22771-9_21

Table 21.1 Situations where out-of-office ABP monitoring may be useful and recommended in Guidelines

	Examples in this chapter	2015 USPSTF [6]	2014 CHEP [7]	2014 ASH/ISH [9]	2013 ESH [8]	2013 ESH/ESC [10]	2011 ACCF/AHA [11]	2011 NICE [12]
In Untreated Patients with								
Elevated clinic BP								
White coat hypertension	Figs. 21.1 and 21.2	X	X	X	X	X	X	X
Non-elevated clinic BP								
Masked hypertension	Fig. 21.3				X	X	X	
In Treated Patients with								
Elevated clinic BP								
White coat effect	Figs. 21.4, 21.5 and 21.6		X		X	X	X	
Drug-resistant hypertension	Fig. 21.7		X	X	X	X		
Non-elevated clinic BP								
Masked hypertension	Fig. 21.5				X	X	X	
Clinic BP that fluctuates considerably over same or different visits	Fig. 21.8		X					
BP variability (24-h)	Fig. 21.9				X	X		
Low blood pressure	Fig. 21.10		X		X	X	X	
Other situations	Figs. 21.11 and 21.12							

USPSTF United States Preventive Services Task Forces, *CHEP* Canadian Hypertension Education Program, *ASH/ISH* American Society of Hypertension/International Society of Hypertension, *ESH* European Society of Hypertension, *ESH/ESC* European Society of Hypertension/European Society of Cardiology, *ACCF/AHA* American College of Cardiology Foundation/American Heart Association, *NICE* National Institutes for Health and Clinical Excellence, *BP* blood pressure

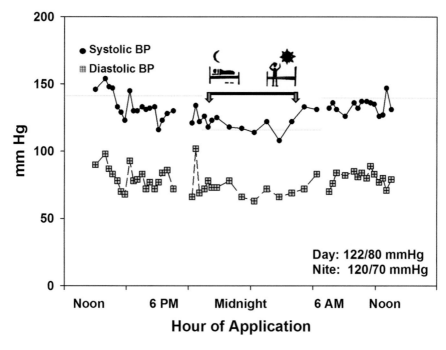

Fig. 21.1 53-year-old man on no medications with elevated office BP. In this and subsequent figures, a faint *dotted line* shows the systolic BP value of 140 mmHg from 0600 h to 2200 h; from 2200 h to 0600 h (corresponding to typical night time) the dotted line shows the systolic BP value of 120 mmHg

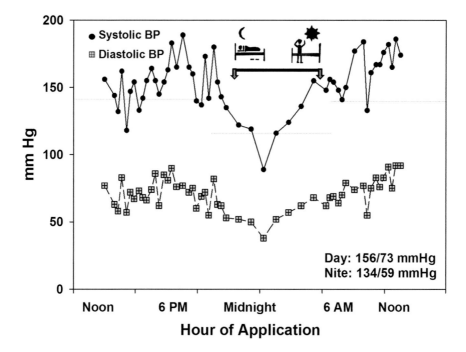

Fig. 21.2 64-year-old man on no medications with elevated office BP

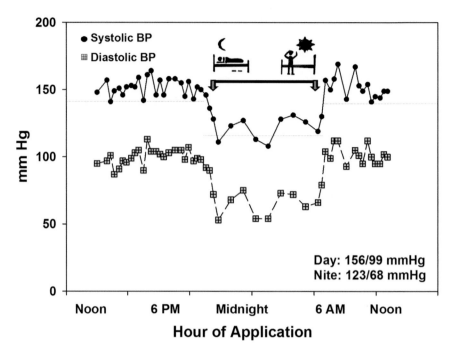

Fig. 21.3 37-year-old man with normal office BP

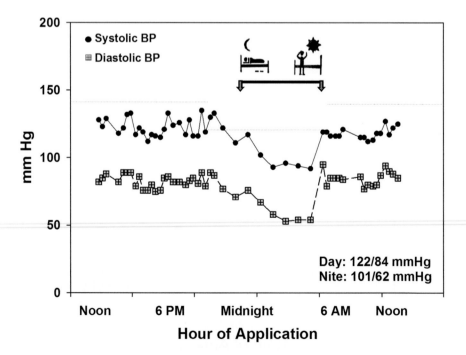

Fig. 21.4 58-year-old woman with office BP>140 mmHg systolic

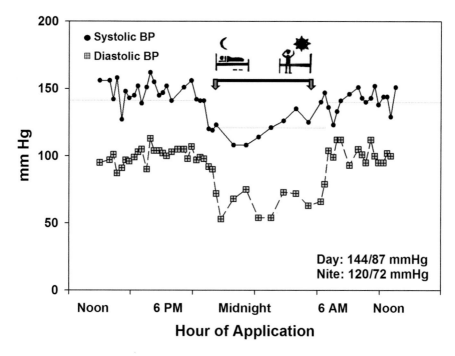

Fig. 21.5 62-year-old woman with office BP > 150 mmHg systolic

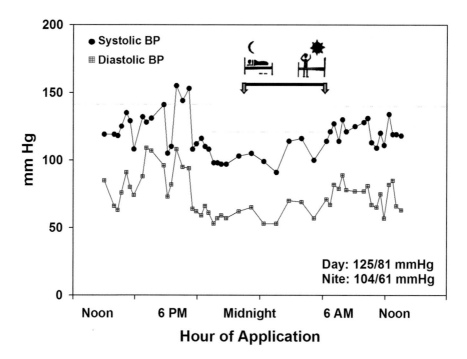

Fig. 21.6 68-year-old woman with office BP 162/100 mmHg

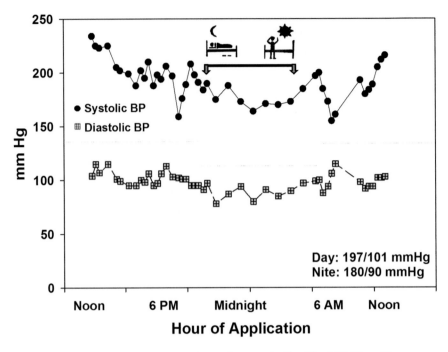

Fig. 21.7 77-year-old man with chronic kidney disease and office BP of 150/88 mmHg

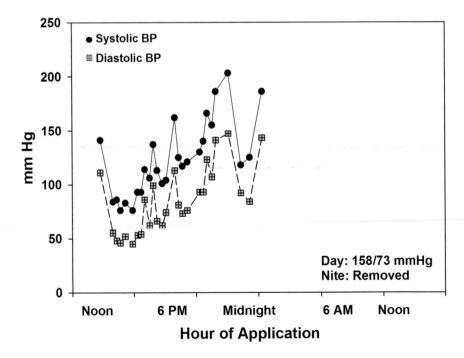

Fig. 21.8 53-year-old woman with erratic office blood pressures

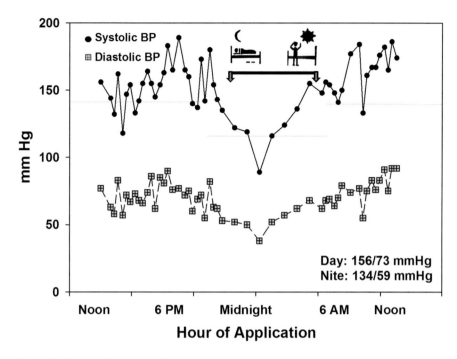

Fig. 21.9 55-year-old woman with pheochromocytoma

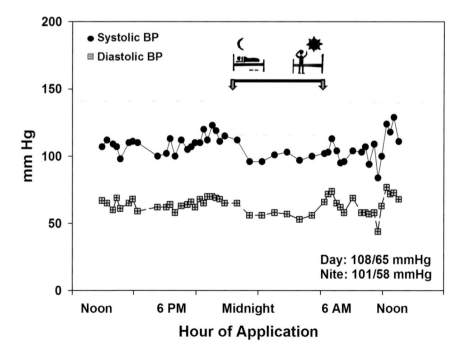

Fig. 21.10 64-year-old woman with dizziness

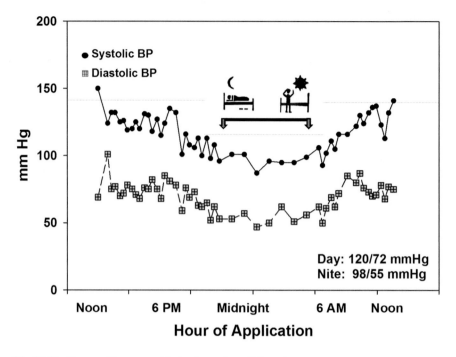

Fig. 21.11 31-year-old man considering becoming a kidney donor

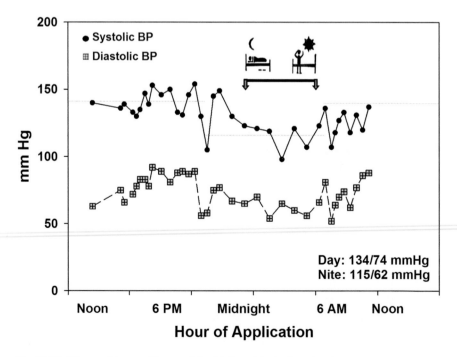

Fig. 21.12 33-year-old man with unexplained left ventricular hypertrophy

Preparing an ABPM Report

It is important to delineate the sleep and awake times, and whether a nap occurred during the period of study. The diary can be helpful, but patients need coaching for diary contents to be of use. In addition to noting times of sleep/awake/naps, it can be informative for the presence of symptoms like dizziness, or extreme fatigue, as a place to record an activity like exercise (treadmill, gym), and also as a place to annotate medication taking, or as a place to note something out of the ordinary which the patient feels may be informative. The use of the diary in the interpretation of ABPM is subjective as there is little in guidance documents outside of recording the time to bed and time to rise for diary usage. In some of the examples in this section, the diary is used to help interpret the 24-h data. Most ABP monitors allow the option of additional blood pressure measurement outside the timed protocol used to configure the automated blood pressure measurement. These extra blood pressures are typically marked with a letter such as an "M" in the raw data section of the ABP report; thus, examining the diary entry around this time may help to link symptoms with blood pressure deviations when clinically appropriate.

Next for consideration is a determination of the number of readings successfully obtained. If one programs the monitor for every 20 min during the day (06:00–22:00 h) and every half hour during the night (22:00–06:00 h), you could anticipate having 60 readings available (not counting the manual readings taken in the office to assure monitor function) for a 24-h ABPM. Opinions differ, but most centers like to see at least 70 % of the expected ABPM readings successfully obtained [1].

Most ABPM programs allow the use of a "caliper" or equivalent capability that lets the operator put in the time a patient went to bed and the time they arose. These summaries are useful for determining the actual daytime and nighttime BP averages (and the average reduction during the time the patient reports as asleep).

It is also useful to examine the overall 24-h raw data in terms of gaps (sometimes patients remove the device for several hours) and for overall variability (see examples below that emphasize these points).

Although there is no universally agreed upon template for an ABPM report, most centers who use ABPM will report the number of successful readings, the daytime and nighttime averages, whether or not the readings appear to be in the "hypertensive range" when white coat hypertension is the clinical question, and any comments from the interpreter of noted patterns in the 24-h ABPM data. When the question is something other than "Does this patient have white coat hypertension," we typically try to address it with additional commentary. A remarkable variety of patterns have been noted in the clinical examination of 24-h ABPM patients.

Each manufacturer of an ABP monitor typically has customizable software that allows incorporation of a potentially large amount of data and graphics into a report. Table 21.2 contains recommendations for what should, at a minimum, be incorporated into the report as suggested by societies that have written guidance documents outlining the value of ABPM.

Table 21.2 Recommendations for what to include in an ABPM report

Patient demographics (age, gender, medical record number)	Number (and percentage) of successful readings
Why the recording was undertaken	Average 24 h, daytime, and nighttime blood pressures
Graphic display of BP and heart rate readings	An impression that addresses the clinical question

Addressing the Clinical Questions

In addition to the standard question, "Does this patient have white coat hypertension?," there are a myriad of other circumstances that complicate the outpatient management of hypertensive patients including:

- Are symptoms reported by this patient corroborated by a blood pressure abnormality?
- Is this person a reasonable kidney donor?
- Is this person's antihypertensive regimen truly controlling their blood pressure?
- Does this person have something in their blood pressure profile that may indicate that I need to do something different in their management?
- Is this person's blood pressure control "all over the place?"
- Do these ABPM data help me to understand why the patient is dizzy, or even pre-syncopal?

What follows next are some examples of the utility of ABPM in managing a variety of patients with blood pressure disorders. Each scenario will include a brief capsule of the clinical question addressed, followed by a 24-h ABPM graphic and a concise interpretation of the ABPM data.

Clinical Examples (See Table 21.1)

In the following examples, the format used is a brief "Clinical:" stem, followed by a graphic of the raw ABPM data. The raw graphed data provide a preferential view of the 24-h output because hourly averaged BP hides variability and can conceal low or high values of BP when they are flanked by relatively normal values. Each example has an "Impression" completing each case.

A Non-medicated Patient with Elevated Office Blood Pressure

Clinical: 53-year-old man on no antihypertensive agents with in-office values >140/90 mmHg on several occasions. He has no known history of CV disease.

Impression: The daytime average of this patient is 122/80 mmHg, which is not in the hypertensive range. He satisfies the criteria for untreated white coat hypertension and his elevated BP at the time of monitor application persisted for about an hour after the first reading; it can take an hour or more for the "white coat effect" to attenuate after monitor application [2]. He does not, however, have sleep suppression evident, and this patient likely requires more vigilance in follow-up. Other chapters in this textbook review the importance of nocturnal BP declines (See, for example, Chap. 6).

Clinical: 64-year-old man on no antihypertensive agents with elevated in-office values of >150/90 mmHg on several occasions.

Impression: In this instance, the daytime ABPM data confirms the diagnosis of hypertension and negates the diagnosis of white coat hypertension. Initiating antihypertensive therapy would be reasonable here.

Unmedicated Patient with Normal Office Blood Pressure

Some patients report elevated readings outside the office despite having what appears to be reasonable BP control in the office; Dr. Thomas Pickering labeled this phenomenon "masked" hypertension [3].

Clinical: 37-year-old man followed for gastroesophageal reflux reports that his blood pressure was high when checked by a friend using their home BP monitor. In prior office visits over the past 2 years, BP values of 120–130 mmHg systolic and diastolic values of 80 mmHg or less were recorded in the office before ABPM was performed.

Impression: Virtually every reading in the ABPM is above 140 mmHg. This un-medicated patient with repeated normal in-office values actually has masked hypertension.

Patients with Elevated Office Blood Pressure on Antihypertensive Drug Therapy

Receiving antihypertensive therapy does not necessarily abrogate a "white coat effect" on the in-office BP. The term "white coat effect" is often used after treatment has been initiated to distinguish the in-office elevation of blood pressure as a finding in a treated hypertensive patient who shows higher levels in-office compared to at home (or by ABPM) compared with "white coat hypertension," which usually implies that the patient is normotensive outside the clinic setting.

Clinical: 58-year-old woman with hypertension treated with a beta blocker. Her in-office systolic BP values are >140 mmHg.

Impression: Her daytime blood pressure is 122/84 mmHg, which represent reasonable daytime blood pressure control. High in-office values are likely a white coat effect that overrides the antihypertensive drug.

Clinical: 62-year-old woman receiving an angiotensin receptor blocker (ARB) and a diuretic for therapy of hypertension. In-office systolic BP values are >150 mmHg.

Impression: This patient had a daytime average of 144/87 mmHg that roughly correlates with in-office values in the low 150 mmHg range, and in-office diastolic values slightly over 90 mmHg. In this instance, this patient does not have white coat effect, but rather treated, uncontrolled, hypertension.

Clinical: 68-year-old woman seen in the office after a recent visit to the hospital emergency department for abdominal pain. In-office readings were 162/100 mmHg on an antihypertensive regimen that included an ACE-inhibitor and a beta-blocker.

Impression: In this case, the daytime pressures of 125/81 mmHg coupled with reasonable reductions in BP during sleep were useful information to the referring provider for continuing the current antihypertensive regimen. There are a few elevated readings in the evening likely associated with a brisk evening walk. The important thing, however, is to consider the average of the awake values rather than the occasional outlier reading.

Patients with Variable Office Blood Pressures on Antihypertensive Therapy

In some cases, the patient displays erratic in-office values, sometimes controlled on medications, sometimes very low, and sometimes quite high. In these situations, home monitoring of BP, if it can be reliably undertaken, may be a useful adjunct to interpretation of BP behavior over time. The example provided next, however, is of such a patient who would not take her BP at home, convinced that "those things don't work."

Clinical: 53-year-old woman on antihypertensive medications with erratic in-office blood pressures

Impression: This patient underscores the challenges in trying to use out-of-office monitoring in some scenarios. She took the BP monitor off at night, so no comments can be made about nocturnal pressure. During the daytime when she did wear the monitor, she had highly variable BP values with systolic readings ranging from: 76 to 203 mmHg and diastolic readings ranging from 46 to 147 mmHg. Her heart rate was also labile with 9 readings >100 beats/min and a range of 73–138 beats/min, supporting the referring providers suspicion of a diagnosis of dysautonomia.

Variability in 24-h BP Profile

Clinical: 55-year-old woman with newly diagnosed pheochromocytoma awaiting surgical removal and treated with the long-acting alpha-1 blocker phenoxybenzamine.

Impression: The averaged value of the systolic and diastolic BPs belies their variability. In her case the daytime systolic pressures (± S.D.) were 156±18 mmHg and diastolic pressures were 73±11 mmHg. The nocturnal pressures were 135±22 mmHg and 59±10 mmHg. The magnitude of these standard deviations—particularly during the night time—is about 1.5–2× what is normally found, and the variability in her blood pressure profile is evident in the Figure.

Patients with Low Out-of-Office Blood Pressures on Antihypertensive Drug Therapy

Sometimes ABPM uncovers low blood pressures outside of the office setting. In many cases, this is done to evaluate symptoms including severe fatigue or dizziness/lightheadedness, which could be related to antihypertensive medications, or to hemodynamic consequence of excessive blood pressure reduction as sometimes occurs after meals [4].

Clinical: 64-year-old woman with occasional symptoms of dizziness. She also has a history of depression and takes fluoxetine daily. The hypertension is managed with an ACE-inhibitor and a beta-blocker.

Impression: Her daytime profile shows average BPs of 108/65 mmHg, with several systolic readings below 100 mmHg. During the time of monitoring, she did not note any episodes of lightheadedness or dizziness. Not shown in the graphic, but evident in the report was an average heart rate of 49 beats/min over the 24 h period. In an instance like this, a reduction in beta-blocker dose could be helpful.

In some treated patients, an ABPM may show several patterns at one time. This next patient is an example of that.

Clinical: 77-year-old man with chronic kidney disease. He was treated with multiple antihypertensive agents. Despite repeated urging, he would not consider doing home blood pressure monitoring. His in-office value for his most recent visit was 150/88 mmHg.

Impression: There are several patterns evident in this patient. First he has a white coat effect. The highest values of his blood pressure were at the time of (and immediately following) monitor application, and the time of removal of the blood pressure monitor. In addition, the average daytime blood pressure of 197/101 mmHg is much higher than the in-office value of 150/88 mmHg, supporting a masked hypertension effect. Finally, he has treated but uncontrolled hypertension.

Uncommon Usages for Out-of-Office Monitoring

Kidney Donation

One of the areas in which ABPM is used is in determining a potential kidney donor's risk for kidney donation. At our center (University of Pennsylvania and the Children's Hospital of Philadelphia), we previously demonstrated that the evaluation process for kidney donation has a significant "white coat effect," especially among potential donors who have "normotensive" blood pressure which declines in an office setting after donation at the 6-month time point [5]. The long waiting times for cadaveric kidney donation have placed pressure on transplant centers to increase the number of living-related or living unrelated kidney donations. One of the principal areas of concern is whether the subjugation of a person with treated or untreated hypertension based on clinic or office levels of blood pressure increases their cardiovascular risk. To address that question, ABPM provides a level of assurance when office or clinic levels of blood pressure are borderline, or elevated above 140/90 mmHg.

Although not required in the evaluation of a person who has come forward as a potential kidney donor, ABPM can be useful in gauging the candidate's blood pressure profile, and this can be particularly useful when the recipient is a blood relative as there may be a hereditary component to blood pressure.

Clinical: A 31-year-old man being considered for kidney donation. In-clinic blood pressures are >140 mmHg with no history of hypertension. He is not on antihypertensive medications.

Impression: This candidate has a clear increase on arriving for monitor application with normal daytime and nighttime systolic blood pressure values (as shown in the lower right inside the graph box). The main times the systolic pressure exceeded 140 mmHg were when the monitor was applied and when it was removed.

Pursuing Causation of Target Organ Effect

We sometimes are asked to do an ABPM on someone with otherwise unexplained target organ effect. One such example follows next.

Clinical: 33-year-old athletic man who upon recent evaluation for chest discomfort was found to have moderate left ventricular hypertrophy on an electrocardiogram, which was confirmed by echocardiography. He is untreated. His prior in-office blood pressures had not been elevated and was 130/82 mmHg at the most recent office visit when referred to a cardiologist.

Impression: The daytime average blood pressure of 134/74 mmHg in this patient makes it less likely that his ventricular hypertrophy is the result of untreated hypertension, and in particular masked hypertension. It may be that a genetic cardiomyopathy is present, or that the pattern of his athletic activity, which includes bench-press weight lifting, should be altered.

When is Out-of-Office Monitoring Not Needed, or Not Useful?

Patients presenting with very high levels of blood pressure (e.g., >180/110 mmHg), whether on treatment or not, are candidates for immediate attention to blood pressure reduction [6–8]. Generally, it is not necessary to confirm these high levels of blood pressure outside the office or hospital, particularly if there is a history of or ongoing target organ damage present. There are occasional extreme white coat effect patients, and in these cases, home blood pressure monitoring is quite useful.

ABPM is usually not useful to pursue symptoms that may be related to cardiac rhythm problems, although recent advances in oscillometric monitoring are improving the ability to measure blood pressure in patients with atrial fibrillation. In patients with symptoms such as loss of consciousness, for example, the blood pressure may be below the limits, the ABPM device can detect or cannot be measured because the pulse is absent.

In a patient with a confirmed diagnosis of hypertension, who seems well-managed and adherent, ABPM adds little beside potential information on the nocturnal blood pressure component. Until there is more agreement on management of this nocturnal segment, little is gained by using ABPM for this instance unless there are morbidities such as unexplained left ventricular hypertrophy, heart failure, or the emergence of chronic kidney disease, complications of hypertension to which blood pressures elevations in the nocturnal segment may be contributing.

In Closing

Out-of-office monitoring with ABPM is useful in a number of clinical scenarios. It provides information on the relationship of symptoms and BP, adequacy of BP control, the circadian profile, and it is unsurpassed as a predictor for cardiovascular risk attributable to blood pressure levels. It is relatively expensive to initiate an ABPM program and requires a moderate amount of staff time devoted to the application and removal of the monitor, as well as the coaching of patients on wearing the device in order to maximize the number of readings obtained. Although reimbursement in the US is generally poor, the provision of this service is a valuable tool to our colleagues in general practice dealing with complex situations in clinical management where the limitations of an office BP are often overcome by the ability to effectively perform out-of-office ABP monitoring.

References

1. Parati G, Stergiou G, O'Brien E, et al. European Society of Hypertension practice guidelines for ambulatory blood pressure monitoring. J Hypertens. 2014;32(7):1359–66.
2. Yanovski A, Townsend RR, Virginia F, Michael C. A psychophysiologic reaction to application of ambulatory blood pressure monitor: fact or artifact? Blood Press Monit. 2011;16(1):29–36.
3. Pickering TG, Davidson K, Gerin W, Schwartz JE. Masked hypertension. Hypertension. 2002;40(6):795–6.
4. Jansen RW, Lipsitz LA. Postprandial hypotension: epidemiology, pathophysiology, and clinical management. Ann Intern Med. 1995;122:286–95.
5. Deloach SS, Meyers KE, Townsend RR. Living donor kidney donation: another form of white coat effect. Am J Nephrol. 2012;35(1):75–9.

6. Piper MA, Evans CV, Burda BU, Margolis KL, O'Connor E, Whitlock EP. Diagnostic and predictive accuracy of blood pressure screening methods with consideration of rescreening intervals: a systematic review for the U.S. Preventive services task force. Ann Intern Med. 2015;162(3):192–204.

7. Dasgupta K, Quinn RR, Zarnke KB, et al. The 2014 Canadian Hypertension Education Program recommendations for blood pressure measurement, diagnosis, assessment of risk, prevention, and treatment of hypertension. Can J Cardiol. 2014;30(5):485–501.

8. O'Brien E, Parati G, Stergiou G, et al. European society of hypertension position paper on ambulatory blood pressure monitoring. J Hypertens. 2013;31(9):1731–68.

9. Weber MA, Schiffrin EL, White WB, et al. Clinical practice guidelines for the management of hypertension in the community a statement by the American Society of Hypertension and the International Society of Hypertension. J Hypertens. 2014;32(1):3–15.

10. Mancia G, Fagard R, Narkiewicz K, et al. ESH/ESC Guidelines for the management of arterial hypertension: the Task Force for the management of arterial hypertension of the European Society of Hypertension (ESH) and of the European Society of Cardiology (ESC). J Hypertens. 2013;31(7):1281–357.

11. Aronow WS, Fleg JL, Pepine CJ, et al. ACCF/AHA 2011 expert consensus document on hypertension in the elderly: a report of the American College of Cardiology Foundation Task Force on Clinical Expert Consensus documents developed in collaboration with the American Academy of Neurology, American Geriatrics Society, American Society for Preventive Cardiology, American Society of Hypertension, American Society of Nephrology, Association of Black Cardiologists, and European Society of Hypertension. J Am Coll Cardiol. 2011;57(20):2037–114.

12. Krause T, Lovibond K, Caulfield M, McCormack T, Williams B. Management of hypertension: summary of NICE guidance. BMJ. 2011;343:d4891.

Index

© Springer International Publishing Switzerland 2016
W.B. White (ed.), *Blood Pressure Monitoring in Cardiovascular Medicine and Therapeutics*, Clinical Hypertension and Vascular Diseases,
DOI 10.1007/978-3-319-22771-9

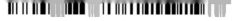

Printed in the United States
By Bookmasters